Not Only the 'Dangerous Trades'

**Feminist Perspectives on the
Past and Present
Advisory Editorial Board**

Not Only the 'Dangerous Trades':
Women's Work and Health in Britain, 1880–1914

BARBARA HARRISON

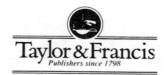

Taylor & Francis
Publishers since 1798

UK   Taylor & Francis Ltd, 1 Gunpowder Square, London EC4A 3DE
USA   Taylor & Francis Inc., 1900 Frost Road, Suite 101, Bristol, PA 19007

© Barbara Harrison, 1996

First published 1996

A Catalogue Record for this book is available from the British Library

ISBN 0 7484 0144 X
ISBN 0 7484 0145 8 (pbk)

Library of Congress Cataloging-in-Publication Data are available on request

Cover design by Barking Dog Art

Typeset in 10pt Times
by Graphicraft Typesetters Ltd, Hong Kong

Printed by SRP Ltd, Exeter

For my mother, Dorothy Croy,
and in memory of Alan Croy and also Elsie Brooks,
who first encouraged me to look at the past

Contents

List of Tables, Figures and Appendix

List of Abbreviations

ASL   Anti-Sweating League
BAAS   British Association for the Advancement of Science
BLPES   British Library of Political and Economic Science
BMA   British Medical Association
BMJ   British Medical Journal
ER   Englishwoman's Review
EWJ   English Woman's Journal
FWG   Fabian Women's Group
ILP   Independent Labour Party
IMR   Infant Mortality Ratio
MOH   Medical Officer(s) of Health
NFWW   National Federation of Women Workers
NUASA   National Union of Shop Assistants
PP   Parliamentary Papers
PRO   Public Records Office
RCL   Royal Commmission on Labour
SPEW   Society for Promoting the Employment of Women
TUC   Trades Union Congress
VA   Vigilence Association for the Defence of Personal Rights
WCG   Women's Cooperative Guild
WEDL   Women's Employment Defence League
WIC   Women's Industrial Council
WIDC   Women's Industrial Defence Committee
WLL   Women's Labour League
WPPL   Women's Protective and Provident League
WTUA   Women's Trade Union Association
WTUL   Women's Trade Union League
WTUPL   Women's Trade Union and Provident League

Acknowledgments

This book has been a long time in the writing. Much of the problem lay in the many distractions elsewhere that are part of contemporary higher education, but also in persuading publishers, although not editors, that a book about working women and health in the historical context was of interest. I am therefore grateful to Taylor & Francis, and Comfort Jegede in particular, for believing in it. There were others who tried on my behalf and gave me encouragment to continue, particularly Michelle Stanworth, Mary Maynard and Haleh Afshar and most recently and importantly June Purvis.

There have also been many people, many of whose names I do not know, who have helped me find my way to the vast array of materials there were to retrieve and read. I have become a firm supporter of the specialist library and archivists who know their subject. In this respect it is hoped that the Fawcett will have an environmentally and financially secure future: Thank you all.

Finally, a word of thanks to all my friends and colleagues, particularly those at South Bank University and at Nescot, who have also had to live through this project. They have been sympathetic to my need for time – although it was never enough – and have been kind enough to help with proofreading and feedback. My postgraduate students at both institutions have helped to maintain my enthusiasm by their own enjoyment and inquisition of aspects of sociological history. There were also all my friends in the *Women and Work Hazards* group over my ten or so years of involvement – too many to name but you know who you are – who between them must share the credit for contributing to a feminist practice in health and safety and women's health. Rob has had to suffer my preoccupations as well as frustrations and anxieties about ever-moving deadlines, so thanks for being there. Friends who deserve special mention for their encouragement are Annmarie, Ann, Jennie, Sue and Stina. I hope you will approve of the finished book.

I take all responsibility for the material and ideas in it. Historical research is trying, time-consuming and often frustrating, but there are many rewards. I will find it difficult not to continue with it. Most importantly, for me this research is a testimony to the courage, hard work and resilience of working women in the face of adversities we can only imagine.

Before I could publish this research as a book, a number of articles and papers were published over the years. Inevitably some of the material in this book, both data and ideas, has drawn on them. I acknowledge my debt to the following:

HARRISON, B. (1989) '"Some of them gets lead poisoned": occupational lead exposure in women, 1880–1914', *Social History of Medicine*, **2**, 1, pp.171–193.

HARRISON, B. (1990) 'Suffer the working day: women in the "dangerous trades"', in *British Feminist Histories*', *Women's Studies International Forum*, **13**, 1, pp.79–80.

HARRISON, B. (1991) 'Women's health or social control? The role of the medical profession in relation to factory legislation in late nineteenth-century Britain', *Sociology of Health and Illness*, **13**, 4, pp.469–91.

HARRISON, B. (1993a) 'Are accidents gender neutral? The case of the industrial accident in Britain, 1880–1914', *Women's History Review*, **2**, 2, pp.253–76.

HARRISON, B. (1993b) 'Feminism and the health consequences of working conditions in late nineteenth and early twentieth-century Britain', in PLATT, S., THOMAS, H., SCOTT, S. and WILLIAMS, G. (Eds) *Locating Health: Historical and Contemporary Perspectives*, Andover: Ashgate.

HARRISON, B. (1995a) 'The politics of occupational health in late nineteenth-century Britain: the case of the match-making industry', *Sociology of Health and Illness*, **17**, 1, pp.20–41.

HARRISON, B. (In press) 'Gender, the State and occupational ill-health: women factory inspectors and the health of women at work, 1893–1921', *Proceedings of the International Conference on Nursing, Women's History and the Politics of Welfare*, University of Nottingham, Nursing Policy Series.

HARRISON, B. and MOCKETT, H. (1990) 'Women in the factory: the state and factory legislation in nineteenth-century Britain', in JAMIESON, L. and CORR, H. (Eds) *State, Private Life and Political Change*, London: Macmillan.

Setting the Scene

Beginnings

My interest in work-related ill-health had more contemporary origins. I have had an academic and personal interest in women's health in general for many years and in the early 1980s I became a member of a small women's group who were concerned about the hazards women faced in their work. The necessity for a separate organization of women for women was the oft-repeated situation that many feminist groups have encountered in other areas of social and political life; the 'work hazards movement' was male dominated and it was difficult for women within it to get women's concerns on the agenda. It was also clear that the trade-union movement, which had long been in the vanguard of the struggle to protect workers from aspects of their working conditions, had often failed their women members.[1] There were many women in non-unionized workplaces, in part-time work and forms of casual labour whose problems were largely unrecognized.

The *Women and Work Hazards Group*[2] worked on three fronts. First, it offered advice to individual women on any aspect of their work with which they were concerned; and while it existed[3] it had a constant mailbag. Second, it aimed to provide information in an accessible form, to document the kinds of hazards or risks to health women faced in relation to work and to make this available as widely as possible. Dissemination occurred through developing written information, holding workshops or meetings and through the making of a film which was finally shown on national television.[4]

The group adopted a political consciousness-raising strategy through its information work and by campaigning on a number of fronts. We wanted those organizations involved with working conditions and work hazards to recognize the particular problems that women might face, but also why it might be more difficult for them to be active in workplace struggles. We also wanted those organizations involved with the politics of health and women's health to recognize that working conditions were an important aspect and needed serious consideration. Our concern with work hazards was, we believed, a necessary component in redirecting health activism away from individual problems and health services to an analysis of why people got sick in the first place and then a political strategy directed at this and other social causes of ill-health. The group was, therefore, part of a wider movement for women's health and a new politics of preventive healthcare that had been developing since the mid-1970s.[5] Whether these grander aims were ever achieved is doubtful. However, all the groups who worked on these issues were successful in giving women information and a basis for action, in raising consciousness and in enabling local groups to effect change. They also ensured that some policies were developed to protect workers' health.

This short autobiographical sketch is pertinent not only because it provided a backdrop for this investigation, but also because these issues have a much longer history, although ideas that history repeats itself are much too simplistic. Women's lives, working conditions, health and activism have often been marginalized, in historically specific ways, which often reveal similar processes of oppression to be present. In the same way that the *Women and Work Hazards Group* had found women's health at work was neglected, I too found this to be the case as I developed my academic interests in historical and contemporary aspects of women's health. In the historical context I thought this might be due to the fact that there was little material available on the various ways in which work might have impinged on women's health status. When I examined the literature on women's work, on women in the family or on feminist activism, it was sometimes included but did not seem to feature as a major topic of investigation: the central interest was always elsewhere. My initial exploration suggested that a lack of primary sources was not the reason for this neglect. Rather, I was looking at a double marginality: that of occupational health and women and occupational health. This project set out to try and decrease that double marginality, while demonstrating its relevance to feminist analysis and practice.

Intentions

The aim of this book is to document the nature, extent and consequences of women's work in the paid labour market on their health in the period 1880–1914. It will examine the direct health consequences – that is those arising from identifiable hazards in the workplace such as exposure to toxic substances and such things as heavy lifting, breathing dusts or poor sanitary conditions. But there are also affects on health that arise from less identifiable cause–effect relationships between a wide variety of working conditions and health, including, for example, levels of pay, the environment, the pace of work and social relations in the workplace, particularly forms of control over work and workers; these also need to be considered. My intention is to examine the widest possible definition of the workplace, work and health relationship. To this extent, although this book is mainly focused on ill-health, it is also necessary to ask questions about the extent to which paid work was also a 'contributor' to health and wellbeing.

In addition to documenting the 'actual' problems of the work and health relationship, the project at the outset had to acknowledge that any assessment of the 'reality' of this aspect of women's lives was confounded by issues of representation. Not only would this be a key methodological issue in the use of source material, but representation would itself be a topic of investigation. This book, therefore, is also about how occupational threats to women's health were constituted and represented in discourse.[6] A substantial proportion of the book is thus devoted to an interpretation of documentary materials as representations, as constituting discourses, and the relation between ideology and material practice. This is an important terrain for historians: such materials not only reflect those domains we wish to study, they also constitute events and human consciousness.[7] There is now an on-going debate among feminist historians about how far we should go in accepting there is any historical 'reality' outside of linguistic signification.[8]

For this study, I considered it essential to consider such signification in order to reach some understanding of how 'problems' are identified and defined in ways that preserve social relations and perpetuate structures of oppression. In fact, it will be argued, it was the discourses on women in paid work and the possible implications of that paid work for their health that was a central constituting discourse of late Victorian and early twentieth-century gender relations.[9] In many areas of social life, some reference to the potentially damaging consequences of women's work was made, although it was most prominent in discussion of work in the paid labour market and in a discourse around national health and 'efficiency'. It was, however, women *at* work as much as the nature of that work that was of concern. So whether it was by choice or necessity, women's participation in the public domain of paid work, even when that work was done at home, threatened the social and moral order. The disorders of the physical body arising from the disordered social roles which women's paid work represented was a dominant metaphor for State intervention and forms of regulation.[10]

This will be especially evident in the discussion of domestic labour, maternity and childbirth and infant care. This topic will demonstrate the extent to which the constitution of women's nature, on the basis of biological difference and thence their social capabilities, was most clearly realized in the arguments about reproduction and the health of others. There would be a specific focus on the effects of work on reproduction – and a converse relationship of women's reproductive biology on the capacity for the physical labours of work – in the debates, investigations and political struggles of men and women at the time. In examining these problems, identified as ones of occupational ill-health and the responses of different people with an interest in them, attention is given to trying to unravel how and why things were perceived as they were, what responses were thought necessary and were made and what were the consequences of ideas as well as actions. This is an essential dimension of understanding how ideologies and structures of women's oppression are articulated and effected in many different domains of social practice.

The rationale for the time period chosen here (1880–1914) has to do with the opportunity it presented for analysing the importance of issues around women's paid work and health in a new social and historical context: the beginnings of State intervention into a number of areas of social and economic life which had traditionally been viewed by members of Victorian society as 'sacrosanct'.[11] There are always difficulties with restricting oneself to a specific time point and any boundaries are always to some extent artificial, since social and historical processes never conform to the schedules of calendric time. There are continuities as well as new contingencies and change. However, despite such limitations, I would argue that in this period the issues of women's paid work and its consequences on health received unprecedented levels of attention. This was associated not only with State intervention, but also with growing trade unionism and feminist activism. Within broad social developments as well as around specific historical events, there was widespread public debate about women and women and work. The preservation of the social relations of class and gender were manifest in this context. The endpoint of 1914 is because the First World War was an event which marked a considerable change in the nation's priorities, disrupted the 'everyday' lives of both men and women and certainly necessitated a different response to women at work. Because the next four years were a rupture in the social fabric and traditional social relations, I felt it would make for a more coherent analysis to stop before, rather than after, the war.

This research was interested in the development of an issue and the variety of responses to it. The time period provides an opportunity to explore State intervention with respect to women's work and women's lives. In this particular respect, to have concentrated on this aspect alone would have imposed a limitation on the research. Although all paid work for women might be construed to be in contradiction of traditional gender roles, it was only some around which the discourse functioned and which were considered for intervention and possible regulation. The discourse around women's work as a 'social problem' requiring State intervention was first, with work in the paid labour market and second, work in the context of manufacture in factories or workshops (including domestic workshops) and some other industrial employments (such as mining). It will be evident, however, that while industry provided a variety of occupations for working-class women in the time period discussed here, it excluded many areas of work in which working-class women were engaged and the increasing number of occupations for middle-class women. While in many respects I have had to work with the constraints of evidence and representations which focused on industrial employment, I also believed it would have been a serious limitation to any understanding of occupational ill-health and paid work to have not attempted to move beyond these. For example, it would have meant the exclusion of the largest single group of paid working-class women workers at this time – domestic servants – and the health effects and potential hazards of any employment. These would have perpetuated the myth that work hazards are primarily associated with industrial (and often also only male) employments, exacerbating other marginal aspects. I have, therefore, tried to examine the consequences of such a focus throughout the book as well as devoting some attention to work outside the industrial sector.

Following this introduction, the book is organized into two main sections, followed by a conclusion. The first four chapters examine the nature of the perceived problems of women's paid work and its possible consequences for health and wellbeing. It documents the extent to which there were aspects of that work identified as causes of ill-health. Although it is not intended to be complete, it aims to offer a more comprehensive analysis of work and ill-health than either a focus on a single type of work or on the social class of women worker would have given rise to. The second part is concerned with responses to 'the problem'. The chapters have been organized around four different interest groups: the State, medical men, women factory inspectors and feminist and women trade-union activists. Where possible, I have included the voices of working women themselves and considered their position. In the conclusion I bring together the specific case of women's work and occupational health with wider analytic and theoretical concerns about gender relations and the political and social structures of gender and class oppression.

Before I begin these two main sections of the book, two others are required by way of introduction or context-setting, first to give an overview of the historical context of women's work in the period and second to provide some conceptual clarification of occupational ill-health.

Women Workers in Late Nineteenth and Early Twentieth-century Britain

Although there are well-known difficulties with using census returns or other official data, they are the only source we have that provide some kind of national overview of the extent and nature of women's employment during this period.[12] The principal weaknesses lie in the extent to which it is likely to underestimate the paid employment of women because of their mobility in and out of the labour market, particularly if they were married, and because both forms of casual employment and homework may have remained unrecorded.[13] It was noted that there was a discrepancy between census returns and Factory and Labour Department or Board of Trade figures, which reflected differences in purpose and then collection and categories of presentation.[14] A second difficulty lay in the categories available. It was only from 1881 that women domestic labourers were returned as 'unoccupied' and one other example noted[15] that it was only after 1891 that 'sick' nurses were demarcated from domestic servants.

The census returns of 1891 as to the employment of women and girls in England and Wales show that women were distributed over 18 occupational classes or groups (see Table 1.1). They were, however, concentrated in three main classes: domestic service, milliners and dressmakers and cotton goods manufacturers. There was also a marked distribution by age: Collet estimated that of the 15–20-year-old group 68.6 per cent were employed.[16] This age distribution remained significant in the 1901 and 1911 census returns. At the turn of the century, women's labour-force participation was very high, at 61 per cent among the 15–24-year-old age group. It fell considerably to 31 per cent in the next age group, 25–34, decreasing further from 35 years. This indicates the importance of marital status in women's work patterns.[17] In 1901, half of all women workers were under 25 years, three-quarters under 35, with those over 35 'a comparative rarity'.[18] Age was also markedly significant within occupations, particularly for the largest single group, domestic servants, where women from 10–25 were in the majority.[19] The seven most common groups and their age distribution can be seen in Table 1.1.

Since the 1881 census returns there had been a decrease in the proportion of women in textiles, while fewer younger women and more older women were in domestic service. In all, as a percentage of the total workforce, the proportion of

Table 1.1 *Women's employment, 1891 census. Ten most important classes by age.
Numbers per 10 000 women 10 years and over*

	10–15	15–25	25–45	45–65
Domestic servants	665	2744	902	479
Milliners and dressmakers	108	732	331	218
Cotton and cotton goods operatives	305	555	258	87
Laundry workers	11	130	164	297
Professors and school teachers	37	245	137	53
Charwomen	2	24	102	213
Tailoresses	32	148	66	58
Worsted goods operatives	87	117	45	16
Woollen goods operatives	32	106	51	21

From Collet, C. (1896) *Statistics of Employment of Women and Girls in England and Wales.*

Remaining categories included nurses and midwives, shirtmakers, shoe, boot and clog-making, drapers, grocers, board and lodging housekeeper, hotel servants and silk operatives.

women was 29.1 per cent in 1901 and 29.7 per cent in 1911, and as a proportion of all women, those who worked represented 31.6 and 32.5 per cent respectively in these same years. Thus women's participation in the labour market remained constant over the period here. In fact there would be little marked change in such patterns until the 1930s and particularly after the Second World War.[20] Such overall patterns obscure many changes which occurred in the kinds of work women did and regional as well as more local patterns of employment. In this period, there was also a substantial increase (161 per cent between 1881 and 1911 according to Holcombe)[21] in women's participation in office work, reflecting a shifting demand for labour in the economy toward new service industries.[22] More women also entered some professions such as teaching. Many of these differences reflected a further important variable in women's participation–marital status.

In her observations on the 1891 census data, Collet noted that there was a north/south divide in women's employment patterns. She argued these indicated different attitudes to work. In the north, where the textile industry had a long history of employing female labour which included married women, work was considered by women as a 'life occupation', not merely a means of support before marriage. The higher wages paid to women (itself related to the early unionization of women alongside men in the industry) enabled them to use their wages for greater comfort. In the south, in contrast, which had a much smaller industrial sector and a larger proportion of domestic servants, Collet suggests that marriage was viewed 'as a release from wage-earning employment'.[23] Whatever the validity of her explanations for different patterns of women's work, the fact that there were different opportunities for work, that women were, therefore, employed in different industries or in different ways within them in different parts of the country, are important for any consideration of how work might impact on their health.

Working women were in a minority and they were still predominately working-class and single. At the end of the nineteenth century it was still not possible to ascertain the extent of married women's employment beyond impressionistic or local studies. Data on unmarried, married and widowed workers was not available until the 1901 census, when widows were included within a category of 'ever married'. In 1911 this group were distinguished. Adelaide Anderson, the Chief Lady Inspector of Factories and a long-term critic of the adequacy of statistical data on women's employment, had told the Interdepartmental Inquiry on Physical Deterioration in 1904 that there were different patterns of employment of married women in specific districts, but it was possible to provide 'only rough estimates of numbers'.[24] Other researchers who have had an interest in married women's employment point out that from 1881 to 1891 the absence of age-structure information also hinders estimates although, by sampling schedules for 1851 and 1871 in Lancashire, Margaret Hewitt obtained estimates of 26.87 per cent and 34.73 per cent among cotton operatives.[25] These figures do not give us much insight into the national picture, however, as it is acknowledged that a characteristic of the textile industry was the large-scale employment of married women. Married women's employment was also high in the Potteries,[26] and in the jute industry in Scotland. In Dundee, women comprised 75 per cent of the workforce in jute: two-thirds of all working women in the city – and of these one-third were married. Unlike the national pattern, the largest group of women workers were aged 25–45.[27]

Other studies of industrial centres suggest that between one-fifth and one-quarter was not uncommon. In their study of Birmingham, Cadbury, Mathieson and Shann found married women comprised 23 per cent of all wage-earning women but the majority worked in 'unregulated trades' with 21 per cent of those in factory work married.[28] Of 85 058 working women in Liverpool in 1901, 21 457 were married.[29] Outside of traditions of employment of married women, there were those which also restricted their opportunity to work by operating a marriage bar. Many industrial companies did so,[30] and it was also a feature of the new middle-class occupations.

By the time we have some census data on the marital status of working women, according to Hakim,[31] it shows that the marital status of working women did not bear any resemblance to the distribution by marital status of all women aged 15–59. Single women were overrepresented and the 'ever-married' and then married underrepresented. Data derived from her tables on participation rates of different birth cohorts by marital status for 1901 and 1911 are shown in Table 1.2. In the 1911 census, out of a female population of ten-plus years numbering 15 million in England and Wales, the total number of working women was 4 830 734. Of these, only 680 191 were married.[32] Only 1 per cent of the largest age group employed, those aged 17 to 20, were married. About 13 per cent of married and 9 per cent of widows were returned as economically active in the early years of the twentieth century (see Table 1.3).[33] Thus the largest category of women workers were single, even where there were traditions of married women working. Factory Department figures for 1907, for example, show that in Blackburn 40 per cent of girls aged 10 to 15 were occupied and 89.5 per cent of the 15–25-year-old age group. Of these, 12 per cent were in domestic service and the majority worked in the mills.[34] The high proportion of single women is related to the prevalence of young girls in the industrial workforce, despite some restrictions on their hours.

Table 1.2 Labour force participation rate for women by birth cohort and marital status, 1901, 1911

Cohort born		Participation rate (in percentages)							
		Single		Married		Divorced/ widowed		All women	
		1901	1911	1901	1911	1901[†]	1911	1901	1911
Born	15–24 years								
1847–1856	1871	57	46	16*	9		32	22	20
1857–1866	1881	64	59	13	11		47	23	23
1867–1876	1891	70	66	10	11		62	31	24
1877–1886	1901	70	74	11	11		66	61	34
1887–1896	1911		73		13		59		65

* Ever married
[†] Divorced and widowed included with married women. 1901 table derived from census tabulation data in Hakim, C. (1979).

Table 1.3 Percentage working women by marital status 1901 and 1911 census

	Single	Married	Divorced or widowed
1901	78	13*	9*
1911	77	14	9

* Estimates: Hakim, C. (1979) p.11.

What is interesting about these data on women's employment is how the development of issues around occupational health, in terms of the discourse about women's employment and the attempts to regulate it and its effects, did not coincide with actual patterns of women's employment. I have highlighted that married women constituted only a small minority of working women, yet it was married women who were a major focus for agitation and legislative intervention. This factor is central to my argument that social purposes, including social control, were responsible for a focus on this group, not a concern with their health *per se*. A further consequence of this attention to married women who worked was that female dependence on wage labour became very problematical for those who occupied different sides of the debate about the desirability of married women in the paid labour market. Census data and other data clearly showed that the assumption that women would have male providers for a substantial period of their lifetime were fundamentally flawed.

The reasons were twofold. First, by the end of the nineteenth century, there were more women than men,[35] in part a consequence of better female survival at birth and greater male migration. Collet[36] observed that in better-off districts of London, women outnumbered men by as many as two to one, suggesting that 'the problem of surplus women' may have been felt more acutely by middle-class women. For women who had not married in the years 25–29, about one-quarter, rising to one-third, would not do so during their reproductive years.[37] For those who did marry, the average length of that marriage was estimated at 20 years. Barbara Hutchins argued that a high proportion of mature women in employment could thus be accounted for by the fact that 'economic self-dependence' was a necessity.[38]

Other commentators at the time also raised the importance of recognizing widows' need for work. For Hutchins, such issues demonstrated how women's lives and employment were related to that of men's. She argues that high male mortality was an issue, raising the question as to whether 'it is necessary so large a proportion of women should be widows at all'. Men also needed 'protection' from the effects of their 'dangerous trades'.[39]

But it was not only not marrying, or the death of a husband, that led to women's dependence on work for wages. It was also a result of men's low wages and/or their casual employment or unemployment. There was a common assumption that married women worked through choice or for 'extras', which was also fallacious. In the Potteries, Hilda Martindale, a member of the women's factory inspectorate, estimated that only 18 per cent of them were not compelled to work out of financial necessity.[40] Studies of homework also revealed the very high numbers of households with little or no income from men.[41] For single women, too, (although, as Collet[42] pointed out, participation can be accounted for by cultural and economic traditions that included expectations that women would work) there were those in all parts of the country who 'needed' work as a means of self-dependence or as a contribution to the household income. The full implications of women's dependence on wages are returned to in many parts of the book, especially as it impinged in a material way on their health and was a contested domain within the discourse. Gender differences in mortality are also pertinent to questions of women's relation to the labour market, as the relatively high participation rates among widows demonstrates.

From 1870 a pattern of greater longevity for women began to be evident. At this time women could expect to have an additional 1.97 years of life and this was to increase from now on. The lower mortality of infants and of women over 45 years contributed most to this pattern. In fact women's increasing life expectancy over men obscured considerable disadvantaged groups of women. There was excess female mortality in the 5–19 year age group and this was the slowest to show a female advantage, while women in their thirties were also more likely to die.[43]

The patterns of women's employment also demonstrate a further disparity between the reality and those issues which were the focus of attention in this period. The largest single area of employment, that of domestic service, was notably not considered for State intervention, although as Chapter 4 reveals, there was some interest in aspects of 'the servant question'. There may be a number of reasons for this. The threat to morals and to health were seen to lie primarily in the factory system, although some kinds of industrial work carried out in domestic dwellings did receive attention and some non-factory areas of employment, especially shop work, were considered early in this period as possibly requiring intervention. Domestic service was also a form of employment that occurred within families and the confines of the private household. There was a general antipathy towards the State's interference with private lives and familial relations so it was unlikely that intervention would have been acceptable to middle-class public opinion. Finally, it was a form of employment whose general conditions remained at the level of individual problems rather than collective grievances that were publicly displayed.

The Labour Market and Sexual Divisions

In considering women's employment patterns, it is necessary to go beyond the attributes of age and marital status of working women. We must explore other characteristics of the labour market and women's work within it that directly and indirectly impinged on their health status. In particular, the sexual divisions within the labour market were a precondition for how the problems of women's employment, including possible health consequences, were responded to. Policies and legislative attempts to regulate either the supply of labour or working conditions will usually be constrained by socioeconomic conditions and factors such as technological development, degrees of complexity in work processes and changing consumer demand. These in turn can effect the changes in demand for skills and labour supply. Gender divisions within the labour market effected and were affected by such factors. Such gender divisions disputes the idea that the work people do reflects some neutral principle of economic rationality. Instead, with its links with political institutions and ideological influences, the market is a mechanism that structures gender-based inequality specifically within the workplace.[44] In contemporary feminism, such sexual divisions and forms of work segregation in particular have been considered crucial dimensions in explaining women's economic disadvantage and their position within the family.[45]

In this period there was evidence of considerable sexual segregation of the labour market. This was both vertical and horizontal: vertical because women were in the worst paid, most menial and unskilled jobs in the labour market as a whole and within particular industries. Women's pay was substantially lower than men's even when they did the same work. Horizontal segregation can be measured in a number of ways but most usually it referred to the extent to which in different occupations men and women were disproportionately represented. In 1901, for example, half of all men worked in all-male jobs, while only 11 per cent of women worked in all-female jobs. Another indicator is to consider what the proportion of men and women are in particular jobs, compared to their proportion in the paid labour market as a whole.

In considering this kind of overrepresentation in typically female jobs or underrepresentation in typically male ones, figures for 1901 reveal that 88 per cent of women were in jobs where more than 29 per cent were women: a 2.7 ratio over that expected, while their ratio in typically male occupations was 0.18.[46] In clerical, shop-assistant and sales work in 1911, women's participation was broadly equivalent to their contribution to the labour force as a whole but such jobs would increasingly come to be occupied by women.[47]

Horizontal segregation is thought to reflect ideas of appropriate work and occupations for men and women based on culturally pervasive ideas of 'femininity' and 'masculinity' and associated social roles. Thus, some work had already come to be regarded as the province of either men or women and this sexual division of labour was believed to be 'natural'. Not only were ideas about what was suitable work for women shared by many women themselves; it was also likely that they accepted that men were entitled to better pay and that their own wages were secondary.[48] In this way sexual divisions and discrimination in the workplace reproduced the separation of the workplace and home, with the workplace as the primary sphere of work for men. Such divisions were also apparent in those industries like textiles or nail- and chain-making where the sexual divisions of former family and domestically based production survived the transition into the factory system.[49]

Sexual divisions in the form of occupational segregation impacted on health and wellbeing in the following ways. If men and women were engaged in different types of work, it meant there would be gender-differentiated risks to whatever hazards might be associated with that work. It has been a common perception that men are at greater risk from their occupations because their work is more hazardous and physically strenuous. There is thus a conflation of 'danger' and 'men' in relation to health risks and work. This assumption has been important in the marginalization of the health consequences of women's paid work – and this period was no exception. Most evidence of occupational mortality does lend support to the view that men are more at risk. Morbidity data also provides support for this contention, although there are considerable limitations with all the official sources of data as an accurate reflection of occupational health problems.[50] However, it is not intended to argue with the validity of the data, rather to point out certain contradictions that arose from gender-specific assumptions about, and responses to, actual occupational health problems. In the period examined here this was most clearly evident in relation to occupationally-related lead poisoning where the incidence for men was greater, yet many regulations were instituted for women only (see Chapter 2). The association of health dangers with men's work could also obscure the same risk to women. This was particularly true of industrial accidents: there were high rates of accidents in areas of men's work, particularly those associated with machines. However, women also experienced accidents at work in a wide range of industries. They were also at risk from machinery, given that it was mainly women and young persons who cleaned them. Here, there was little evident concern with accidents to women, nor were women factory inspectors given responsibilities for them.[51] The association of men or women with particular occupations and the attendant health risks led to the possibility of either gender being given undue attention or having their interests ignored. Laundrywork, which until the early twentieth century was mainly women's work and where they remained predominant, employed more men as it became more mechanized and factory-based.[52] In relation to increasing regulation instituted in the 1890s and contrary to demands made, laundries were excluded, yet in other industries where women were in the minority, although employed in particular processes, legislation was introduced to deal with them specifically. Thus there was no necessary relationship between 'protective' legislation or other health and safety regulations and the gendered differences in occupational risk.

Sexual segregation of work and work processes was not fixed, however. It depended on local labour markets and job opportunities. Lewis[53] points to the example of brick-making, which in areas of mining or heavy industry was a women's job, whereas where women were employed in cotton manufacture, brick-making was a male preserve. To this extent the attribution of work as 'naturally' gender-specific was adjusted to local circumstances. This was also evident in health risks. In the Potteries, for example, where there was a well-defined sexual division of labour and processes that exposed both men and women to the possibility of lead-poisoning, women were thought to be particularly at risk.

This did not mean that all processes in which they worked came to be regulated. In majolica-painting, for example it was never entertained that women should be restricted because it was considered to be 'natural' work for women that men would never be able to do (see Chapter 2). Further, whether or not women were perceived by men to be a competitive threat to their jobs, which some analysts have argued was an important dimension of attitudes to restriction,[54] also requires consideration of such local features. Contemporary activists also engaged men's opposition in these terms (see Chapter 8).

Sometimes women could be 'allowed' to take over men's jobs. There was no threat of undercutting because new forms of employment became available for men, as in the Leicestershire hosiery industry when boot-and-shoe manufacture became available,[55] or where technological change redefined the skill level of jobs as in the deskilling of spinning in late nineteenth-century mills.[56] This suggests that a combination of labour markets and skill supply, consistent with gendered notions of work, could also determine whether intervention would be demanded or considered.

The lack of employment opportunities for women in the factory system, combined with the practical difficulties they encountered in relation to their domestic responsibilities, also resulted in a predominance of women in small workshops and forms of homework (see Chapter 3). The precise amount of homework at this time is difficult to ascertain because of its casual, unregulated and 'hidden' characteristics. But as workshops were brought within the remit of factory regulation by the 1891 and 1895 Factory Acts and by local authority surveillance of environmental and sanitary conditions, it is likely that homework increased.[57] The employer benefited from the fact that little capital was required and workers bore some of the costs. This particular aspect of the segregated labour market had major implications for women's health. Yet despite the fact that the 'sweated trades' were a focus for reform of the industrial system, ultimately it was low pay and economic efficiency, rather than health, that essentially prompted action.[58]

Occupational Health and Industrial Disease

Knowledge about the occupational basis for ill-health and disease was in its infancy. Even within those professional groups which had a responsibility for public health in its widest sense, only a few national and local figures took an interest in these questions (see Chapter 6). This had a number of consequences. First, that ideas and knowledge tended to develop as a result of people's personal observations of a workplace, including those of the workers themselves. These were then communicated in response to particular circumstances. One such context was official enquiry. Whether or not health consequences were addressed was often in relation to whether this question was central to the enquiry's purpose. Thus we can find witnesses being rigorously questioned on their health status in one enquiry and hardly raised at all in others.[59] Equally in the work of factory inspectors, and in specific campaigns with political objectives, injury to health would seem to enter the discourse as a context of justification, that is, in order to reach desired objectives.

Although some use was made of what 'expert' knowledge did exist, the assumptions of health risks associated with work remained at a very general level. Typically, the tenor of the discourse was that aspects of work were 'injurious to health', or led to 'weakness' in undermining physical strength. There was rarely any mention of how or why such health consequences arose. Outside of specific investigative work that was oriented to particular conditions and the accumulated knowledge that developed about specific work-related morbidity, this generalized argument about health operated more as a social and political strategy than a preventive health one.

There were difficulties in doing more than this, given the problematical nature of establishing cause–effect relationships: whether symptoms or illness were occupational in origin or derived from other possible causes. In medical practice the establishment of the particular agent responsible for observed pathology has been a necessary basis for the 'appropriate' targeting of therapeutic intervention and preventive activities. Identifiable occupational 'diseases' have fallen within the 'medical model' in this way. The possibility that a 'cause' can be found was (and still is) essential to establishing that work was responsible, if, for example, a worker was to be entitled to compensation. In the case of accidents, this is usually unambiguous, although who was responsible for the accident might not be. Accidents came to be viewed in this context as 'disease'.[60] With other 'diseases' the link might also be relatively unambiguous, as in exposure to poisons or bacteria. The measurement of occupational ill-health has involved using indicators such as required notifications, mortality rates or compensation claims which have been associated with a limited range of illness. Such a 'medically-oriented' model of illness has generally been found wanting in understanding contemporary patterns of health[61]. These have relevance to the specific case of occupational health and ill-health.

When we move from the 'disease' concept of occupational ill-health, the task of identifying the relationship becomes more difficult as forms of acute and chronic morbidity have varying degrees of specificity. There will be a wide range of symptomology and perceived or experienced wellbeing that may be psychological as well as physical. What is responsible for these outcomes is more complex. It is rare that any one specific aspect of working conditions will give rise to a single outcome, but rather that a number of features of work will interact to produce debility or its converse. There will be contingent as well as alternative causes operating. For example, the pace of work may only result in negative. wellbeing, if that pace is externally imposed. Unfortunately, it is not just the operation of factors in the work-place which interact in this way. The circumstances in which people live can also contribute to whether health will be undermined in the workplace.

These arguments are relevant in this historical context because they were aspects of a discourse available to historical actors about occupational ill-health. More specifically it is evident that there were a multiplicity of factors and a com-plexity of cause–effect relationships which required all the facets of women's lives to be considered in relation to their health and wellbeing.[62] In turn this had con-sequences on how the problems of working conditions were defined and responded to. Inevitably such arguments were not only a reflection of the actual difficulties involved in establishing health outcomes, but part of 'duelling discourses' each of which hoped to win the argument. These were inseparable from the pursuit of moral, social and political objectives.

Equally, in the same contexts, there were often attempts to arrive at consensus. In the more obvious example of factory mothers and infant mortality (see Chapter 3) social purposes were evident in debates about intervention. They were also there in all aspects where links were made between women's health and their participa-tion in the paid labour force, including middle-class women's work (see Chapter 4). But despite the fact that health dimensions featured in discursive representations of the 'problems' of women's work, it was evidently difficult to envisage either the scale of occupational health problems or an effective remedy to deal with possible risks (see Chapter 5). For women themselves, many occupations required them to stand most of the day for long hours. These could be associated with specific symptoms such as leg ulcers and varicose veins. Such conditions also contributed to a sense of strain, feelings of exhaustion, headaches and loss of appetite, yet these were rarely perceived as ill-health in their own right. Single remedies were often pursued, such as regulating the hours of work, but this in itself made little impact.

The following chapters aim to describe and explain the paradox within pre-ventive strategies pursued in relation to occupational ill-health at this time, exem-plified by the 'dangerous trades'. As Chapter 2 will demonstrate, while it was possible to remedy the identified cause of the problem, such as lead, phosphorous, asbestos, arsenic and other substances, by elimination, this was rejected in favour of regu-lations introduced into specified industries to control working conditions to the extent that the risks would be minimized. Ironically, it was in the case of the 'dan-gerous trades' that general conditions were improved, even though the sources of disease remained present, while in the many industries without such identified 'dan-gers' these same aspects of working conditions were not regulated and continued to undermine health and wellbeing. Finally, in identifying links between work and ill-health, it is important to take account not just of the physical environment and the nature of work processes and work organization, but also the social relations and meaning of work. For women, such considerations as their lack of control and power in the workplace also have a health dimension.

This introduction has given a personal background to the investigation and has developed both a descriptive and conceptual context for the detailed chapters that follow. There are important theoretical and empirical issues which have not been discussed here, particularly those related to developing a feminist analysis of women, men and the State in relation to work and health. These will be discussed in the conclusion.

Notes

1   There was considerable feminist activism around trade unionism itself, especially of women's absence from positions of power. See, for example, Coote and Kellner (1980) *Here This Brother: Women Workers and Union Power*; and Beale (1982) *Getting it Together: Women as Trade Unionists*.

2   The *Women and Work Hazards Group* was an associate group of the British Society for Social Responsibility in Science, whose campaigns extended over a wide range of political and social concerns about the production and use of knowledge.

3   The group finally ceased to exist in 1990, but there were groups such as City Centre who continued to support occupational health issues for some women workers.

4   The film *Bitter Wages* was produced by the group and directed by Audrey Droisen, with financial support from the Greater London Council (GLC) Women's Committee. It was broadcast by Channel 4 on 14 June 1985.

5   In 1981, a number of women's health groups organized one of the largest women-only conferences on the social causes of women's health in Islington, London.

6   By discourse I mean those linguistic forms and practices which are intended and heard to give meaning within social contexts. As such, discourses are forms of social knowledge, formalized topics that people acquire, share, disseminate and critique. As such, discourse is a social practice that has a material basis and both knowledge and ideology are achieved through and by it. Forms and content of meaning in discourse are also a function of and exercise power. See the many works by M. Foucault, but especially *Power/Knowledge: Selected Interviews and Other Writings* (1980) edited by Colin Gordon; Dant (1991) *Knowledge, Ideology and Discourse: A Sociological Perspective*.

7   Canning (1994) 'Feminist history after the linguistic turn' p.370.

8   I return to this debate in the conclusion, but significantly this view is pursued by Joan Scott. See especially her 1988 collection of essays *Gender and the Politics of History*.

9   There are others who would argue with this as a centralizing discourse of women's oppression. Others see sexuality occupying this role, including State policy and the law, for example, MacKinnon (1989) but at this time, in my view, it was the relationship between economic and family life that was crucial. Sexuality was important, but less so.

10   For an examination of how the disordered metaphor operated around women's health in another context, see Verbrugge (1988) *Able-bodied Womanhood*.

11   This particular term is one used by Jane Lewis (1986c) in 'The working-class wife and mother and State intervention', but many commentators have argued there was a sea-change of opinion at this time (gradual rather than dramatic) including contributors to Langan and Schwartz (Eds) (1986) *Crisis in the British State*.

12   Higgs (1987) 'Women, occupation and work in nineteenth-century censuses'; Hakim (1985) 'Social monitors: population censuses as social surveys'. There were a number of locality-based studies which are also useful sources of information about women's employment patterns, notably Booth (1895) *Life and Labour of the People of London*;

Cadbury, Mathieson, Shann (1906) *Women's Work and Wages: A Phase of Life in an Industrial City* (on Birmingham); Harrison (1904) *Women's Industries in Liverpool*, although such local studies reflect an emphasis on industrial employments.

13 Hakim draws attention to some of these problems in her 1980 paper *Census Reports as Documentary Evidence: The Census Commentaries, 1801–1951*. Most overviews of women's work in the period and the time and recently also draw attention to such weaknesses, for example Lewis (1984) *Women in England* p.146.

14 Collet (1896) *Report on the Statistics of Employment of Women and Girls in England and Wales* and Hutchins (1909) 'Statistics of women's lives and employment'.

15 Davies (1980b) 'Making sense of the census in Britain and the USA: the changing occupational classification and the position of nurses'.

16 Collet (1896) 'Report on the statistics of employment of women and girls in England and Wales'.

17 Hakim (1979) *Occupational Segregation* p.4.

18 Ibid., p.10.

19 Collet (1898) 'The collection and utilisation of official statistics bearing on the extent and effects of the industrial employment of women'.

20 Hakim (1979) p.25.

21 Holcombe (1973) *Victorian Ladies at Work* p.216.

22 Anderson (1988) 'The white blouse revolution' p.4.

23 Collet (1896)p.96.

24 See her *Memorandum on the Employment of Mothers* (1904) PP XXXII.

25 Hewitt (1958) *Wives and Mothers in Victorian Industry* pp.15–16.

26 See Hewitt (1958) ibid., and *Report of the Interdepartmental Committee on Physical Deterioration*, (1904).

27 Gordon (1987) 'Women work and collective action', p.29.

28 Cadbury, Mathieson and Shann (1906) *Women's Work and Wages*.

29 Harrison (1904) *Women's Industry in Liverpool*.

30 See Rose (1992) *Limited Livelihoods*.

31 Hakim (1979) *Occupational Segregation* p.11.

32 Hutchins (1915) *Women in Modern Industry* p.83.

33 This is tentative because of the change in category. It could still be an underestimate.

34 Cited in Hutchins (1909) 'Statistics of women's life and employment' p.25.

35 Hutchins (1909) cites 1901 data of 15 729 000 males to 16 799 000 females, an excess of over one million.

36 Collet (1902) 'Educated working women', in the essay *Prospects of Marriage for Women*.

37 Lewis (1984) *Women in England* p.4.

38 Hutchins (1909) 'Statistics of women's life and employment', p.16.

39 Ibid., p.17.

40 *Report of the Interdepartmental Committee on Physical Deterioration*, (1904). PP XXXII.

41 Cadbury and Shann (1907) *Sweating*.

42 Collet (1898) p.96.

43 For a detailed discussion of gender differences in mortality at this time see Johansson (1977) 'Sex and death in Victorian England' and Shorter (1983) *A History of Women's Bodies*.

44 See Scott (1986) 'Industrialization, gender segregation and stratification theory' for a development of this argument.

45 Many examples could be cited here, but see Hartmann (1976) 'Capitalism, patriarchy

and job segregation by sex'; Walby (1986) *Patriarchy at Work*; Walby (Ed.) (1988) *Gender Segregation at Work*; Bradley (1989) *Women's Work, Men's Work*; Lown (1990) *Women and Industrialisation*.

46   Hakim (1979) *Occupational Segregation* pp.28–9.

47   Ibid., p.27.

48   Lewis (1984) *Women in England* pp.162–73.

49   Lewis (1984) *Women in England* pp.173–6.

50   Standardized mortality ratios, an accepted measure of differential occupational mortality, has not been able to provide comparative evidence because women's occupations were not recorded on death certificates until recently. However, higher death rates generally occur in male-dominated industries. Morbidity poses similar problems although analyses suggest considerable chronic occupational morbidity: see Doyal (1979) *The Political Economy of Health,* pp.66–75. Recently, analyses based on women's occupational morbidity suggest that different occupations are implicated in high morbidity: see Arber (1991).

51   I have noted the consequences of this in relation to the industrial accident in this period, where there were more accidents to men, but those occurring to women received little attention. See Harrison (1993a) 'Are accidents gender-neutral'?

52   Malcolmson (1981) 'Laundresses and the laundry trade in Victorian England'.

53   Lewis (1984) *Women in England* p.162.

54   See Walby (1986) *Patriarchy at Work*; Rose (1988) 'Gender antagonism and class conflict'.

55   Osterud (1986) 'Gender divisions and the organisation of work in the Leicester hosiery industry'.

56   Rose (1992) *Limited Livelihoods*.

57   For an overview of homework in this period, see Pennington and Westover (1989) *A Hidden Workforce*.

58   Morris (1986b) *Women Workers and the Sweated Trades*.

59   For example in some enquires there was a specific brief to examine health consequences, as in the lead industries, in the *Royal Commission of Labour Reports on Women's Work (1893–4)*, and in matchmaking. In others, such as the *Report of the Select Committee on Homework 1908*, this was not the case.

60   Figlio (1985) 'What is an accident?'

61   There are too many examples to mention, but for a development of this critique the following have been frequently cited: Freidson (1970) *Profession of Medicine*; Doyal (1979) *The Political Economy of Health*; Illich (1976) *The Limits to Medicine*.

62   For an overview of women's health issues in general in this period, see Harrison (1995b) 'Women's health'.

Part I

The Problem

Chapter 1

Suffer the Working Day: Women's Work and Endangered Health

Despite a relative absence of professionally based knowledge about occupational disease and ill-health, the fact that work did make women sick was recognized and documented. There was as Beatrice Webb described it 'the same dismal refrain', about earnings, hours of work and sanitary conditions.[1] There seemed to be little that mitigated the litany of wrongs of the industrial system and its consequences in this case for women. In this chapter some of these aspects, which exemplified the possible health consequences for women within the labour market, will be examined. First, a brief analysis of women's pay is followed by a more detailed examination of three aspects of working conditions – hours, sanitary conditions and issues about ventilation and temperature. The chapter concludes with examples of the exercise of male power over women.

Barely Enough to Survive: Wages

The amount of money workers take home from their employment has been fundamental to the material basis of health and ill-health. It is therefore essential to consider this particular kind of deprivation which many working-class people experienced at this time, as a consequence of both class- and gender-based discrimination. While working-class people's lives were a constant struggle to maintain some kind of existence, for women, whose entitlement to subsistence-level pay was itself in question, the consequences of inadequate wages were even more devastating. Clementina Black, the trade unionist and social feminist activist, concluded in 1889 that low wages were at the 'root of working women's problems', a problem which at this time she considered to be a product of extreme economic competition so that 'if people must work or starve, there will be found some people who will give them work at a price just above starvation'.[2] In the mounting agitation around 'sweating' pay was given special prominence and the House of Lords Select Committee on Sweating concluded as much in its report of 1890.[3] When proposals for the elimination of sweating were considered much later, in the first decade of the twentieth century, the most prominent involved an attack on low pay and the establishment of the 'minimum wage'.[4]

In discussing pay in this section, I focus first on the evidence of wage levels and differentials between occupations and men and women, as well as features of the labour market and work organization which impinged on these, particularly the doctrine of the 'family wage'. Second, in recognition that such wage levels were a crude indicator of disposable income, the particular problem of 'truck' is discussed: that is, the system of payment in kind, as well as fines and deductions from wages which were common in many areas of women's work. Finally, brief reference is made to the campaign for a 'minimum wage' as the basis for the elimination of 'sweating' and the consequences of Trades Board legislation to this effect on women's pay.

It was in the domain of pay that gender divisions which permeated through the class structure were most evident. Sweating and low pay were a result of the sexual division of labour. This operated through divisions within the labour market which determined the suitability of kinds of work for women and men – and thereby women's eligibility. This structuring of the labour market and the management of labour was accompanied by judgments about the social value of women's labour which deemed it to be less than men's, even when women were employed in the same or similar processes. In many instances, however, this structuring took the form of ensuring that men and women did not work in the same processes on the basis of such factors as appropriate skill, strength and machine type and who should operate them.

An important basis of these labour-market sexual divisions was the ideology of 'separate spheres': a division between paid work as appropriately the domain of men and women's primary responsibilities in the domestic sphere. The 'family wage doctrine' or the 'male breadwinner norm' lay behind the idea that men should be paid a wage sufficient to maintain his family members and that accordingly there was no economic necessity for married women to work. Thus differential entitlement to pay become a focus for both male and female activism.

According to Seecombe,[5] in the nineteenth century there was a shift in the prevailing wage form from a joint to an individual payment and in the predominant subsistence norm of a living wage in the form of a living wage from a 'family wage' to 'adult breadwinner wage'. The significance of this distinction for Seecombe is that in the latter women and children did not constitute part of the workforce for that wage. However, other writers have also used the term 'family wage' in this context but they have noted that there was a change in form when wages were removed from a context of family labour.[6] Traditions of family labour and women's employment were important determinants of male attitudes to married women's work, and the extent of women's own active resistance to forms of discrimination.[7] There has been considerable debate among feminist and social historians about the pervasiveness of the idea of the 'family wage' and the part it played in either gender- and/or class-based politics including 'protective' legislation. There is a consensus that the 'family wage' involved male control over women's labour; it was an ideal which some working-class men and male political élites used in strategies to exclude women[8] and married women in particular from paid work. As such the 'family wage' was also an important site of feminist resistance.[9] That it would be 'imperfectly realised in practice' and therefore should be treated more as 'myth'[10] or an ideal within political rhetoric does not undermine its significance in the gendered structuring of work and entitlement to its economic rewards.

Because women were not expected to be in paid employment, or thought to need money to support themselves either fully or in part, or to have dependants, but rather to be economically dependent on men, male and female wage differentials could be maintained. The defense of both the 'family wage' and male and female pay differentials at this time reveals the long history of the concept of women who work for 'pin money'. Gender-based pay differentials in turn reinforced the lower economic value and social worth of women's work and confined them to low status, unskilled work usually then designated as 'women's' processes.

One of the constant problems for investigators and activists in this period was that such deeply entrenched ideas and the structures which maintained them contradicted the increasing evidence and knowledge about the reality of working women's lives and their economic circumstances. Ultimately there was a failure to deal with the problem because the gender divisions which gave rise to it frequently remained unchallenged. In reality there were many problems with the achievement of a 'family wage'. First, the assumption did not reflect the realities of men's bargaining position in the workplace and their own relative lack of success in achieving wage levels that would provide subsistence-level pay for their 'dependants'.

In 1911, Bowley estimated there were 2.5 million adult men who earned less than 25s a week working full-time.[11] As part of her campaign work around family allowances, Eleanor Rathbone's study of prewar subsistence wage levels revealed that using the standard of 35s per week, 74 per cent of men earned less than this, and using 25s, 32 per cent when in full work.[12] In any case, as she argued in her attack on the 'family wage', even if a man was earning there was no guarantee he would provide for his wife and children.

These two aspects of male wages, then, often required women to enter paid work in order to try to achieve earnings to sustain family life. There were also non-unionized men, men with illness and disabilities, as well as considerable numbers who relied on casual employment who brought in little if any income.[13] Second, the majority of women workers were not married and for many women, both working and middle-class, the need to support themselves alone necessitated paid employment.[14] The paradox was that the use of the 'family wage' argument in male trade-union strategies, whether exclusionary in intent or not, was that over the country as a whole only 10 per cent of the women's workforce were married.[15] In some areas, such as textiles, where there was a tradition of married women's work, this was much higher. In any case there were both cultural traditions as well as formal marriage-bars in operation which continued to restrict married women's employment. Some argued that competition from women 'drove down men's wages'. This could only have been the case if all women were targeted and in some cases this was so. But the use of the doctrine in relation to married women must be seen primarily in terms of a reassertion of patriarchal control in the domestic sphere.

Data on pay presents us with many difficulties. Generally we have to rely on anecdotal evidence, enquiries into specific trades or areas of women's employment and statistical evidence which, despite its more systematic basis, still had numerous flaws which cast doubt on its accuracy. That said, a consensus emerges as to typical levels of pay across a variety of women's employment. These show some universal features: that women's pay was lower than men's although the ratio may have varied; that these differentials did not change much over the decades considered here or thereafter; that opportunities for higher wages were very limited; and that differentials between 'middle-class' occupations and 'working-class' work were evident but were not of any magnitude. As Chapter 4 reveals, some areas of middle-class non-manual professional work did pay better but many others paid little more and sometimes less, for example, some clerical work and nursing. In this sense, lesser eligibility was a problem for all women regardless of their class origins. It allowed activists to pursue a political platform on the basis of gender as a class.

An example of more systematic enquiries were those conducted under the auspices of the Board of Trade. In 1906, for example, a census of wages and hours of labour of persons employed in all industries was undertaken. This voluntary return probably only covered about half of the wage-earning population and represented 'better' employers. The census covered women over the age of 18 in full-time employment and wages were calculated on the basis of one particular pay week. In reporting this data, Mallon[16] concluded that the cotton industry 'stands out conspicuously as showing a relatively high level of earnings' at least within textile and clothing industries, with only 3 per cent earning less than 10s a week. In clothing this figure was 21.6 per cent. Different trades and different localities (with the two often associated) showed different patterns. Average rates could be very misleading about the experience of many women workers whose earnings fell below this. It could also obscure widespread poverty in certain areas, particularly in Ireland. In clothing, as one example, there were apprentices who received no wages at all; among milliners this accounted for 43 per cent.

In general, those in workshop employment earned less, but increasing factory employment did not necessarily bring about better pay. In laundries, for example, there was only one penny difference in average wages between those which by virtue of using mechanical power were defined as factories and those which did not – 'hand-laundries'. In any case since much factory work paid on a piecework basis, this produced its own differentials. In turn even if opportunities were there to earn more, there was the additional pressure involved in the requirement of increased speed. The 1895 Factory Act did secure a claim for the textiles pieceworker to a definite contract as to her prospective earnings on any given piece of work and in 1901 and 1903 this was extended to other industries. Unfortunately this did not provide any protection against 'driving' – setting contracts at higher levels for agreed rates.

There were estimates of the minimum sum necessary for a woman living independently of relatives to maintain herself in 'decency' and a low standard of comfort. These pointed to a figure of around 14s 6d to 15s but this probably assumed that women shared the knowledge and means to spend the money in the same way as those who made the calculations. In any event such an inexact standard, in the clothing industry alone, would leave 111 681 on wages that were grossly inadequate. For the majority of working-class women enough food and warmth was difficult to attain.[17] Such calculations fail to tell us about the particular difficulties posed by seasonal fluctuations and layoffs or short-time working.

One of the worst abuses in late nineteenth-century employment was the operation of 'truck', or payment in kind. The 1881 Act, which first made it illegal, defined it as 'the entire amount of the wages earned by any artificer shall be actually paid to such artificer in the current coin of the realm and not otherwise'. However, commentators[18] noted that allowable exceptions, differential interpretations and signed agreements which were permitted under the legislation, meant the practice continued and so provided little protection for workers.

The payment of wages in kind operated in several ways. At its most simple it involved providing board or lodging and meals and charging the cost of these against the girl's or woman's wage. This was commonly found in some forms of clothing manufacture and in shop work. As most commentators noted the presumed cost did not usually match the quality of what was provided. The worst extreme of 'truck' was a system of paying workers in goods, commonly food and clothing usually from a store owned by the employer. Again, prices were inflated.

The operation of this latter system in relation to outwork in Ireland occupied a considerable amount of women factory inspectors' time and energy. Lucy Deane reported on embroidery work in Donegal where women obtained virtually 'little or no profit' from their work, nor any control over 'the fruit of their work which had to be spent in the shop of the agent who distributed it'.[19] It was difficult to deal with such practices even after 'truck' came under legislative control, although women inspectors devoted considerable energy to try to bring about prosecutions and an end to the practice. As Adelaide Anderson, the Chief Lady Inspector, reported in 1899, after spending a fortnight in Dungloe as a private resident, the 'law breakers represent the wealth and carrying power of the community'. The men on the Bench were representatives of local trades, to add to their deep-rooted suspicion of British officialdom.[20] Similar practices to those in Ireland were common among glove-makers in Somerset and knitters of fishermen's jerseys in Cornwall.

Inspector Gould described the practice of 'truck' in 1890 as 'pernicious':

> Wherever it has existed it has pauperised the working-class, reducing them to the condition of slaves, destroying their independence and placing them entirely at the power of the master, out of whose clutches they can never escape.[21]

Although he is not speaking specifically about women, their relatively greater lack of power in the workplace made them particularly vulnerable to these forms of abuse. Gould was not the only official to describe the operation of 'truck' as pernicious or harassing. In 1898,[22] deductions were made from the wages of young match-workers to pay for their parents' rent arrears.

The other abusive practice was the operation of systems of fines and deductions. Fines were monetary deductions for contravention of particular rules or small breaches of discipline, typically for any slips in punctuality. In some cases the latter would result in being 'locked out'. When wages were based on piecerates, this resulted in considerable loss of earnings. Miss Paterson, a woman factory inspector, suggested that these rules 'seem to be designed to exercise a kind of terrorism over the workers by the threats of undefined punishment to be imposed at the discretion of some subordinate official'.[23]

Fines were also levied for 'mistakes' or damage that occurred during the production process. The women factory inspectors described the case of a biscuit factory where labellers were paid at the rate of 1d per 12 tins, which involved putting labels on four sides and the top. If they damaged one label they would be fined 1d, thus the next 12 tins would in effect be done for nothing.[24] In steel-pen manufacture where wages of 2s 6d for 90 gross of pens were paid, women were regularly fined 6s to 7s for waste. Because the wages were so low they were constantly in debt, paying fines by instalment. In the 1902 report, inspectors mention a woman who was in debt for 18 months as a result of being fined in a single batch of machined shirt collars.[25] There was also a practice in some firms where workers had to buy damaged goods, sometimes through a system of raffles which further depleted low wages.

There were other deductions besides fines. These were for the costs of materials which many women had to provide in order to do their work. The worst excesses were in domestic workshops and forms of homework, where the employee had to pay for lighting, power, if used, and equipment. Again, women inspectors described these costs as 'numerous and harassing' where in one year[26] they cite examples of workers paying for carriers and cleaners and the replacement part for a machine. Sometimes employers were accused of dishonesty in charging women more than the retail price. To describe these dealings as abusive does not seem excessive because they frequently operated on the basis of arbitrary rules and the exercise of mainly male power vested in foremen and employers on a vulnerable workforce. As women inspectors observed, 'not merely was starvation pay for women and girls prevalent . . . but the employers had almost uncontrolled power to fix and alter rates for unorganized workers'.[27] These widespread practices 'render almost impossible any attempt to ascertain the wages actually earned'. It was possible these could be lowered by as much as 15 per cent.[28]

The operation of 'truck' was brought under some legislative regulation in 1896 with effect from 1897. The provisions essentially encompassed fines and deductions. They required employers to specify and display a standard set of rules and the penalties for contravention, to keep a register of fines and to issue receipts. This gave some relief, although it seemed that many employers considered that as long as they had displayed them their obligations were complete. In 1901 women inspectors found that girls in a corset factory had been fined for dancing to a harp in the dinner hour, 'allegedly in contravention of a rule that "due order and decorum be maintained"'.[29] Equally, as with most other areas of legislation, the words 'reasonable deductions' were used which allowed subjective judgments of employers to prevail. The regulations did not prevent lock-out for lateness and in many cases this continued to result in the loss of a half-day of work.

Investigations and campaigns around 'sweated labour' from the late 1880s through to the early decades of the twentieth century identified low wages, excessive hours of labour and the insanitary state of work places as primary conditions of sweating. It was also recognized that particular groups, by reasons of their sex, age or infirmity and without the benefit of trade-union organization, were vulnerable to this kind of exploitative form of employment. A more detailed examination of homework as a form of 'sweated' work is in Chapter 3.

Because low pay was identified as perhaps the most fundamental characteristic, it requires some discussion here. Although in the early twentieth century there were differences of view as to legislative remedy for 'sweating', eventually there was a consensus around the 'minimum' wage. This was implemented in the Trade Boards Act, 1909. It was based on the belief that if low pay was the problem, then payment had to be targeted. As one of the leading campaigners, Clementina Black, argued, 'The cure of underpayment needs to be applied at the point of payment; and the establishment of a legal minimum wage is the most direct method of application.'[30]

Far from providing a solution to the structured inequalities that had always been reflected in the idea of the 'family wage'; the setting of minimum rates by Trades Board simply reinforced its legitimacy. Dealing with minimum rates in predominately women's trades perpetuated differential pay rates and an association of men's work with the maintenance of family life. The 1909 census on wages and hours of work revealed that fixed minima did succeed in moving some traditional 'sweated' industries out of that category, although pay at the Trade Board's rate was often still low and well below the level necessary for any reasonable level of material existence. In 1906, in jam and food preserving, the minimum level set was 10s 11d per week, little different to rates in the previous century.[31]

While it is clear that there was an identification of certain trades, many of which were small factory workshops, domestic workshops and in particular forms of homework, with 'sweating', it can be argued that all women's employment at this time exhibited features of 'sweating'. It is these features and their relationship to health that this chapter now turns.

All of the Day and All of the Night: Hours of Work

Before the 1880s hours of work were the principal focus for trade unionists and others with an interest in the reform of the industrial system. Although there had been a concern with the employment of women, but more especially children, this was within the context of limiting hours of work. In the early 1840s, when the first attempt to introduce the 10-hour day failed, Lord Ashley had noted the 'evil effects on women and the demoralisation on the home life produced by long hours'.[32] In 1844 women's hours were reduced to 10.5 hours per day, plus 1.5 hours for mealtimes. Women and children were prohibited from cleaning machinery at the end of shifts and from remaining in workrooms at mealtimes because of the likely evasion of mealbreaks, although this latter aspect continued to be a major source of evasion.

The 1878 Factory Act explicitly established the principle of 'protective' legislation in respect of women's employment.[33] Although this Act was the first to restrict women and children in relation to the 'dangerous trades' by forbidding the taking of meals in workrooms where such processes were carried out, it was the actual hours of work that were the legislation's main focus. The Act set a limit of no more than 4.5 continuous hours of work in textiles and 5 hours in non-textiles without a half-hour break for meals. It made the requirement that they could only be employed within a specified 12-hour period: 6.00 am to 6.00 pm or 7.00 am to 7.00 pm, or 8.00 am to 8.00 pm on weekdays and until 4.00 pm on Saturdays, to a maximum of 60 hours per week.[34]

The problem was that not only were these still long hours but women's actual working hours rarely conformed to them, because the legislation allowed for exclusions and exemptions and for overtime. Legal overtime, for example, brought the average working week to 66 hours. As a result, one contemporary socialist feminist, Barbara Hutchins, argued: 'the regulation of women's hours especially presents a particular chaos of conflicting principles which are inexplicable without historical clue'.[35]

The chaos to which Hutchins referred was a direct product of a morass of methods permitted under the legislation which allowed the contravention of limits on the hours which women would work, particularly in relation to different classes of workplace and work. This was to have an impact on the ability of officials to detect contravention of regulation, or enforce compliance with it. There were obviously many areas of employment where more than 60 hours were worked.

In her report to the Royal Commission on Labour, Clara Collet noted that shop assistants often suffered from anaemia, indigestion and headaches as a result of their long hours, hasty meals and lack of rest-breaks. Typically they would work from 8.30 am until 8.00 pm weekdays and from 8.30 am to 11.00 am on Saturdays with only 15 minutes for dinner and 10 for tea. Some women also worked on Sundays to clean the shop and prepare the windows for Monday, reporting that this could take until 2.00 am.[36] Barmaids and waitresses were observed by another Assistant Lady Commissioner to work as long as 105 hours a week in holiday hotels. They often started at 5.00 am and finished at 3.00 pm, worked from 9.00 am to midnight on Saturdays and also on Sundays.[37]

The hours and conditions documented in the early 1890s continued to be at the forefront of shop-girls' grievances as seen by one who worked 83 hours a week for 7s 6d and food per week. In a letter to the *Glasgow News* in 1910, she wrote: 'There are many such as I, starving ever hopelessly in obscurity and weariness, with no choice between submission and dismissal.'[38] Shop assistants, as with many other women workers, found themselves subject to long hours as a consequence of widespread evasion and exemptions (see Chapter 4).

Exemptions were granted to jam-making and food-preserving, as well as fish-cleaning, salting and curing, on the grounds that they were 'emergency processes' necessitated by the industry's seasonality and the perishable nature of the materials. Arguments similar to these, such as 'materials likely to be spoiled by the weather' or 'sudden pressure of unforseen orders' were relatively easy to use as grounds for requesting exemptions, even though there was a limit of three days in any week and 30 days in any year that could be applied for.[39] In the first decade of the twentieth century, such arguments were mounted with respect to whether to regulate hours in florist shops. One official report noted 'that I do not think hostesses will be satisfied with any decorations which have lost their beauty'.[40] However, in addition to those legitimately obtained exemptions, there were ways these could be used to contravene the legislation still further. A common practice in industries such as those involving fresh produce was to move workers from process to process, since the rules were often specific to particular ones. Women factory inspectors found girls employed in pouring hot jam, who the previous afternoon had been candy-peeling and the previous night bottle-washing. In such industries, they reported, some young women worked seven days a week for a total of 86 hours. They found one young woman who had worked continuously for 36 hours.[41] One inspector reported receiving complaints that girls of 13 were working from 6.00 am until midnight, 'not only on five but six days a week. But we are powerless to intervene because the process in which these girls are employed is a privileged one: that of cleaning and preparing fruit.'[42]

In fish-curing and processing, an important source of employment for women in Scotland, one inspector found girls of between 13 and 15 employed from 6.00 am to 6.00 pm in regulated processes and then in exempted ones until: '"well, I've not been working after midnight" one girl of 14 said to me'.[43] Printing and Christmas card manufacture were also employments where women were switched from regulated processes by day to others by night. Newspaper-folding was often done by women print-workers at night.[44]

In addition to particular processes there were whole industries excluded from hours-of-work regulations. Perhaps one of the most problematic in this respect, as well as the other conditions associated with it that also remained unregulated, were laundries. Laundries were an important area of work for women. They varied from a form of homework to domestic workshops (usually known as hand-laundries) through to 'steam' laundries and factory establishments.[45] Following the 1891 Act, laundry workers found they were condemned to continue working a 14-hour day. With mounting agitation on their own behalf and by women unionists – the Women's Trade Union League (WTUL) in particular – they eventually gained some relief in the 1895 Act, although this excluded institutional laundries.

Women factory inspectors continued to document and comment on the problems posed by the lack of regulation in laundries. In her 1898 Report, for example, the Chief Lady Inspector argued:

> The immensely long hours, the absence of any conditions such as meal times, other than there shall be a half hour every five hour spell, and the extraordinary manner in which overtime is at present worked, combine to make the inspection of laundries more difficult than any other trade under my notice.[46]

There were examples of young women who worked 60 hours a week ironing, folding and starching and who were then required to work three to four hours cleaning floors, work benches and machinery. Other women moved from washing

*Figure 1.1   Carshalton Laundry, reproduced by permission of Hulton Deutsch Collection
Limited.*

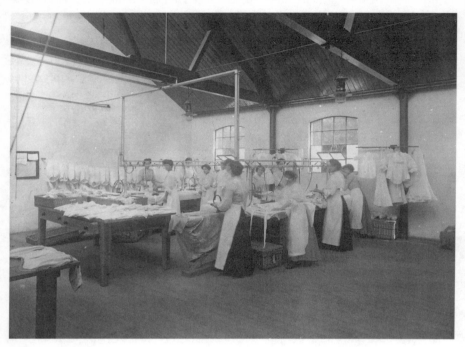

and ironing in one laundry to work in another.[47] Miss Vines gave an example of
one ironer who started at 7.00 am in one laundry and finished work at midnight in
another.[48] In one hand-laundry visited by a woman inspector, a woman packer and
sorter had been driven into hospital with sores on her legs from standing every day
of the week from 8.00 am to 10.00 pm with indefinite meal times. On Sundays she
gave parcels to customers for the entire morning.[49]

One of the problems was the trade's insistence that laundry was brought in
on a Monday to be ready for collection by the weekend. This met with scathing
criticism by campaigners that work should be so disorganized in the interests of
'the one-shirt brigade'.[50] It was little wonder that laundresses such as Linda Mayhew,
who worked 15 to 24 hours at a stretch and up to 86 hours a week, earned the title
of 'slave of the washtub',[51] or that Gertrude Tuckwell, the trade-union activist,
argued that the main defect of legislation on hours was that exemptions meant that
women could be asked to work nights following days with no limit 'save that set
by physical endurance', particularly when in these circumstances 'infringement is
so hard to detect'.[52]

It was not just exemptions but also evasion which led to long hours of
work, including illegal overtime, contravention of meal breaks and other devices
which served to lengthen the working day. One way of doing this was the practice of
many employers in clothing manufacture, especially in small workshops, to 'secrete'

workers away in upstairs bedrooms. There were many complaints from the workers themselves from the outset of the women's inspectorate, particularly because it would probably go undetected by the normal inspection routines. One such complaint from 'a work girl' to the Factory Department confirmed the practice:

> . . . another thing, Sir, after the hours you allow employees for overtime, we are sent up into the bedroom to work, and told to say it is our own dresses we are doing should the inspector call, and most of us dare not refuse, as I like many others depend upon my work for my board.[53]

Another asked the women inspectors 'Dear madam. Will you kindly inform me how far your powers extend as to visiting bedrooms in search of girls who may be secreted there during illegal hours.'[54]

This practice was specifically referred to in the campaigns of the 1880s and early 1890s to appoint women as factory inspectors. It was argued that male inspectors would not be able to enter and 'inspect bedrooms',[55] and women inspectors eventually engaged in considerable detective work at nights to uncover examples of such illegal overtime. Rose Squire remembers entering a bedroom in Manchester after 2.00 am and finding 'two girls disguised as bolsters behind a woman in bed, all fully dressed, working aprons and thimbles complete'.[56]

A slightly different method of achieving longer hours was to require workers to take work home. In 1913, a newspaper report gave the example of a 15-year-old girl machining gentleman's white linen collars from 8.30 am to 6.30 pm with a quarter-hour for dinner, who then took a gross home and worked a further two-and-a-half-hours after tea.[57] Inspectors also observed women leaving workshops carrying work to be done at home in the evening. This practice led to a view of legislation as increasing homework, although others countered that it was defects in production.[58] Illegal overtime of this kind was perceived to be a problem by women workers, campaigners and those officials with responsibility for regulation alike. In 1896,[59] for example, women inspectors received 108 complaints about illegal overtime, 24 about employment in mealtimes, and a further 23 for half-day, holiday or Sunday employment.

However, the granting of legal overtime concerned inspectors as well as workers. Inspectors shared a view with those that sought reform of the industrial system that 'overtime [was] injurious to young persons and women employed' but that it was also 'unnecessary to the successful management of business'.[60] Throughout the 1890s, the WTUL argued that overtime was unnecessary, inefficient and injurious to all workers. But, despite the campaigners and workers' own desires to work less, there were problems. Among the arguments used by activists who remained opposed to legislative limits on hours of work for women and young people, as a form of a discriminatory restrictive practice, was that it would result in men displacing women. Such arguments were in part fuelled by employers' assertions that legislating for women's hours would result in substitution. Collet, who had noted that women did not seem to complain about their hours as often as men, also noted there were some employers who said they would replace women.[61]

But there is little evidence that such restrictions actually led to loss of work for women. Employers would also have had to pay men more and thus any material difference in profitability in doing so was probably minimal. This would depend on the degree of sex segregation existing within the work concerned. In some industries, where there was a tradition of night work, such as printing, it was difficult for women to enter, but the work done at night had traditionally been done by men in any case. In fact there were probably advantages for men in hours-of-work legislation for women, since it frequently meant that their hours were also reduced.[62]

For women, there was often a fear that fewer hours would result in reduced pay, especially when many women were paid on a piecework basis. This also resulted in increasing pressure on work-rates. Complaints made by workers about hours indicate the climate of fear and intimidation that existed in many establishments, compounded by their dependence on the work and wages. Inspectors frequently commented on the difficulties of obtaining prosecutions because of the 'extreme reluctance' of potential witnesses to give evidence and 'that their very natural and by no means ill-founded fear of dismissal makes women more willing to put up with such hardships which the law expressly protects them from'.[63] The 'anti-protectionist' feminists continued to express scepticism of inspectors' observations of 'pale, tired and weary women' as being 'one-sided',[64] arguing that: 'The chief temptation of the British workwoman is to work too long, to be ready to give up holidays. That which has hitherto been regarded as a virtue has been turned into an offence.'[65]

Women did complain about their hours of work. The WTUL organized a rally of 3000 laundresses in Hyde Park in 1891 and there were a number of strikes by women during 1910 to 1911. At the same time it must be acknowledged that women often did not feel able to protest, for reasons which were rooted in their social and economic position. There is little evidence that this lack of complaint was because they regarded their long hours as a 'virtue'.

The problems caused by long hours were compounded by the shortness of mealbreaks: in some shift systems these amounted to only half-an-hour (the legal minimum in regulated employments). By the time women washed up and got to the mealroom it was even less: 'One seems hardly out of the workroom before one is back in it again with all one's dinner down one's throat.'[66] In many cases, opportunities to move from the workstation were rare, especially in the clothing trade and shop work. The returns of the factory department revealed that there were frequent complaints about the lack of a properly specified mealbreak. Inspectors constantly referred to the undermining of health which occurred to those who spent their working day in one room doing sedentary work. Even so, some mealrooms were judged to be 'seriously objectionable', often underground, stuffier, darker and more insanitary than the workrooms themselves.[67] Miss Sadler also pointed out that women and girls in the clothing trade were either forced to stay in their workrooms or go out in all weathers to some place in the neighbourhood for cheap food.[68]

By themselves, the hours of work were punishing enough. But there were also aspects of the type and organization of work and conditions of the workplace that either exacerbated the consequences of long hours, or where the effects were made worse by long hours of exposure. For laundryworkers, as in other industries, the

Figure 1.2   Bobbin winding in a Lancashire cotton mill, reproduced by permission of Mary Evans Picture Library.

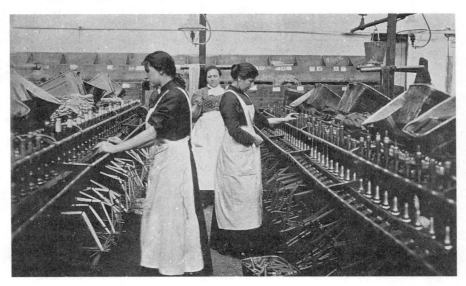

long hours were spent standing, in a poor working environment in terms of temperature and humidity, with unsanitary facilities. Lucy Deane's 1900 investigation of laundries revealed that laundresses were more four times more likely than women in general to suffer from ulcers of the leg; twice as likely to suffer from phthisis (pulmonary tuberculosis) and also had an excess of rheumatism and bronchitis.[69] It was the combination of these circumstances that led not only to a propensity to pulmonary complaints, but also to varicose veins and uterine displacement: the latter 'embitters the lives of far more women than is generally known and is particularly prevalent among laundresses'.[70]

In textile and cloth factories, standing was singled out:

> in all this time, in most cases the women are on their feet . . . breathing an unnaturally heated air, sickened by the disagreeable smell of oil and size, the ceaseless din of machinery in their ears, dust, fluff continually ready to invade the system.[71]

In these factories there were further problems related to the speed and pressure of work and in many processes its unremitting and monotonous character. Some of the ambivalence of cotton operatives to shorter hours was on the basis of fears that the same amount of work would be extracted in the shorter period of time. This may have accounted for some of the opposition women in the cotton industry had shown to the Ten Hours Bill earlier in the century,[72] and some considered such fears justified. So 'While the hours of work have been little shortened since 1874, the strain of the work has considerably increased through increased speed at which the machines run.'[73] Women factory inspectors repeatedly cited that 'driving' occurred to increase the speed of production. Trade unions reported instances of women 'breaking down' through the strain. They pointed to the high rates of claims for paid sickness allowance for those women eligible under the 1911 National Insurance scheme.[74] The consequences of strain on health and efficiency was encapsulated by one mill worker in 1914 as: 'we feel when we get through to the dinner hour that we have got through as much work as a woman's physique will stand. All the other four hours we are taking it out on our bodies.'[75]

By 1914 there had been no reduction in the legal hours of work. Some attempts in 1913 to reduce textile factory hours to nine, with further limits on overtime, did not succeed in becoming law. In 1914 demands for increased productivity were being made for another reason. Women inspectors became anxious that the 'special circumstances' of wartime work should not undo what had been achieved to date, however little that might have been. At the outset Adelaide Anderson, as Chief Lady Inspector, was adamant that hours of work should be strictly defined, with clear sanctions for evasion, 'to overcome any belief that the Factory Acts were in abeyance'.[76]

Hours of work represent the clearest example of the industrial exploitation of human labour, of what Marx saw as maximising the extraction of surplus value (profitability) from those whose only bargaining power in the workplace was to be able to sell their labour. For women, with even less bargaining power than men, the position was worse.

There were other factors which, even if legislation had been more effective in tackling the problem of working hours, also contributed to the overall time worked and the consequent strains on working women. Many women and girls walked long distances to work. Even a distance of one or two miles took time and required women to wake and set off early to be ready for the start of the working day. Many walked as far as six miles. Women inspectors pointed out that most women who worked in London's West End walked on average up to three miles for a 8.00 am start.[77] The consequence of such journeys were that women and girls would often spend their sedentary day in wet clothes, with only gas jets for heat and light. The journey home also had to be made at the end of the day. In the detailed investigations into some deaths from lead-poisoning, this factor was viewed as contributory to the likelihood of succumbing to the poison. Harriet Walters, a young enameller, was considered to 'have been enfeebled by her practice of walking to her work without having tasted food' and then working at her dangerous employment 'til the dinner hour'.[78]

There was also what has come to be known as the 'double day' with respect to women's work. On top of journeys to and from work and the length of the paid working hours, women still had their own domestic work to attend to. This burden was particularly acute for married women who shouldered the main responsibility for this in working-class households:

It should not be forgotten that many women and girls have domestic work to do after their day's work in the mill is over, and the high standards of comfort or 'housepride' in Lancashire make this a considerable addition.[79]

One factory inspector in reporting on an accident to a laundry worker noted:

> Sometimes one feels one dare not contemplate too closely upon the life of
> our working women . . . She told me she left home at 5.15 am, walked
> two-and-a-half miles to the factory, stood the whole day at her work and
> then at 6.00, sometimes later, started to walk home again, and then had to
> prepare her meal, mend and do her housework. This case is typical of
> thousands of women workers.[80]

Again, it was not simply hours that created strain in these circumstances but hous-
ing conditions and the state of general sanitary facilities available that frequently
thwarted women's best attempts to make their homes comfortable. It is not surprising that, unlike the more sympathetic view above, many middle-class visitors and
investigators would find women who appeared to have given up, or whose efforts
at cleanliness remained invisible. Unfortunately, such circumstances were often
seen as a consequence of a 'preference for factory life' and a lack of housewifery
skills rather than as a result of the material conditions of most working-class homes
and communities. Feminist and other supporters of a woman's right or 'need' to
work gave some sympathetic attention to the 'double day' but did not question
Victorian social values that promoted the domestic sphere as women's. As middle-
class feminists and labour activists increasingly supported the strong maternalist
ideologies of the early twentieth century, the double day was seen as solvable
within 'minimum wage' legislation which it was hoped would remove the necessity
for women to do paid work at all.

Hours of work remained a salient issue in the reform of industrial working
conditions at this time. It was the most common of the complaints which workers
themselves made about their conditions, and it formed a major aspect of the regulatory apparatus, with most prosecutions arising for breaches of hours regulations.
This in itself might indicate other processes at work, such as the fact there was
already a strong tradition of both trade union activism, and legal control of conditions which focused on hours. This would serve to amplify hours as something to
be complained about. In addition, given the difficulties of what could be regulated
over the range of poor conditions, and consensus about disruption to capitalist
interests, then hours may have been an obvious choice. This is to suggest that some
kind of 'halo' effect operated to keep hours on the political agenda, even if from
the 1880s it was not to occupy such prominence in regulation emanating from
official circles. As Adelaide Anderson so succinctly put it in retrospect: the control
of the dangerous and injurious trades is in complete contrast to the stagnant condition of legislation on hours.[81]

A Matter of Decency: Sanitary Conditions and Provision

Hours of work already had a place on the political agenda and were to remain an
occupational health threat during this period. This was less so in respect of those other

aspects of working conditions whose link to health and well-being were hardly articulated. In the second example considered here, that of sanitary conditions in the workplace, there had been at least from the 1830s onwards an increasing concern with 'public health'. A developing expertise was associated with the employment of public-health specialists including medical officers of health as part of local government administration. They had the main responsibility for pursuing health policies. Gradually a number of controls were introduced to deal with matters such as effluvial removal, the disposal of waste, food adulteration, milk supplies and street-cleaning.[82] The effects of dirt and disease were not particularly discriminatory about the class of its victims. This undoubtedly contributed to the important role which sanitary science and administration acquired in the nineteenth century. However, despite improvements by the end of the century in health indicators such as mortality,[83] sanitary conditions in British towns and in relation to dwellings and workplaces left much to be desired. It was not surprising that on investigation working conditions were often revealed as extremely insanitary and conditions in dwellings or domestic workshops could be liable for the spread of infection.[84]

Alongside hours of work, this area of working conditions provided for the major source of complaint and contravention of legal standards as and when they were established – although it must be said these were limited. In part, this may be accounted for not only by the prominence of 'public health' issues in administrative circles generally, but also because, as Wohl suggests,[85] until the 1890s a large proportion of the work of factory inspectors was with sanitary aspects. I would also contend that a sanitary model, in terms of an emphasis on environmental conditions and personal cleanliness, was the predominant focus of prevention in late nineteenth and early twentieth-century discourse. It would also be evident in political strategies, both regulatory and educationally, around occupational health, even when specific industrial diseases were established and became the focus for intervention.

With respect to women workers, the issue of sanitary conditions was not solely one of the traditionally defined public health threats. Sanitary conditions were viewed as contravening accepted standards of 'decency'. The notion of decency encompassed what was considered 'acceptable' within ideas of womanhood and femininity. References were often made to women's 'sensitivity' and need for 'privacy' and there were concerns about the 'delicacy' of relations between the sexes. Thus sanitary conditions were at one and the same time a threat to health and to morals. Poor sanitary provision was considered 'debasing to women'.

In the Assistant Lady Commissioner's Reports to the Royal Commission on Labour, 1893–94, reports on women's workplaces found problems of both sanitary provision and cleanliness in nearly every case. In one of her reports, May Abraham considered that morality was most threatened by insufficient sanitary accommodation: 'the same closets being common in some mills to men, women and children'.[86] She describes the 'filth and offensive odours' of lavatories cleaned 'twice a year'.[87] In another of her reports, an employer admitted conditions were bad, 'so bad it was unwise on my part to wish to see it' but that employers expressed reluctance to improve accommodation 'as it would certainly be damaged by operatives'.

Here there were mills infested with rats, dirty drinking water and toilets open to the road without doors which women did not use.[88] The reports of the women factory inspectors continued such themes with constant examples of where sanitary provision did not meet acceptable standards of morality and decency.[89] These included lack of privacy with accommodation directly off workrooms or spinning sheds, often without doors or with glass doors and no bolts, as one inspector suggested 'for the purposes of the improper supervision of decent and respectable women'.[90] Women frequently had to walk through male workrooms or male-operated machines to reach them and all too often there was no separate accommodation for women at all.

A visit to 40 textile mills in 1897 found that 20 had no separate accommodation and 34 the most 'appalling conditions'.[91] In another example:

> I notified a case of defective accommodation for women in a rubber factory, having found it to consist of one dry closet containing six pails, unseparated by partitions, unprovided with doors or with any artificial light, unpaved and with the ground in front of the seats in a very wet and muddy condition. The whole interior showed no signs of having at any time been lime-washed and was very filthy.[92]

In 1895, the Women's Inspectorate reported receiving 68 complaints about the lack of separate sanitary accommodation or insufficient or defective provision, but they reported a total of 425 to local authorities. In addition to the 234 that were defective (which included the two categories above) there were 73 cases of overcrowding, 82 of 'want of cleanliness' and 28 without ventilation.[93] By 1896 referrals totalled 669.[94] This reference to referral highlights a particular problem for factory administration in relation to their ability to achieve improvements, because the administrative base for regulatory arrangements was not located within the Factory Department.

The 1891 Factories Act brought a change in the administrative responsibility for sanitary conditions in factories and workshops, removing this from the factory inspectorate to local authorities. Within local sanitary authorities there was already a body of expertise in the form of sanitary inspectors and medical officers of health to do this kind of work. Thus factory inspectors were to report or refer instances requiring attention to these authorities. The reality was less than satisfactory. The local authorities were already overburdened by existing responsibilities and there was a time lag, if not a permanent problem, in having enough staff to carry out such extended duties on top of the pressure created by the expanding town population. There was also evidence of both lack of knowledge and lack of will in carrying out such responsibilities, as the 1893 Report confirmed. One medical officer of health (MOH) 'did not see his way at present to any inspection', while another 'did not intend to do so for his present pay'.[95] In smaller towns and rural areas inspectors reported that sanitary authorities 'seemed entirely ignorant of their powers and duties', and one medical officer of health agreed there were sanitary deficiencies but 'he did not personally press it'.[96]

This lack of will was in many cases a result of the lack of independence of local sanitary authorities as political bodies. In the case of one textile mill, the sanitary authority responsible was composed mainly of mill owners and the chair was one of the 'worst offenders'.[97] In another case where sanitary officers had sought improvement, the owner had taken no action because he believed 'the local sanitary inspector to be in the pay of plumbers, and he did not intend to improve his accommodation'.[98] Thus the intention of the Act in recognizing the expertise in sanitary matters created a dual responsibility between reporting and action that simply delayed any attempts to effect change.

The potential for any genuine 'dual inspection' was limited by a failure of sanitary inspection to deal with factories and workshops at all – but given that any typical industrial district might have around 4000 workshops alone this was hardly surprising. Women factory inspectors discovered that it was at best months and at worst years since factories had been inspected. It was in rare instances that inspectors developed good working relationships and these were with women sanitary inspectors in some districts in London.[99] More often, for women inspectors their frustration with what were terrible conditions and their own lack of power on the face of little and slow action was understandable. As Lucy Deane described it:

> over and over again, the same objectionable features are to be met with . . . There appears little or no diminution of the difficulty and often direct opposition which has to be encountered to obtain elementary codes of decency.[100]

Adelaide Anderson noted how much of their time was used up in revisiting a 'notified' factory and in repeated efforts at corresponding and conferring with local authorities to try to raise standards.[101] Rose Squire remembers it as, 'the most distasteful and troublesome of all our tasks, to fight and struggle against the apathy of sanitary authorities and the determination of employers to oppose expenditure'. Her view of the dual-inspection arrangements were that they were 'wasteful, irritating and ineffectual'.[102] For operatives, it seems they concluded that in the case of suitable sanitary arrangements and facilities it was 'nobodies business'.[103]

There was some provision for factory inspectors to prosecute cases, if they discovered something serious and nothing had been done – and they did have some success in the magistrates' courts when this happened. But there was a constant difficulty here of establishing what could be deemed 'suitable' provision and they certainly found employers who offered quite wide interpretations. Otherwise they worked with persuasion although, as one inspector commented, patience was needed: 'It is not in ten minutes that one can convince an employer who puts the women's conveniences alongside of men at work and has no fastening on the door "so that time may not be lost".'[104]

The provision of sanitary accommodation was only one dimension, although undoubtedly the worst, of the lack of sanitary facilities. Over and above this many problems remained outside factory regulation as a means for securing some kind of improvement. There were few examples of provisions for maintaining personal cleanliness, such as wash-basins or running water, let alone soap and towels. Even where these were required, in the 'special rules' for specified 'dangerous trades', these were often inadequate and in a filthy state. One trade-union activist noted that in lead factories, for example, she had found:

> the baths so foul from use that additional danger was incurred by washing in them, or that no towels were supplied, so that the bather's own clothes were the only means she had of drying her body (and these were permeated by dust).[105]

Facilities for hanging (and drying) clothes, or changing into work clothing were a long time coming, although women trade-union activists joined women inspectors in their campaigns to improve these aspects of the workplace. Consequently in mills, for example, 'common decency' continued to be contravened: 'it is the shame that young girls and women in these days should have to do in the mill, what they would not do in front of their brothers', reported *The York Post* in 1912.[106] More often women did not have work clothes to change into and they ended up working, often standing, all day in wet clothing. Clothing could be wet as a result of walking to work, but there were numerous factories where wet floors were commonplace and long skirts acted as capillaries for carrying damp to the body. Wet floors were seldom clean. Laundries were problematic in this respect, as were bakehouses, aerated water-bottling and food-preserving factories. There was no provision for water to run off the floors, which were often dilapidated and uneven.[107] Adelaide Anderson noted in the final chapter of her review of the work of the inspectorate[108] that women had become increasingly impatient for improvements in provisions for personal cleanliness and hygiene. She argued that considerable gains could still be made to improve the welfare aspects of factory life. These would include wider aspects than those considered here, and there were other factors which impinged on the state of the environment besides sanitary conditions. Some of these are considered in the next section.

Hot and Cold and Fresh Air

There are two dimensions to this discussion: the first concerns lack of access to fresh air and effective ventilation to remove vitiated air, as well as dusts and fumes. In the latter case it was recognized that these could be the source of industrial disease and respiratory illness. The second concerns the temperatures in which women were expected to work: extremes of hot or cold could undermine their health.

Ventilation was not a new problem. Harrison and Hutchins[109] had observed that as early as 1795 medical opinion had recognized the debilitous effects of hot and impure air. Later still, in 1861, Sir John Simon, the MOH to the Privy Council, noted this connection in his Fourth Report.[110] In the report he claimed that 'the accumulated evidence that ill-adapted attempts at general ventilation, together with non-ventilation made up to that time the most potent single cause of injury to workers'.[111]

The 1864 Factory Act required that factories 'should be kept in a cleanly state and shall be ventilated in a manner as to render harmless so far as is practicable any gases, dust or their impurities generated in the process of manufacture that may be injurious to health'. Further requirements for extractor fans in grinding and polishing were laid down in 1875 and 1878. An 1884 government report on cotton operatives commented that the constitutional tendencies to rheumatic, phthisical and dyspeptic ailments 'cannot fail to be intensified by working continuously in an ill-ventilated atmosphere'.[112] Despite this early recognition and regulation, problems continued to be laid at the door of inadequate ventilation and in particular to a lack of knowledge, inspection and enforcement.

The two factors of ventilation and temperature were frequently interrelated in factories at this time because of the lack of anything approaching ventilation science. The use of open-roof skylights or open doors or windows caused cold temperatures and draughts. Clara Collet had commented on this feature in factories in Bristol in her report to the Royal Commission on Labour in 1893.[113] She observed that in most cases, where there was no means of ventilation except open windows, women preferred 'a close atmosphere and warmth to toothache, stiff necks and rheumatism brought on by draughts'. In 1894, Miss Paterson, emphasised the elementary knowledge of ventilation when she reported that she had 'been gravely assured that a door leading from one room to another equally crowded, served the purpose of ventilation for both'.[114]

The either/or equation of warmth or fresh air made it difficult for workers to accept the desirability of ventilation *per se*. Dr Thomas Arlidge wrote in 1892:

True, there is on the part of many workers a morbid dread of fresh air, but this is no doubt the result of experience with draughts, and also owing to the extreme susceptibility to cold developed by long continuance in closed rooms.[115]

Such experiences were often encountered by inspectors, who also found such objections unsurprising when the means of ventilation is a skylight above their heads 'through which cold air falls like an avalanche upon their heads'.[116] Skylights, Lucy Deane concluded, were the 'most useless of all forms of ventilation' given the English climate.[117] Vitiated air resulted from the use of gas jets for heat. Persistent quinsy in a brush-works was considered to be caused by the combined effects of low temperature and impure air. Girls in a military embroidery factory were observed to look 'cold and pinched with blue fingers, with only gas lights overhead for warmth'.[118] Women factory inspectors received letters complaining about the lack of heat in workrooms:

Dear Miss, can anything be done for us machinists to get a little warmth. Many of us have no parents or homes of our own, so we are not so very well fed or warmed. We don't want anything unreasonable, only just to be warm enough to work.[119]

And:

> Dear Miss Martindale, would you kindly see to the heating of our room in the Ornamenting department . . . the girls are like frozen meat and their [*sic*] is such a bad smell especially on a Monday morning with no ventilation.[120]

The provision of proper heat for cold workrooms would have been the simplest way to improve ventilation, but for many women it was not the extreme of cold that was the problem but heat. Hot workrooms were frequently associated with steam and thence with wet clothing. This could lead to experiences of cold and related morbidity in both hot and cold conditions. Problems of heat, steam and humidity arose in relation to cotton manufacture. Legal controls on moisture were introduced in 1889,[121] but complaints persisted and there were accusations that excessive steaming was particularly damaging to health. Both weavers and some doctors testified to this effect to the 1897 Committee of Inquiry into the working of the 1889 Act.[122] Among them was the MOH for Blackburn who claimed steaming contributed to the town's high mortality.

There was considerable disagreement about the extent of health impairment and a concerted attempt by committee members to undermine the legitimacy of weavers' arguments. Workers described women emerging from mills at the end of the day as 'exhausted and tired out' with 'the fronts of their dresses open fairly gasping for breath'.[123] Doctors reported patients with 'fainting and sickness' and rheumatic symptoms. They accepted that complaints made to them of 'lassitude and malaise' had foundation. They also supported the committee's own conclusion that there was insufficient evidence to prove that weavers in humidified sheds were more unhealthy than other cotton operatives. The report concluded that accusations of workers being 'steamed to death' were exaggerated and indicates that women's complaints were not taken seriously, for example, expressing the perception that 'steaming' existed in women's minds; that they simply 'followed the leader'. 'Hysteria' was even suggested, a disorder that some thought was associated with 'shamming'.[124] Women continued to complain. As one worker described it more than ten years later: 'at times one has the feeling of being out in a shower of rain. I have never had such a feeling in the lungs as steaming produces, one's bones ache.'[125]

In addition to cotton-cloth manufacture, there were other weaving industries with similar conditions. Lucy Deane commented specifically on the possible consequences for the constitutions of young girls: 'those scantily clad little figures, their faces often beaded with perspiration who pass to and fro' in both cotton and flax spinning and weaving.[126] Laundries were also workplaces where steam and high temperatures prevailed. Clara Collet reported that temperatures in the high 70's and 80's with high humidity were common. In one laundry she found 78° in the mangling room, 78° at the entrance to the ironing room and 86° near the boards, with 75° in washrooms.[127]

There was one area of work where measures around ventilation were recognized as essential to reduce the health risks to workers: this was in dusty processes and in particular those trades specified as 'dangerous' under the 1891 Act. Here the provision for 'special rules' included regulations on the provision of ventilation in rooms where dangerous processes were carried out. Unfortunately, the level of ignorance about both the means of ventilation and the principles underlying it were once again evident. Fans in spinning mills were seen to extract air from one room and unload it into another. The incidence of poisoning in both the lead- and match-making industries, two of the designated 'dangerous trades', indicated that fumes and dust were being propelled into neighbouring workrooms not subject to the 'special rules'.[128] Such circumstances continued to place women at risk even if they were not directly employed in dangerous processes.[129] Single fans were positioned so that the air was blown back by window draughts. One indication that ventilation might not be effective in its own right at protecting workers from the inhalation of dusts was that women were also required to wear protective clothing, including masks. There was controversy about women's lack of compliance in wearing masks, but there was also considerable evidence that they were often unsuitable, uncomfortable and insanitary. However, emphasis on the control of 'industrial disease', probably gave some impetus to the science and engineering of effective ventilation. The Chief Medical Inspector for Factories considered that the use of fans and especially exhaust ventilation had brought about a reduced incidence of poisoning.[130] From the late 1890s, factory inspectorate reports contained many technical drawings of ventilation systems. They were indicative of an increasing emphasis on changing practice through education that developed during the twentieth century.

As with all other areas of regulation looked at so far, there was a continual problem with the use of vague terms such as 'adequate' or 'sufficient', without some measurable standard or criteria as to what this might be. In 1902, a special Departmental Committee was appointed to investigate ventilation.[131] It recommended that the traditional standard, based on cubic space per worker, be replaced by a standard of purity of 12 volumes per 1000.

The health consequences of inadequate ventilation and 'vitiated air' were in many respects difficult to separate from the consequences of extreme heat and cold, an exacerbation of the likely exposure to infectious diseases and the transmission of dusts and fumes and organisms. The 1902 Committee considered the health effects were 'somewhat obscure', but that 'loss of appetite, headaches, general symptoms of discomfort and sickness' all seemed to the associated with it.[132] The lack of control over dusty processes in general had the most important implications for health. Phthisis or consumption (TB), although showing evidence of decline as a cause of mortality, was the largest single killer of women at this time,[133] although it was not specific just to workers or the working-classes. Social and environmental conditions undoubtedly also contributed. In some studies, however, there was evidence that deaths from phthisis were much higher in workers. It certainly took a greater toll than exposure to poisons such as lead, as was evident in the Potteries. The 1910 Committee Report concluded there were 30–40 excess deaths from lung disease to every one from lead-poisoning although, as the Committee also pointed out, such deaths often followed years of chronic illness and these workers would have had little benefit from regulations to reduce dust.[134]

The fact that at the end of the century it was pottery workers who had the highest occupational mortality indicates the extent to which dust was a feature of nearly all work processes.[135] One group of workers vulnerable to an extremely dusty process were china scourers, 'always women, belonging usually to the rougher, more ignorant, and reckless of their sex' who spent their long working hours in 'clouds of dust'.[136]

The issue of effective ventilation and the adequacy of working temperatures were viewed mainly as problems of indoor work. But many women were engaged in outdoor work. They were at the mercy of the climate, having to work in all weathers, often without any form of shelter or protection. Angela John describes how women engaged in pit-brow work remembered 'bitterly cold winters, and snow and rain drenching them', where 'the lunch break might have to be spent drying out wet clothes and trying to get a little warmer.'[137] There was also a view that open-air work brought distinct advantages and that such women were healthier than those in sedentary, confined factory conditions. Oliver, a prominent occupational health physician, reported that 'London dust women seemed hale and well-coloured',[138] as did Emily Hobhouse in her investigation of these women in the East End.[139] In the debates about the possible restriction of pit-brow work for women, advocates of the work and women themselves used arguments about the value of 'open air' working to counter-attack those about the physical strength required and its unsuitability for women. However, the idea that pit-work was a 'health resort' for former mill-women, as Arthur Munby, one of the petitioners, claimed was, as John rightly argues, an example of an over-generalized and over-romanticized idea of the work involved and neglected its considerable dangers.[140]

There were other industries where women were exposed to extreme weather or wet conditions. Fish curing, a seasonal and peripatetic employment for women in Scotland, involved some outdoor processes, and living as well as working conditions were extremely poor. Tin plate manufacture, also often outdoors or under basic shelters, required women workers to immerse plates in large baths of sulphuric acid. Some indoor work was also very wet, especially aerated water bottling, fruit preserving and jam making, and laundries. On top of this women often lifted heavy weights or performed hard manual labour for long hours. In this respect women's working conditions often provided a lethal cocktail, but as Wohl argued, had they been able to return to 'healthy homes' at the end of the day perhaps such a heavy toll would not have been exacted.[141]

The Oppressive Power of Men at Work

It might be thought that the exercise of male power over women in the workplace is not an issue of occupational health, or if we take those problems which we readily identify in this way today such as sexual harassment, that these are recent problems. This section demonstrates that such assumptions are incorrect. More importantly, it reinforces the argument that it is not just social conditions but social relations in the workplace which impact on health and wellbeing. In addition to examples of direct violence in the workplace that may cause injury and the other forms of coercion that can occur with respect to the operation of 'truck', it is the lack of control over aspects of one's own situation, whether or not it is consciously sought, that can be damaging.

The period considered here reveals that at any time when women remained in subordinate social positions to men, the exercise of male power was a feature of their lives. Young workers were also frequently subject to violence, as Rose Squire noted:

> A complaint reached me when in the West Riding of brutal treatment of little girls by the overlooker in a spinning mill and even by the master himself. It seems scarcely credible that nowadays little 'Doffers' should be knocked down by grown men, violently struck on the head and shoulders, their heads pushed down upon the spinning frame.[142]

Women's reports for the Labour Commission and the factory department also noted the extent to which overlookers used 'objectionable' and 'loose and violent language'. One overlooker was found guilty of making immoral proposals to married women and using indecent language to another, following a strike over the issue in the cotton industry.[143] Lambertz[144] has documented the extent to which harassment of this kind was to be found in the cotton industry. Observations of male behaviour were often linked to broader discussions of morality in the context of women's working conditions. Inspectors considered that greater threats to morality came from poor sanitary arrangements. But the intimidatory nature of such an environment served as a further reminder to women of their lack of power and social worth.

The exercise of male control also entered into what women could earn and what kinds of conditions they would be required to work under. This led women activists in labour questions and women factory inspectors to lay considerable store by women occupying supervisory posts and positions of authority. In the case of women inspectors the arguments they and their supporters advanced drew on gender as offering the underlying credentials. Their own experience seemed to support the case, 'the eagerness with which women have received me as a woman' as one inspector described it.[145] It was argued that workers would gain confidence, develop self-help and forms of self-expression with the help of inspectors 'of their own sex' and from leading women organizers. The Evidence to the Royal Commission on Labour in 1892[146] noted that women rarely communicated with men or women. However, opportunities for women supervisors were often a product of male management strategies to maintain gender divisions. Rose, for example, describes the extent to which a 'paternalist' firm, such as Cadburys of Bourneville, maintained strict sexual segregation that served to restrict women's work opportunities (married women were excluded altogether) and reinforced gendered family relations.[147]

The exploitation and abuse of women workers was not a male prerogative, however. It was often women who occupied positions of control in some forms of manufacturing (in particular clothing) and who were at the receiving end of factory inspectors reprimands or prosecutions, not always providing examples of good practice! In some cases they did: Emily Faithful's women's printing works had explicitly set out to provide women with better conditions of work than elsewhere in the trade. But outside of such noteworthy examples, there were very few women in positions of responsibility.

If pay and working conditions were damaging to women's health, there was only marginal recognition of this in State intervention. In some cases, there were improvements in the general environment of the workplace, but these were often only as a by-product of dealing with different problems, such as the approach taken with respect to industrial poisons, with an emphasis on cleanliness and ventilation. Inevitably, the concern with 'the dangerous trades' led to the neglect of developing knowledge of other ways in which working conditions 'caused' ill-health and also technologies that might have helped prevention. In part this neglect related to the difficulty of dealing with women workers. Some conditions would have led, albeit unintentionally, to interference with both the organization of production and with men's labour and conditions and, in the case of pay in particular, with the priv-ileged position men held within the labour market. There was little evidence that male activism sought such improvements on their own behalf, although their sup-port for 'protective' legislation for women might have had that desired result. Thus, fundamental improvements in the basic conditions of work were sidelined in the political priorities of maintaining male power over women workers in the work-place and men's position as 'breadwinners', and over their wives and daughters in the working-class family. The lack of recognition given to the realities of many women's dependence on work rather than men meant that it was likely that strat-egies would be pursued to exclude them from such undesirable conditions rather than to change the conditions themselves.

Notes

1   Webb (1902) commenting on the *House of Lords Select Committee on Sweating, Fifth Report* (1890) in her *The Economics of Factory Legislation*, 'The Case for the Factory Acts' p.7.
2   Black (1889) 'The organisation of working women', p.699.
3   *Report of the House of Lords Select Committee on Sweating (1890) Fifth Report*, PP XVII.
4   See Morris (1986b) *Women Workers and the Sweated Trades* for an overview of this campaign, discussed in more detail in Chapter 3.
5   Seecombe (1986) 'Patriarchy stabilised: the construction of the male breadwinner norm in nineteenth-century Britain', pp.53–4.
6   In fact the concept of the family wage is more commonly used. See Mark-Lawson and Witz (1988) 'From family labour to family wage'; Benensen (1991) 'The "family wage" and working women's consciousness in Britain 1880–1914'; Dyhouse (1989) *Feminism and the Family 1880–1939*; and Lewis (1984) *Women in England 1870–1950*. It is this concept that analyses of women's position *vis-à-vis* the labour market and the Welfare State after this period have also tended to use.

7   See, for example, Mark-Lawson and Witz (1988) and John (1984b) *By the Sweat of their Brow* on coal-mining; and Benenson (1991) on the textile industry.

8   In addition to those studies cited above, see Walby (1986) *Patriarchy at Work*; Rose (1988) 'Gender antagonism and class conflict: exclusionary strategies by male trade unionists in nineteenth-century Britain'. Exclusionary tactics were also used in middle-class and professional occupations: see Witz (1992) *Professions and Patriarchy*.

9   See especially Benenson (1991) for an analysis of the activism of women cotton and other textile workers.

10 Mark-Lawson and Witz (1988) p.155.

11 See Thane (1982) *The Foundations of the Welfare State* p.53.

12 Rathbone, E. (1924) *The Disinherited Family* pp.16–17.

13 This is supported by studies of the time, such as Bell (1907) *At the Works*; Reeves (1914) *Round about a Pound a Week*; Beatrice Webb's work for the Commission on the Poor Law (1905–9).

14 The 1911 census reveals 327 737 working women, consisting of the widowed, the deserted and the never-married, with no men to give them support.

15 Hewitt (1958) *Wives and Mothers in Victorian Industry*.

16 Mallon (1915) 'Women's wages in the census of 1906', in Hutchins (Ed.) *Women in Modern Industry*.

17 Mallon (1915) p.227.

18 Fox and Black (1894) *The Truck Acts*.

19 *Annual Report of Her Majesty's Chief Inspector of Factories* (1898) *Report of Women Inspectors for 1897*, PP XIV, p.108.

20 *Annual Report for 1899* (1900) PP XI.

21 *Annual Report of Her Majesty's Chief Inspector of Factories* (1890–1) *for the Year 1890*, PP XIX.

22 *Annual Report for 1898*, PP XII, 1899.

23 *Annual Report for 1896*, PP XVII, p.72, 1897.

24 *Annual Report for 1901*, PP XII, p.190, 1902.

25 *Annual Report for 1902*, PP XII, p.190, 1903.

26 *Annual Report for 1896*, PP XVII, p.72, 1897.

27 *Annual Report for 1902*, PP XII, pp.60–1, 1903.

28 Fox and Black (1894) p.11.

29 *Annual Report for 1902*, PP XII, 1903.

30 Black (1907) *Sweated Industry and the Minimum Wage* p.210.

31 Mallon (1915).

32 Cited in Hutchins (1902) 'The historical development of the Factory Acts', in Webb (Ed.) *The Case for the Factory Acts*.

33 See Harrison and Mockett (1990) 'Women in the factory: the State and factory legislation in nineteenth century Britain', in Jamieson and Corr (Eds).

34 Abraham (1897) *The Law Relating to Factories and Workshops*; Hutchins and Harrison (1903) *A History of Factory Legislation*.

35 Hutchins (1902) 'The historical development of the factory acts' p.107.

36 Collet (1893–4) 'Report on the conditions of work in London', in *Reports of the Assistant Lady Commissioners for the Royal Commission on Labour*, PP XXXVII, pp.550–1.

37 Eliza Orme, *Report on Conditions of Work of Barmaids, Waitresses, Book-keepers Employed in Hotels, Restaurants and Public Houses and other Places of Refreshment*, ibid.

38 Cutting in the Gertrude Tuckwell Collection, reel 1, section 39.

39   Abraham (1897).
40   Judge Ruegg (1909) *Inquiry into the Application of the Factory and Workshops Act to Florist Workshops.*
41   *Annual Report of Her Majesty's Women Inspectors 1898*, PP XII.
42   Miss Tracey in the *Annual Report for 1897*, PP XIV, p.106.
43   Miss Paterson in the *Annual Report for 1900*, PP X, p.389.
44   *Annual Report for 1897*, PP XIV.
45   See Malcolmson (1981) 'Laundresses and the laundry trade in Victorian England'.
46   *Annual Report for 1897*, PP XIV, 1898, p.107.
47   *Annual Report for 1899*, PP XII, 1900.
48   *Annual Report for 1900*, PP X, 1901, p.386.
49   *Annual Report for 1896*, PP XVII, 1897, p.68.
50   See Anon. (1902) *Life in the Laundry*, a Fabian tract.
51   *The Saturday Journal*, 22 August 1898, in the Gertrude Tuckwell Collection, reel 2.
52   Tuckwell (1902) 'The limitations of our current factory laws', in Webb (Ed.) *The Case for the Factory Acts.*
53   *Annual Report for 1893*, PP XXI, 1894, p.22.
54   Ibid., p.11.
55   See, for example, the numerous delegations to the Home Department in the early 1890s, in PRO file HO45/9818/B8031.
56   Squire (1927) *Thirty Years in Public Service* p.69.
57   Reported in *The Daily Citizen*, 12 September 1913, in the Gertrude Tuckwell Collection.
58   Black (1902) 'Some current objections to factory legislation for women', in Webb (Ed.) *The Case for the Factory Acts.*
59   *Annual Report for 1896*, PP XVII, 1897, provides just one example of the proportion of complaints and prosecutions about hours of work.
60   May Abraham in the *Annual Report of 1894*, PP XVI, 1895.
61   Collet (1893–4) *Report on the Conditions of Work in London*, PP XVII.
62   Rose Squire (1927) suggested this was the case at the time. Other historians have subsequently supported this view.
63   Miss Tracey in the *Annual Report for 1897*, PP XIV, 1898, p.161.
64   See, for example, Boucherett and Blackburn (1896) *The Condition of Working Women and the Factory Acts.*
65   *English Women's Review*, 15 January 1896, in a report on working women and the Factory Acts.
66   As one witness told Clara Collet in her investigations for the Royal Commission on Labour.
67   See Lucy Deane's reference to these issues in the *Annual Report for 1900*, PP X, pp.396–7.
68   Ibid., p.397.
69   In the *Annual Report for 1900*, PP X, 1901, pp.391–5.
70   Anon. (1902) *Life in the Laundry* p.7.
71   Hutchins (1915) *Women in Modern Industry* p.110.
72   Morgan (1992) 'Women, work and consciousness in the mid nineteenth-century English cotton industry'.
73   Hutchins (1915) p.184.
74   Annual Report of the Central Committee of Weavers Amalgamated Union, cited in *The Factory Times*, 29 May 1914, in the Gertrude Tuckwell Collection.
75   Ibid.

76 *Annual Report for 1914*, PP XXI, 1915–16, p.449.
77 Miss Sadler's example in the *Annual Report for 1900*, 1901, PP X, p.365.
78 'Report on the death of Harriet Walters', in the *Report on the Various Lead Industries*, PP XVIV, 1893–4.
79 Hutchins (1915) p.59.
80 Miss Tracey (1915) cited in Hutchins, *Women in Modern Industry*, p.289.
81 Anderson (1922) *Women in the Factory* p.148.
82 Wohl (1983) *Endangered Lives* presents a good overview of public-health concerns and the relative roles of State and local administration.
83 There is still an ongoing debate about the contribution of public health to health improvements. See, for example, Szreter (1988) 'The importance of social intervention in Britain's mortality decline *c*. 1850–1914: a reinterpretation of the role of public health'.
84 This was particularly so in relation to homework and 'sweated' workshops. *The Lancet* investigated one such outbreak in 1888 and it was a major factor in setting up the House of Lords Inquiry into Sweating in 1890 (see Chapter 3).
85 Wohl (1983), Chapter 10.
86 Abraham (1893–4) *Report on Conditions of Work in Textile Mills in Yorkshire*, PP XXXVII, p.649.
87 Ibid., p.653.
88 Abraham (1893–4) *Report on Conditions of Work in the Cotton Industry of Lancashire and Cheshire*.
89 These terms feature in most reports about sanitary issues. See, for example, Adelaide Anderson's report in the *Annual Report for 1894*, PP XIX, 1895.
90 Miss Tracey in the *Annual Report for 1903*, PP X, 1904.
91 *Annual Report for 1897*, PP XIV, 1898.
92 Adelaide Anderson in her *Annual Report for 1900*, PP XI, 1901, p.364.
93 *Annual Report for 1895*, PP XIX, 1896.
94 *Annual Report for 1896*, PP XVII, 1897.
95 *Annual Report for 1893*, PP XXI, 1894, p.366.
96 Both examples are taken from the *Annual Report for 1897*, PP XIV, 1898.
97 Miss Squire in the *Annual Report for 1897*, PP XIV, 1898, p.99.
98 May Abraham in her *Report on Cotton the Industry in Lancashire and Cheshire for the Royal Commission on Labour*, p.664.
99 *Annual Report for 1900*, PP X, 1901, mentions such joint work.
100 *Annual Report for 1896*, PP XVII, 1897, p.286.
101 Ibid., p.283.
102 Squire (1927) *Thirty Years in the Public Service* p.47.
103 May Abraham in her *Report on the Cotton Industry in Lancashire and Cheshire for the Royal Commission on Labour*, p.664.
104 *Annual Report for 1895*, PP XIX, 1896, p.98.
105 Dilke (1895) *The Industrial Position of Women* pp.9–10.
106 'The metamorphosis of the mill-girl', in *The York Post*, 26 November 1912, the Gertrude Tuckwell Collection.
107 *Annual Report for 1898*, PP XII, 1899, provides some examples of these conditions.
108 Anderson (1922) *Women in the Factory*.
109 Hutchins and Harrison (1903) *A History of Factory Legislation* p.10: a reference to the work of Dr Thomas Percival.
110 *Fourth Report of the Medical Officer of Health to the Privy Council for 1861*, PP XXVII, 1862, pp.31–2.

111   Ibid., p.13.
112   *Report on the Effects of Heavy Sizing in Cotton Weaving on the Health of Operatives*, PP LXII, 1884, p.9.
113   *Report on the Conditions of Work in Luton and Bristol, Royal Commission on Labour*, PP XXXVII, 1893–4.
114   *Annual Report for 1894*, PP XIX, 1895, p.15.
115   From his 'The hygiene, diseases and mortality of occupations cited in the *Annual Report of 1896*', PP XVIII.
116   *Annual Report for 1896*, PP XVIII, 1897.
117   Ibid., p.288.
118   Ibid., p.290.
119   Squire (1927) *Thirty Years in the Public Service* p.47.
120   Martindale (1944a) *From One Generation to Another 1839–1944*, p.98.
121   The Cotton Cloth Factories Act 1889.
122   *Report of the Committee to Inquire into the Working of the Cotton Cloth Factories Act of 1889*, PP XVII, 1897.
123   Ibid.: *Evidence of David Shackleton of the Darwin Weavers Association* p.69.
124   For a variety of contemporary views on 'hysteria' see Jalland and Hooper (1986) *Women from Birth to Death* pp.95–108. 'Shaming' was not the only explanation.
125   *Daily Dispatch*, 8 March 1910, in the Gertrude Tuckwell Collection.
126   *Annual Report for 1896*, PP XVIII, 1897, p.290.
127   Report on the *Conditions of Work in London Royal Commission on Labour*, PP XXXVII, 1893–4.
128   Evidence to this effect was found by Clara Collet in her investigation of the match-making industry in London, for the Royal Commission of Labour, PP XXXVII, 1893–4, and in the various *Reports of Inquiries into the Lead and Match-making Industry*.
129   This was especially so in match-making, where women were mainly employed in the boxing of matches. This was not considered to be as dangerous a process as dipping. See Harrison (1995a) 'The politics of occupational health in late nineteenth century Britain' and Chapter 2.
130   Legge (1914) 'Industrial Poisoning: Five Years' Notification', in the *Annual Report of His Majesty's Inspector of Factories*, PP XXI, 1914–16.
131   Haldane and Osborne (1902) *First Report of the Departmental Committee to Inquire into the Ventilation of Factories and Workshops*, PP XII, 1902.
132   Ibid., Appendix 1.
133   See Shorter (1983) *A History of Women's Bodies*; Johansson (1978) 'Sex and death in Victorian England'.
134   *Report of the Committee of Inquiry (1910)*, PP XXIX. Comparative evidence compiled by Dr Reid on pottery workers and artisans in the same district.
135   Wohl (1983) *Endangered Lives* p.275 and pp.280–2.
136   Arlidge (1892) *The Hygiene, Diseases and Mortality of Occupations* pp.310–11.
137   John (1984b) *By the Sweat of Their Brow* p.178.
138   Oliver (1902) *The Dangerous Trades* p.280.
139   Hobhouse (1900) 'Dust women', *The Economics Journal* pp.411–20.
140   John (1984b) *By the Sweat of Their Brow* Chapter 6 for a full discussion of health aspects; pp.177–80 on Munby's opinion.
141   Wohl (1983) *Endangered Lives* p.278.
142   *Annual Report of Her Majesty's Women Inspectors for 1900*, PP XI, 1901, p.362.

143 *Annual Report of Her Majesty's Chief Inspector of Factories for 1894*, p.31; *Report of Miss Abrahams on the Textile Industry in Lancashire* for the Royal Commission on Labour, PP XXVII 1892–3, pp.649–50.

144 Lambertz (1985) 'Sexual harassment in the nineteenth-century cotton industry'.

145 *Annual Report of Her Majesty's Women Inspectors for the Year 1896*, PP VII, 1897. The inspector who commented thus is Miss Paterson.

146 *Royal Commission on Labour*, PP XVII 1892–3, Minutes of Evidence Group C, Vol. Q, 4368, Minutes 6830–2.

147 Rose (1992) *Limited Livelihoods* pp.41–5.

Chapter 2

The 'Dangerous Trades'[1]

The 1880s and more especially the 1890s witnessed a new development in the agitation around the possible threats to health posed by working conditions in factories and workshops. Although there was factory legislation from the 1830s, its scope was still minimal. Opinion was generally against such State interference in this as in other areas of social and economic life.[2] In marked contrast to the earlier period, there was now a call for the State to take a more proactive role, intervening in and regulating industry in order to protect workers from the worst excesses of conditions found in most industrial workplaces.

This chapter considers one important dimension of this change in attitude towards State interference and the State's response to the problem of working conditions: the 'dangerous trades', those industries or processes that were thus legally defined under the 1891 Factory Act. The 'dangerous trades' not only indicated changes in the role of the State with respect to workers and industry. The identification of these 'dangers' at work provided the conditions for it.

Conceptualizing 'Danger'

The dominant model of occupational ill-health up until the 1880s had been based on hours of work and a 'public health' oriented model emphasising general sanitary and environmental aspects of working conditions that could undermine health. However, there was often little knowledge of the ways in which these were responsible for ill-health or disease. This was equally the case with other possible causes arising from dusts and other substances to which workers were exposed. There were some exceptions, notably in the work of some medical officers of health[3] and Factory Commissions such as the Children's Employment Commission 1864. These identified particular industries, such as lucifer match-making, as giving rise to specific health problems.

This recognition of identifiable dangers was incorporated into the 1864 Factory Act, where children, young persons and women were forbidden from taking meals in workrooms where 'dangerous processes' were carried out. The idea of danger as specific to classes of worker, rather than to aspects of industrial production, was incorporated into this early regulation. The 'protective' principle was further extended and entrenched as a result. From then on there was evidence that beliefs about risk in relation to danger encompassed the view that it was not only age-specific but gender-specific. Consolidation of these regulations came in the

1870s, but nothing further happened until 1883 when there was investigation into and then legislation for one particular industry: the manufacture of white lead.[4]

The reports and regulations of the White Lead Act signalled an explicit recognition of identifiable 'dangers' specifically to the health of women who worked in particular processes and/or in certain industries. While white-lead manufacture was the main area to be considered in this light in the 1880s, from now on trades that were considered to be a danger to health, life and limb – lead-poisoning included – were to be a major preoccupation of those concerned with working conditions and health in the late-nineteenth and early-twentieth centuries.

The designation of particular kinds of work and work processes which resulted in exposure to hazards such as fumes, dusts, organisms and machinery, was considered a departure from previous thinking about occupational ill-health, as one medical expert on occupational disease noted in 1892:

> the observations of Medical Officers of Health in so far as they have seen them have proved barren . . . an indication that the importance of noting industrial diseases and estimating their influence on public health and mortality has not yet been recognised.[5]

To some extent, therefore, calls for State intervention paved the way for the development of a consciousness that Dr Arlidge noted above had been generally absent. The possibility of designating trades for the purpose of regulating their dangers required some identification of 'causes' of observed symptomology and illnesses. These then needed to be considered as 'industrial diseases'. Debates about such a constitution contributed in turn to the development, albeit slowly, of expertise and knowledge about such 'diseases'[6] (see Chapter 6).

In addition to and alongside developing medical expertise about industrial ill-health, the 'dangerous trades' received formal recognition and definition with the regulatory framework of factory legislation. This occurred in Schedule 8 of the 1891 Factory Act. This authorized the drawing up of special rules or measures as appear to be 'reasonably practicable':

> as the Chief Inspector of Factories sees fit, where the Secretary of State certifies that in his opinion any machinery or process or particular description of manual labour used in a factory or workshop is dangerous or injurious to health, or a danger to life or limb either generally or in the case of women and children or any other class of person.[7]

Special rules specified many requirements on both employers and workers about such things as cleanliness, ventilation, protective clothing and inspection.

The schedule provided an operational definition of the potential for trades to be designated. It also set up a distinct regulatory framework that significantly departed from other areas of factory legislation. Because it invested power in the Home Secretary, on the advice of the Chief Inspector of Factories, it by-passed the need for any of the proposed rules and regulations – and future additions or amendments – to have parliamentary approval. This might have seemed advantageous, given the slow passage of most of the Factory Acts and the consequent delay in effecting changes. At the same time, there were those who were critical of such anti-democratic interventionist measures, especially because the schedule also confirmed that these might be particular workers. Those feminists who opposed any legislation affecting the employment of a disfranchized group also had supporters on this issue in the House of Commons. Stuart Wortley MP complained to the House that the schedule:

> not only applied to the employment of women, and was directed, possibly, at restricting, if not prohibiting, their employment in certain industries; (and) . . . went further . . . to withhold this kind of cognisance and control from the house.[8]

In practice, however, there were limitations to these powers. The schedule did not give the Home Secretary the right to prohibit certain classes from engaging in certain processes altogether, as he complained to the House in 1895.[9] The constant use of investigation and official enquiry as a precedent to any regulation also slowed its pace and may have been important in preventing the more radical alternative remedies available to the State. A further major limitation on the Home Secretary – perceived as a problem because it also delayed regulation – was that the schedule provided for employers' rights to arbitration on any proposed rules, and for a limited period workers too. Employers often used this provision and, perhaps more than any other factor, it served to frustrate Home Secretaries and to leave workers' exposed to hazards. Although they often threatened legislation to withdraw this right, they never actually did.[10]

There are other points to note about the conceptualization of the 'dangerous trades' within the schedule. It was evident from opposition to its unique regulatory powers that the regulation had a context within a perceived 'need' to protect women and children in particular from the effects of the 'dangerous trades' and set further precedents for the establishment of differential risk. As a result, although men's work was subject to some regulation, there were many examples where it was not, even when women and men worked in the same industry or processes. Thus there was an implicit requirement to establish women's special susceptibility to risk and thence to regulate the work in which they were engaged. This would have consequences for the occupational health of both women and men. Finally, the schedule's use of the term 'reasonably practicable' was to cause the same difficulties of implementation and enforcement as the terms 'suitable' and 'appropriate' did elsewhere in the language of regulation.[11]

If the specification of risk in relation to classes of worker was to be problematic, so too was the idea of what constituted a danger to health, life and limb. The definition within the schedule seemed to be a broad one, but in practice it required a focus on the control of exposure to specific substances and machinery. Work processes or the organizational aspects of work were regulated only in so far as they were implicated in exposure. Thus, despite the advantages that might have accrued from a medical model of industrial disease, it would also deflect attention away from a wider range of occupational health risks and where specific and direct effects were identified at the expense of a gradual deterioration in health. The problem was, as the physician Thomas Oliver noted at the time:

> it would be well if we could have some clearer conception of what is implied both by industrial disease and 'dangerous trades' for there is scarcely any trade or occupation that is not attended by some risk or another.[12]

Only some of these risks could be attended to in turn.

To establish whether or not a particular trade or process might be eligible for regulation under the schedule often required investigation and extensive enquiry. This drew initially on existing inspection expertise within the Factory Department and their use of medical experts, although labour women activists such as Gertrude Tuckwell of the WTUL became increasingly involved. In 1892, the first four scheduled industrial poisons and their related trades were those where existing knowledge and some prior regulation had already designated 'danger': lead, phosphorous, anthrax and arsenic.

In 1895 the Home Secretary set up the Dangerous Trades Committee, which met on a continuous basis until 1899. As with other investigative committees, it drew on a mixture of medical and factory expertise – including May Abraham, one of the first women inspectors.[13] This committee investigated the possibility of 'danger' in miscellaneous trades, either on their own initiative or through referral, that 'had not been dealt with elsewhere'.[14] There were areas of work already well-established within the definition of 'dangerous trades', so these were subject to continued enquiry in their own right.

This was particularly so with lead and phosphorous, two trades that dominated the discourse on the 'dangerous trades' with respect to women and, despite early regulation, remained persistent causes of ill-health. They provide examples of how the principles of 'protective legislation' worked with respect to 'industrial disease' *per se*. For these reasons, lead and phosphorous are examined as case studies later in this chapter. In all, the Dangerous Trades Committee investigated 26 trades. They found 17 in need of regulation, not all in the areas of women's employment.[15] Although the existence of such a committee might indicate some urgency for the need to identify and proceed with regulation, there were complaints that this was not evidently the case. Harold Tennant MP, the Committee Chair, complained to the House in 1900 that to date only two sets of rules had been adopted, 'and at this rate it would take 34 years to put the whole into force'.[16] Notwithstanding the legitimacy of such complaints, before 1895 16 trades had been regulated and more were added. In some cases voluntary codes were called for and this was a considerable hindrance to any enforcement.

The 1895 Factory Act extended the regulation of the 'dangerous trades' in two ways. First it increased the role of medical inspection, giving certifying surgeons (whose chief responsibility to date had been for children) responsibilities in relation to the investigation and notification of cases of industrial poisoning and accidents and the periodic inspection of adults in scheduled industries. Second, the notification of cases of poisoning was now a legal requirement for all medical practitioners. In 1898, the Factory Department appointed a medical inspector who was to investigate and report annually on these matters. Although notification was unreliable, it began to provide better information on the extent to which various trades might endanger health. The 1895 Act is thus important because it indicated that henceforth reliance would be increasingly placed on 'fitness' for work as a way of ameliorating the damaging consequences of exposure to danger.

Women in 'Danger'

Once again it was women investigators, initially in their work for the Royal Commission on Labour and then in the women's factory inspectorate and women's labour organizations, who provided information about those areas of women's work that might meet the definition of 'dangerous trades' under the 1891 Act. There were other important ideas of 'danger' that entered into political discourse about women's work. It was not just that there might be occupational hazards which affected women in particular, but that there was also a general 'danger' to women's health from their employment in factories and workshops. The identification of specific 'dangers' confronting women who worked would then become a powerful reinforcement of the idea that women should not be working at all. The extent to which the discourse conflated these two ideas of 'danger' is important to an understanding of the success and failure of interventions to restrict women's work and/or protect their health. While many inspectors and reformers campaigned vigorously for extensions of the legislation to include more trades or more extensive regulations, they also experienced considerable frustration that this would also leave untouched many aspects of working conditions that were equally if not more damaging to health. As Rose Squire reported in a chapter she wrote for a medical text on the 'dangerous trades':

> no description can convey any adequate impression of a fur-pulling room, whether it be occupied by one or fifty workers – the universal grey, the haze of floating hair, the sickly disgusting odour of uncleaned skins – it must be seen, felt and smelt to be understood.[17]

And while fur-pulling was recognized as one of the 'worst' occupations engaged in by women at this time, it was never subject to regulation.

Most contemporary commentators argued that there was a particular labour market for the 'dangerous trades'; that because the work was viewed as 'dangerous' and associated with very poor conditions, only those who were desperate would choose to work in them. There was no indication that the choice was based on higher wages or 'danger money'[18] since the work was still low-paid. Women were often desperate because their economic and domestic circumstances, including their locality, provided few alternative forms of employment.

In general such views once again elaborated the situation of many working-class women, without economic support from men either because they were single, widowed or had husbands who were out of work, ill and/or disabled or at the mercy of casual employment. It also indicated the lack of power many women workers had over the work they did and its conditions. The 'dirty repulsive nature' of fur-pulling which Rose Squire described attracted mainly old or middle-aged women in distress from the poorest classes.[19] Oliver, discussing the employment of women in lead-mills stated:

> Women working in dangerous processes led rather a casual life and took to the trade as a last resort, owing to the idleness, illness or death of their parents or husbands. They were mostly of the poorest class, were often ill-fed and ill-clad.[20]

The idea that there might be a distinct pool of labour for the 'dangerous trades' had consequences. First, it required that some recognition be given to the fact that poverty sometimes led to desperate forms of employment for women, although they did not always perceive the choice of work in these terms, nor did they always share 'official' perceptions of the work as 'dangerous'. It is difficult to disentangle women's 'needs' from the context in which they expressed their views, such as when officials questioned them about their health at work in dangerous trades – and the content of those opinions. A recognition of women's work in relation to the impoverishment of many working-class families worked both for and against them. On the one hand, arguments that occupations worked selectively, in that 'weaker vessels are constantly recruited to those fields of employment least able to foster development', could be used to reinforce the arguments that work continued a downward spiral of physical degeneracy.[21] It was frequently argued that married working women had primary responsibility with regards to this. On the other hand, it forced a certain realism into demands for, and official considerations of, restrictions or prohibition of women's employment. It was probably an important factor in limiting such intervention.

Finally, the extent to which poverty determined the labour-market supply for dangerous forms of employment served to complicate the extent to which 'experts' could unequivocally determine that the illnesses which workers suffered were due to the harmful effects of their work. Thus, it was often argued that women would not succumb, for example, to lead-poisoning if the conditions they brought with them to the workplace were not so bad. As Adelaide Anderson told the Committee on Physical Deterioration in 1904: 'I have seen more change in the surrounding of the factory for the better, than I have in the actual condition of women and girls.'[22] If women were vulnerable in these terms, however, then this vulnerability might also be a reason for restricting their employment in the 'dangerous trades'.

'Dangers at Work'

As well as lead manufacture and industries where lead was used, and match-making associated with the use of white or yellow phosphorous, there were a number of other areas of women's employment that were observed and sometimes classified as endangering their health in similar ways. Some of them were included in regulation while others were not.

In 1897[23] women inspectors reported on the effects of mercurial poisoning in hatters and furriers. This was associated with the various processes of carrotting, in which the natural grease is removed from the fur of rabbit pelts. The mixing of the liquor, scrubbing the fur and then handling the skins in the drying stoves and dampening the skins to make them pliable before shaving the fur from the pelt, all involved exposure to fumes containing nitrate of mercury. In carrotting rooms there were no precautions to prevent the inhalation of fumes. As a result women suffered muscular tremors, anaemia, sore gums, offensive breath and blackened teeth. The symptoms of mercurial poisoning lie at the origin of the metaphor 'as mad as a hatter' indicating that symptoms of disorientation and nervous dysfunction also occurred. Mercury was scheduled in 1898.

There were other fumes that also worked in this way. India-rubber works came under investigation because they were associated with women's ill-health. The conclusion reached on the pungent vapour that dried the nose and throat was that it was unpleasant but not dangerous, although given conditions in the industry it would in time undermine health.[24] Bisulphide of carbon, used in vulcanizing, had more dramatic effects which led to peripheral neuritis, vomiting, dizziness and paralysis. Reports of girls staggering home and falling into a drunken-like sleep without eating their supper were common. One example is given in the 1895 report of the women's inspectorate:

The mother of one girl, whom I saw in her home tells me that she never expected to see her daughter the same girl again, that she sits down in a stupor or extremely drowsy condition in front of the fire, whenever she come home, refusing food, and that she can only be got to bed by being carried there, while if aroused she gets wild and excited. All these and other symptoms are the affects attributed to poisoning by bisulphide of carbon.[25]

In 1910 inspectors reported a case of a girl who had been dismissed from an india-rubber works for 'insobriety and rowdyism' after she had been exposed for two-and-a-half hours in excess of the time allowed.[26] She had developed hysteria and near insanity.

One very strenuous form of work involving fumes was tin-plate manufacture. 'Pickling girls', Rose Squire reported, were the 'roughest, dirtiest and unhealthiest'. They had to load and unload cradles that dipped iron plates into tanks of sulphuric acid. 'Heavier, dirtier or more unlikely work for women and girls could scarcely be imagined, yet hundreds are employed.'[27] They suffered smarting and sometimes blackened lips, nausea and giddiness and feelings of being 'stifled'. Yet she found that many of them believed the pickle gave them an appetite and helped to ward off infection. The condemnation by women inspectors of this trade as one unsuitable for women was, however, because it also exposed women to the weather, deafening noise, hot, sharp metals, heavy lifting and, in common with other workplaces, a lack of sanitary facilities.

Of the many dusts which were thought to cause harm to workers, the women inspectors paid increasing attention to asbestos. In 1906 Adelaide Anderson reported that of all the injurious dusty processes of which she had received complaints, 'none I believe surpass in injuriousness to the worker, the sieving, carding, and spinning processes in the manufacture of asbestos'.[28] This was eight years after the injury done to the respiratory organs by this particular jagged type of dust particles was identified under the microscope. Inspectors reported rooms full of dust circulating and settling. One spinner, reported to have died of consumption at the age of 24, was found to have worked for six years spinning asbestos. For three years she had had symptoms of a hoarse cough and she had been completely unable to work for the last ten months of her life.[29] Given what we now know about the latency period between exposure and the development of this form of cancer of the lung-lining, the toll which this particular industry took on women's health at this time remained invisible. The observed mortality and morbidity represented only a small proportion of eventual sufferers. It reveals the problem of relying on incidence and prevalence as a basis for introducing regulation.

Bronzing[30] was another process that involved the inhalation of dusts. Inspectors frequently reported finding women with the dust in their hair, on their hands, faces and lips and with symptoms of anaemia, loss of appetite, nausea and headache. The printing industry, where it was primarily used, was concentrated in towns, often in ill-ventilated basement workrooms. A special report on printing works in 1907[31] suggested there should be limits on the use of bronzing in hand-processes, noting that with increasing mechanization such use was essentially unnecessary. However, despite technological developments in mechanizing production in many industrial sectors, the development of appropriate machinery or its introduction into the workplace often lagged behind. For example, women inspectors were still commenting on the failure of machine production to develop adequate safety guards well into the twentieth century.[32]

Processes which created dusts were widespread in flax- and linen-milling, cotton and clothing industries, brass-finishing, ivory button-making and pearl button-grinding and boring, to name only some which were thought to be 'dangerous'. Dusts whatever their source or nature posed a threat to health and played a role in the continuing toll of respiratory disease in this period. Within the framework of the 'dangerous trades' regulations, however, only specific dusts were of interest. Silk dusts were investigated by the Medical Inspector of Factories after girls had complained of 'coughing up worms'.[33] In silk debris he found the horny skin of the pupa case of the silkworm together with portions of the larvae![34] A more common bacteriological hazard was anthrax, which had been one of the first scheduled in 1892. Despite regulation, cases rose. This fact, along with its rapid course of action and potentially fatal outcome, continued to cause concern. In 1897 the medical inspector reported 23 cases. In 1899 there were 55 and, by 1907, 67 cases with 22 deaths.[35] Women were at risk because they worked with imported hides, skins or wool which harboured the bacteria. But even if they did not work directly in such industries, some were found to be at risk from cleaning and mending their husbands' contaminated clothes. In 1914, six cases occurred to women not working in the industry.[36] Despite the fact that anthrax was scheduled early and the requirements to notify provided evidence of a continuing toll, like many 'dangerous trades' effective limitation came late, in this case not until 1919.[37]

One process referred to the Dangerous Trades Committee by women inspectors was the licking of labels for reels in thread mills, a process that occurred elsewhere in packaging and bottling. Many younger women and girls doing this work suffered from swollen glands. Some labels were found to contain copper and lead. There was also a complaint called 'stamp-lickers tongue', a form of blood-poisoning resulting from infections entering wounds on the tongue. Some medical experts thought the constant use of saliva in this way might stunt growth. The committee heard evidence from one woman who completed 45 gross of bobbins a day, sticking tickets at each end. This is all the more extraordinary since human licking could have been easily eliminated by the provision of an artificial means of dampening the label. For this reason the committee concluded that there was no need for special rules as the practice 'was now considerably reduced'.[38]

Finally, it is important to discuss those trades where the danger was not to health and life, but to life and limb: that is, the risk of accidents. For women workers, only one such trade was scheduled in this category – aerated water-bottling in 1896. Bottles were filled under pressure and there were cases of injury caused by bottles bursting and sending glass fragments flying. Bottle-wirers, sighters (those looking for impurities) and bottle-labellers were most at risk. Clara Collet noted cases of women who had lost eyes and who had facial injuries requiring stitches. It was not surprising, she argued, that bottle-sighters who had to hold bottles up to the light for 10 hours a day should occasionally knock them, causing them to burst.[39] Thus although more men than women worked in this industry, more accidents occurred to women (absolutely and relatively) because of the processes in which they worked. Unfortunately, while accidents to women in this industry were recognized, elsewhere they received scant attention.

I have argued elsewhere[40] that this was one consequence of perceptions of who was at risk from particular occupational hazards linked to a sexual division of labour, that both associated accidents with machines and machines with men and made accidents more prevalent among men.[41] But women were exposed to machinery even if they did not work with them, as in moving near them and cleaning them. The number of shuttle injuries to women in mills was evidence that not working with machines did not protect them from their effects. Inspectors observed scalping injuries from shafting, including one case where the knowledge of first aid was so poor the scalp was left in the shaft for an hour.[42] Women also used machines in their work: mangles and irons in laundries, stamp presses in pen manufacture and sewing machines in the clothing industry. The extent of their exclusion from the discourse around accident causation and prevention was also evident in practice, as indicated by the removal from women inspectors of any powers in this respect other than to report accidents to their male counterparts. In 1909, their developing expertise was finally recognized by returning to them responsibility for accidents first in laundries and then in clothing manufacture.

'White Cemeteries'

This was a name used by women workers for white-lead works, according to the *Daily Chronicle* in 1892.[43] For them it encapsulated the fact that many workers in the manufacture of white lead died as a result of their work. Given the dramatic symptoms of lead-poisoning, often with a fatal outcome, it is not surprising that this industry and others in which lead was used became synonymous with the 'dangerous trades'. These symptoms of lead-poisoning could be acute or could result in chronic morbidity and disability. They included colic, constipation, violent diarrhoea, anaemia, fits, delirium, paralysis and blindness. Cirrhosis and insanity could result. As with many other kinds of exposure to toxic substances, onset could be sudden or it could have a long latency period. Attacks were in some cases singular, in others recurrent. Lead was used in a number of industries in which women worked: in the manufacture of white lead, bricks and tiles, artificial flowers and cosmetics, in dyeing, lithographic transfers and most prominently in the potteries where lead was used in enamels and glazes. In most of these industries – and certainly in white-lead factories and the Potteries – more men than women were employed. For example in 1895, 43 738 men and 27 137 women were employed in the Potteries, about 7000 of whom were employed in lead-based processes. In the same year, 1889 men and 610 women were employed in white, red and orange lead manufacture.[44]

However, it appeared that women were disproportionately at risk of lead-poisoning. More men than women suffered overall but the relative rates for women seemed to be greater. It was a common perception that women were at greater risk and this perception served to make lead-poisoning a gender-specific occupational health problem, particularly for the period considered here.[45] As Adelaide Anderson claimed in her evidence in 1909 to the committee investigating the health of operatives in the Potteries,[46] concern with poisoning was not only because earthenware and china employed a large number of women and girls but:

> because of the peculiar importance of the conditions and health problems
> for women . . . and whether through a) special constitutional susceptibility
> or b) lack of sufficient nourishment or c) exposure to special risks, women
> are proportionately suffering more plumbism than men.[47]

It is important to consider how these ideas developed and their consequences for intervention in women's work in the lead industries. Outside of mine-work earlier in the century[48] and in the pit-brow protests of the 1880s,[49] it was in the lead industries that calls for the total exclusion of women were most vociferous and, in part, successful.

In the early 1880s the Home Department initiated two enquires conducted by Sir Alexander Redgrave, the Chief Inspector of Factories, into the manufacture of

Figure 2.1 A group of white-bed women from the white lead works in Newcastle from *The White Slaves of England, reproduced by permission of Hulton Deutsch Collection Limited.*

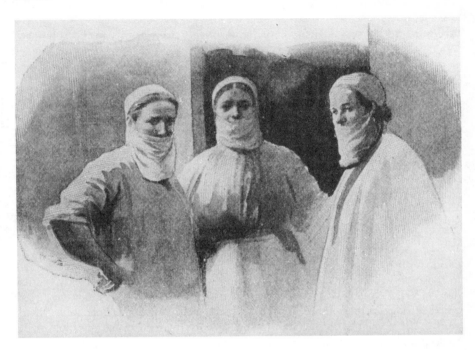

white lead. The first considered the need for regulation.[50] The second was initiated after communications from the Guardians of Poor Law Unions of cases of lead-poisoning in their infirmaries.[51] Here they had noted there were more women than men, but the Guardians and Redgrave in his report considered that these differential rates were caused by labour conditions. Redgrave concluded that it was not necessary to restrict the employment of women – but the possibility of women's greater susceptibility to lead was now firmly on the agenda.

The White Lead Act 1883 was a forerunner for the regulative approach that was followed with respect to the 'dangerous trades' in the 1890s. It laid down standard rules for employers who wanted to be licensed manufacturers. These included the provision of washing facilities, a mealroom and an acidulated drink; a requirement for 'efficient ventilation' and, for women, baths, overalls, head-covering and respirators were to be provided. Thus the rules embodied a preventive principle of protecting workers from work hazards and that women required more protection than men. Critics of the Act noted that nothing had been done to modify the methods of production. *The Times*, for example, suggested:

> It would be more practical to forbid poor and ignorant men and women being employed in an occupation dangerous to health and life, and to compel the substitution of machinery . . . and more useful and easy to

enforce than one which directed the inhabitants of Poplar and Gateshead to clean their teeth before eating, and to be careful to brush away all the dirt from under their fingernails.[52]

According to the two contemporary commentators on women's work, Bulley and Whitley, despite 'the establishment of a sort of hygienic police, which is maintained in the best works with a view to enforcing regularity in the matter of baths', poisoning continued in white-lead works.[53]

Throughout the 1880s and into the early 1890s, criticism of the Act mounted. There was evidence of continued suffering and death, not only in white-lead manufacture but also in other industries. In 1892 under Schedule 8 of the 1891 Act, white-lead works, paint and colour works and enamelling of ironware were scheduled as 'dangerous trades'. This was immediately followed by an extensive enquiry initiated by the State. In 1893 two committees were set up. One reported on various lead industries[54] and the other on labour conditions in the Potteries[55]. At the same time Assistant Lady Commissioners appointed to investigate women's working conditions and the effects on health and morals led to a report by May Abraham on the white-lead industry and by Clara Collet on the Staffordshire Potteries.[56]

The scale of investigation was unprecedented. These enquiries proceeded on two main lines: first, an emphasis on regulation which would eliminate the threats to those engaged in 'dangerous' work with an emphasis on cleanliness, ventilation, protective clothing and the extent of compliance by workers and employers with the rules in these domains; and second, whether or not people were 'fit for work'. The pursuit of this second line of enquiry returned to the question of the 'susceptibility' of women and allowed prohibition to be considered, or if not prohibition then some restrictions and medical surveillance.

The White Lead Committee of 1893 thus recommended excluding women altogether from certain processes and young women from firms using the 'Dutch Process'.[57] The Potteries Committee, which had been more concerned with the health damage of dusts than with lead, proposed nevertheless that married women should be excluded from lead processes particularly because of the effects on pregnancy and the unborn child. In the event it was not until 1898 that any such recommendations were implemented, with the exclusion of women from the 'dangerous processes' in white-lead factories and the requirement for medical certification on age and fitness before employment and 'recovery' after illness.

The perception of 'susceptibility' requires further discussion. Even before the official requirement of 1896 to notify cases of poisoning, which provided some confirmation that there was a higher attack rate in women[58] and that they were, therefore, more susceptible, there were debates in this context about the data and the phenomena itself. Some people thought it might not be a question of sex alone, but an interaction of sex and class or some personal idiosyncrasy within a more vulnerable group. At the same time there was little supporting clinical evidence. Medical witnesses were divided on the issue and their judgment in any case seemed based mainly on impression, experience and supposition.[59]

There were also continual problems with the statistical evidence. In his first report the Medical Inspector of Factories acknowledged that there were difficulties in deciding whether symptoms were caused by lead. Although he conceded that 'it is likely to be more females than males' who suffered, because there was no information as to the age distribution in employment, 'we cannot say whether relatively females under 30 are attacked in greater numbers than males at a corresponding age'.[60] The data on repeat attacks indicated that men were more likely to suffer from chronic plumbism, but that may have been because women left work after a first attack of the illness. We also know that although notification was a legal requirement, it did not always occur. The use of medical journals such as *The Lancet* and *The British Medical Journal* to advertise the requirement did not guarantee it reached all medical practitioners. The figures on notification included cases counted more than once, while others were successful in concealing illness. Despite doubts about the data and the lack of consensus as to its cause, degree of risk or protection, the discourse continued to reproduce a constitutional susceptibility in women. Inquests on deaths in the industry, particularly those of women, were given considerable press publicity and further served to amplify a gendered vulnerability.

There was a growing view that women's particular 'susceptibility' was related to their reproductive biology. Commentators referred to the high rates of miscarriage, still-births and infertility among women lead-workers. Committee members on various enquiries pursued questions about reproductive health. We should not be surprised by such a line of questioning, since late nineteenth-century conceptualizations of women's health rested on the pathological nature of reproductive biology: it was thought the menstrual cycle and the organs of the uterus and ovaries resulted in disordered bodies and minds.[61] In evidence to the White Lead Committee one witness who had argued there was no difference in mortality between Newcastle and Chester, where women and men were respectively exclusively employed, was interrupted by the Chair: 'You have of course special physical matters connected with females that are more difficult to control.'[62] High rates of miscarriage, still-birth and early infant deaths were the norm for most working-class, women whether they worked in lead or not, although later investigations in the Potteries suggested that higher rates did exist among young women who had worked with lead before and after marriage, although the data once again was contentious.[63] The specific issue of lead as a reproductive hazard is explored in Chapter 3, but requires brief mention here because it was inextricably part of beliefs held about general susceptibility.

In 1897 two members of the women's factory inspectorate, Mary Paterson and Lucy Deane, undertook a special enquiry in the Potteries. They spent time investigating the pregnancy histories of 77 married women. This revealed that 15 had no children or miscarriages, 8 had 21 still-born children, 35 had 90 miscarriages and of this group 15 had not had any live children born. They concluded: 'the effects of lead upon the nervous system, however, are less striking and general than its effects upon the bloodmaking and reproductive functions. For this reason . . . woman from her constitutional idiosyncrasy is more liable than man to be impressed by lead.'[64] This view of 'the pernicious influence' of lead on women's reproductive system was emphasized by Dr Thomas Oliver and Professor T. Thorpe in their report[65] of a State-initiated enquiry in 1898 into the substitution of carbonate of lead as a means of reducing the dangers of lead in pottery manufacture. Figures from Oliver's own Newcastle Infirmary and poisoning notification were used to confirm their belief in female susceptibility.

But more important evidence from their point of view was the decline in female poisoning as a result of exclusion. Inevitably there would be different patterns of poisoning as men replaced women. But was this confirmation of female susceptibility? An overall diminution may only have indicated that women were now less exposed to danger. Support for this view is contained in the figures, as there is an almost direct transference of male and female numbers rather than an overall decrease in poisoning. As the medical inspector concluded: 'substitution and the excess of male lead poisoning in white lead manufacture suggests the greater susceptibility to lead of women to be much exaggerated'.[66] However, it was evidently difficult to let the issue go. Oliver himself argued:

> Admitting for the moment that susceptibility is equal in the two sexes, and the fact too, that in both illness may be severe, still I unhesitatingly *assert* that in the main the symptoms are neither so severe in men, nor does the malady run so rapidly to a fatal determination as it does in women.[67] (*my emphasis*)

Under these circumstances official reports continued to countenance that there was a special case for the protection of women from the effects of lead. Although the 1899 report did consider substitution of a 'fritted' lead[68] of low solubility to be possible, they did not consider the prohibition of lead to be likely. Restriction on the work of women, but not their exclusion from the potteries altogether, was recommended, with increased 'safeguards'.[69]

I suggest that whether or not there was some 'real' differential risk of poisoning cannot be disentangled from the social constitution of that risk. Beliefs about vulnerability or risk will themselves serve to create such differentials in diagnostic and reporting decisions and, in a sexually segregated labour market, will be conditioned by where women worked. Although regulation did not include the more extreme demands for women's total exclusion from such industries, it did reflect a view that they required protection. In 1903, a woman inspector was placed in the Potteries for six months of the year. In the same year, women were excluded from mixing and weighing raw materials for glazes. The question of exclusion was returned to once again during the committee enquiry of 1909–10 into the health dangers from lead and dust to workers in earthenware and china.

That an enquiry was once again considered necessary after nearly two decades of regulation was an indication of the general failure of the State's strategy in combatting lead-poisoning. Notifications of poisoning rose toward the end of the 1890s from 1030 cases in 1896 to 1258 in 1899. Although there was a decline early in the next century, notifications and deaths both continued to fluctuate. By 1910 these had fallen to 505. They then rose again to 587 in 1912.[70] By 1914, of the 648 factories under regulation in relation to pottery and china manufacture, only 109 used non-lead glazes.[71]

Regulation failed to be implemented: in the latter case it was hindered by employers' prolonged use of arbitration. Poisoning continued to extract a toll on health and lives. There was stronger agitation for a prohibition on the use of lead in manufacture, but in its 1910 report the committee still did not recommend it. Instead it put its faith in the increasing surveillance of workers and ensuring adherence to regulation. Although it expressed doubts about the susceptibility argument, concluding that 'lead poisoning can largely be accounted for by defective conditions of labour' and 'undue pressure of work', they did concede there might be reproductive damage. However, 'the danger to women working in lead processes . . . should be greatly mitigated, if not actually removed by very strict observance of the proposed precautions'.[72] Gertrude Tuckwell, a committee member, disassociated herself from the final report because of its failure to prohibit lead. In her separate memorandum, she accepted there were risks to women. Exclusion might be the answer 'had it not been that a definite alternative exists by imposing limitations on the use of material instead of on a class of worker'.[73]

The enquiry gives us some insight into how women lead-workers themselves may have perceived the risk. The use of experienced symptomology was pursued in relation to women witnesses. It included those most commonly thought to be associated with poisoning – a bad taste in the mouth, pallor, headaches, constipation, loss of appetite, stomach aches and an irregular menstrual cycle. For women there was a distinction to be drawn between what they saw as 'normal' everyday illness and the 'lead', although these often included the same symptoms. One witness was asked 'Why do you not think the headache you suffer is due to the powder?' 'Well, Sir, all people suffer from headaches.'[74] When questioned about their pallor most replied that they had 'always been that way'. There were difficulties for some women in recognizing terms applied to poisoning as being consonant with their symptoms. Bertha Homer, when asked if she had ever had any colic, replied 'only indigestion'.[75] Mary Mack said she had never had illness: 'I have been sick in myself from sick headaches and bad stomach, but I have never been bad with the lead.'[76] Mary Ann Wood told Oliver she did not 'think it a very healthy occupation, but I do not find it makes any difference to me whatsoever'.[77] However, she confirmed she had no appetite in the morning, a disagreeable taste in her mouth and felt sick after taking food. She attributed her stomach pains to hunger (which may well have been the case, given that bread and dripping and tea was all her breakfast consisted of), but it may also indicate the extent to which women either did not know these were possible symptoms of poisoning or were reluctant to make that connection.

That women did experience sickness and illness, whether due to work or not, is further evidenced by their testimony to long and sometimes frequent periods of sick leave. Elizabeth Jukes, an enameller, had worked for three different firms in three years and had had to leave one firm several times for two to three weeks at a time.[78] Some protection might also have been afforded to women because of working on a casual basis. Mary Jane Mill had only worked for 18 months in the last five years when her husband was unemployed.[79]

Some improvements did occur, although the dramatic decline in poisoning in

1914 was a result of changes in manufacture necessitated by the First World War. Improved ventilation and medical surveillance were thought by the medical inspector to have been the most effective measures.[80] Ultimately the simplest and most effective solution would have been the prohibition of lead. But carbonate of lead was not excluded from manufacturing until 1921. The position of the State in this respect is discussed in more detail in Chapter 5 in the context of general State intervention into working conditions. Certainly, it was not surprising that a morass of rules and regulations that were often contested, not implemented and only partially enforced, failed to deliver what their protagonists had hoped for.

It was also a constant refrain that the best intentions of employers, officials, doctors and the State could be undermined by individual workers themselves. In relation to lead-poisoning, as in other 'dangerous trades', there was a perception that carelessness, 'ignorance, prejudice and obstinacy marred the good efforts of manufacturer and State',[81] a contention that other parties to the political struggles around working conditions, especially women activists, disputed. But an ideological belief in the culpability of workers for their misfortunes and a preventive approach that all too frequently focused on biological as well as on social weaknesses, served to deflect attention from the need to ban lead. As a result, women and more especially men continued to suffer lead-poisoning; and women had restrictions put on their employment as well as increased surveillance of their health and ultimately their role in society.

'Match-girls': The Other Story

Phosphorous poisoning also resulted in a dramatic, disfiguring and often fatal disease – phosphorous necrosis. It had been identified as an industrial disease in Vienna in 1838, seven years after match-works were established. Conditions in British match factories had been highlighted as particularly poor by factory commissioners earlier in the century.[82] However, the match industry has more often been identified with the strike of 1888. As one of the first strikes by unskilled women workers, it has been seen as significant in trade-union history.[83] This was a strike about payment and systems of fines and deductions, rather than directly about working conditions and health, although activists linked to the strike, such as Annie Besant, were aware of and also articulated these problems.[84] Despite this, or perhaps because of it, the match industry and its attendant health risks occupied a particularly prominent position in activism around and official responses to the 'dangerous trades' in the 1890s.

Bryant and May, who had been the focus of workers' earlier grievances, were also to be one of the major sources of disquiet over a continuing incidence of necrosis.[85] The prevalence of 'phossy jaw', as phosphorous necrosis became known, was considerably less than lead-poisoning and it was confined to one industry. The match-making industry was located in a few major centres: notably, London, Liverpool and the Midlands and employed mainly women and children. In 1897, 25 factories employed 4152 people, of whom 2015 were women and 1067 young female persons.[86] But women were not usually employed in the dangerous processes of mixing the phosphorous-based paste, dipping and drying. The majority of women were employed in boxing, but both women and young girls still succumbed to phosphorous necrosis.

Outside the industry's inclusion in the 1864 provision to prohibit women and children from eating food in rooms where dangerous processes were carried out, there had been little regulation of the match-making industry before the 1890s. This may have been because of a view within the Factory Department that the problem was minimal if it existed at all. In evidence to the 1876 Factory Commission, Alexander Redgrave, Chief Inspector of Factories, suggested 'necrosis has entirely ceased'. In 1892 his successor considered the 'evils of the trade to be much exaggerated'.[87] At almost the same time it was one of the four 'dangerous trades' to be scheduled and was therefore subject to special rules about cleanliness, ventilation, the separation of dangerous processes, certified fitness before employment and cases of toothache or swelling to be medically examined and reported.

The scheduling of the match-making industry might have been a response to evidence provided by *The Star* in early 1892 of a case it had discovered of phosphorous necrosis.[88] The Factory Department reconsidered its position, indicating that the allegations that 'there were others' (cases) were substantially correct, although the disease was not widespread.[89] Alexander Redgrave confirmed he had uncovered seven cases at Bryant and May that were being treated at home.[90] Even so, there was hardly an epidemic, but the industry continued to come under scrutiny. Clara Collet, who investigated a number of companies for the Royal Commission on Labour, noted that conditions were variable. She called on the expertise of the socialist Tom Mann, also a Commission member, to emphasize the problems which she thought arose from deficiencies in ventilation. In his letter reporting on Bryant and May and Palmer and Sons, he noted 'that there was a decided lack of anything like scientific ventilation' so that fumes were frequently carried to other parts of factories. 'The rule of thumb, and a bad and ugly thumb, appeared to me to be the stamp of both firms' he concluded.[91] Collet was also sceptical of employers' denial of cases. She personally interviewed victims, some of whom had disfiguring surgery, via Dr Garman Bryant and May's own physician.[92]

Despite the relatively few cases of phosphorous necrosis that were found, if not recorded, the cases continued to have a high profile in the political arena of State intervention. It was an awful disease. It started as a kind of influenza, alongside toothache. The pain eventually spread to the lower jaw and frequently to the whole face, throat and throat glands. Inflammation of the gums and cheeks and putrid abscesses developed (an aspect according to testimony that made it very difficult for sufferers or their relatives to deal with the disease). Treatments involved extractions and often surgery which might remove diseased facial bones. It was not surprising that cases remained hidden from view, or that sufferers would hide symptoms for fear of the disease and its consequences. As Rose Squire recalled in her autobiography:

In a certain town I dug out cases of men and women, hidden away in the slums – piteous cases they were. One woman had completely lost her lower jaw, a young girl at earlier stages was constantly in great pain while her suppurating jaw bone was gradually decaying.[93]

It may well be that this spectre of an identifiable 'industrial disease' was a powerful weapon in the political struggles around working conditions and the effectiveness or otherwise of State regulation. One case was one too many and it is interesting that employers were the only group who seemed to have used the small numbers involved as a defence. The fact that it was a small industry and that sufferers and deaths were relatively small-scale did not diminish its importance or the attention it received. The industry was also constantly in the public domain as an example of 'sweated' outwork or homework, with women and children making boxes. Lady Dilke, a trade-union activist, reported that the weekly average earnings 'in this miserable industry, stand as far as I can judge, at something under seven shillings for 84 hours of labour'.[94]

As in the case of lead, enquiry continued to take place throughout the 1890s. In 1893 the Chemical Works Committee of Inquiry had been asked to investigate lucifer match-making. They concluded that 'despite few visible cases . . . the danger from the disease exists to all workers where white or yellow phosphorous is still used'.[95] In 1898 the women's factory inspectorate conducted a special enquiry into match-works and traced several unreported cases of phosphorous necrosis in Gloucester.[96] Lucy Deane and Rose Squire emphasized the dangers that resulted from the fact that this industry had all the characteristics of a 'sweated' trade. Wages were so low, they claimed, that 'sufficient food and clothing are impossible unless some of the necessities of life are supplied by relatives and friends' – and many match workers were orphans or had relatives to support themselves. In this context the 'silent endurance of extraordinary suffering' and a general apathy toward the protective measures provided could be observed.[97] The report underlined the poverty of the classes from which many 'dangerous trades' recruited and the difficulties this might create for the kinds of preventative strategies being pursued. It also confirmed the continuing concealment of cases.

After the 1892 disclosures of cases of phosphorous necrosis by the press, this line of investigation was pursued by a variety of papers throughout the 1890s. It was part of a wider campaign in which many became involved, to discredit the actions of both employers and the State in the improvement of working conditions. In 1898 Bryant and May were once again in the limelight, charged with three cases of failing to notify under the 1895 Act. The *Daily Chronicle* described the case as one of 'the worst breaches of the Factory Acts to be brought to court'. In the House of Commons, MP Harold Tennant described it as 'a conspiracy to defeat the bringing to the State the cause of death' although he argued this was not unique to Bryant and May.[98]

There was also a strong suspicion of collusion between medical practitioners and employers to conceal cases, although equally likely was 'the unaccountable ignorance' which the women inspectors found among medical practitioners about the disease.[99] Direct evidence of intimidation by threats of lost income was found in relation to one of the cases at Bryant and May. A Mrs Lean, whose son had died of phosphorous necrosis, was told 'if I called another doctor in, the pay (ie the sick pay from the firm of 29 shillings a week) would be stopped'. The firm also admitted in a letter to Mr Henderson, a factory inspector, that in the case of Alice Skeeles her allowance had been stopped because 'she declined to continue care under our doctor'.[100] Employers and doctors defended their position and continued to argue that the problem was only a minor one. The State, however, decided that given the level of agitation it needed to be seen to act. In a minute dated 14 June 1898, the Secretary of State wrote in relation to the match industry:

> There is so much feeling on this subject that probably a short bill confined to this industry could be passed just now. A Committee puts off the difficulty til [sic] a time when the excitement has cooled down and when legislation will have become more difficult.[101]

A committee was set up and reports commissioned on the scientific, medical and dental aspects of the question, from Professor Thorpe, Dr Oliver and Dr George Cunningham of the London Dental School.[102] Despite the attention paid to the use of phosphorous and its effects, the frame of reference was still firmly set within the prevailing preventive strategy of improved cleanliness, ventilation and medical, including dental, surveillance. In the preamble to setting up the enquiry, for example, some emphasis was given to whether phosphorous could be 'readily and effectively removed from the hands by soap and water'. Both employers and workers, the report concluded, were less than diligent in observing the rules, but with further improvements here as well as in structural arrangements and mechanized production, illness could be prevented. Prohibition was considered as a possibility, but arguments about consumer preferences (for the 'strike anywhere match') and foreign competition were accepted as ruling out this option. In any case it was seen to be unnecessary as other measures would work.

In the enquiries into lead-poisoning, questions of gender-based susceptibility were central to the discourse about risk and prevention. Did questions arise here, too, especially as in relation to all the 'dangerous trades' there was a strong argument in favour of excluding women? I suggest the possibility of gendered risk was always raised, even if there was little evidence to support it. Match-making was no exception. Women did not work in the dangerous processes, but they were evidently at risk from them, both because in the process of boxing, matches frequently flared and burned, releasing the fumes and because fumes from other areas of the factory entered the rooms in which the women and young girls worked. However, there did not seem to be any disproportionate risk.

Because of the nature of the symptoms in the teeth and mouth, there was agreement that necrosis had links to dental health – but there was less consensus on the nature of that relationship. Although necrosis was thought to develop through the action of phosphorous on the jaw, it was not clear whether this was a local action or whether it was absorbed into the body system and promoted decay initially to the teeth and then elsewhere. There was also doubt about whether the poison entered by the inhalation of fumes or whether it was by the direct absorption

Figure 2.2 Bryant and May: cutting and packing, reproduced by permission of Mary Evans Picture Library.

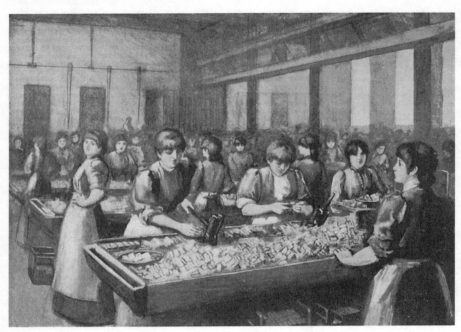

of paste: that is, from hand to mouth. In most expert discussion, the favoured theory seems to have been inhalation, especially as there were sufferers who had not been exposed to the paste. There were puzzles, however, in the fact that only a few workers exposed to the fumes seemed to succumb to the disease, including those in the 'dangerous processes'.

Differential susceptibility was a potential explanation. In general, however, this susceptibility was thought to lie in the dental health of the worker prior to onset, or their general constitutional health. The state of workers' teeth as a predisposing factor, and not just a disease outcome, consequently became something to be considered in the regulations. This may have been more practicable than an acceptance of the broader constitutional theory which would have required more radical change to broader social conditions.[103] It was accepted that workers in the industry came from extremely poor backgrounds and that they were not in full health on arrival.

The possibility of a gender difference was only partly accepted. Thomas Oliver concluded that 'as regards phossy jaw neither sex is spared, nor is there any difference in the severity or location of the malady. Men who dip, girls who cut down and those who fill boxes suffer all alike and equally *once the disease has taken hold* (my emphasis).[104] He emphasizes that the course of the disease itself is similar in men and women, whereas dental opinion was inclined to the view that women were more susceptible because the state of their dental health was poorer. In his report George Cunningham addresses this issue, providing evidence from his own investigations. In one study of 945 workers in five factories he concluded that the teeth of 35.5 per cent of the men and 67.5 per cent of the women working in phosphorous and 69.5 per cent of men and 89.6 per cent of women not working in phosphorous to be 'in an extremely bad condition'.[105] He concluded:

> On the whole my contention is that the teeth of women are in a worse condition than those of men at a corresponding age employed in match factories . . . it would therefore appear that women are more liable to the disease than men. But I am unable to say the distinction is very marked . . . the difference such as it is, results, I think, entirely from the fact that the diet of men is more nutritious than that of women.[106]

However, this form of susceptibility did not provide grounds for exclusion, especially given the industry's reliance on women. In fact, it was argued that men might materially be more at risk because of their location in the dangerous processes and the more permanent nature of their employment. It was concluded that the solution to the problems of dental health as a predisposing cause was best dealt with by dental inspection and dental treatment.

The control of the match-making industry as a designated 'dangerous trade' thus exhibits many of the same features as the lead industries. The main preventive strategies focused on giving factories and workers rules and regulations that would ostensibly protect them from the hazards and ensure as far as possible that they were 'fit' enough to work. Despite requirements to improve structural arrangements and provisions for ventilation and cleanliness, the legislative approach left production methods largely intact – and in the case of match-making also its requirement for women's labour. Even after the 1906 Bern agreement to prohibit white or yellow phosphorous because other safer forms were now available and in use elsewhere,[107] the British government failed to act. A further investigation in 1907[108] revealed a necrosis death at Morelands. In 1908 a Bill was finally introduced and both white and yellow phosphorous were prohibited from 1910.

Regulating Danger: The Reality

In the light of these case studies and other examples of trades which were perceived to be 'dangerous to the health, life and limb' of those who worked in them, an assessment is necessary of the preventive strategies enshrined within regulation and the discourses which both supported and countered such approaches. Inevitably some problems arose because there were other political and ideological purposes that had to be served by State action and which were pursued by other parties concerned. These political purposes and responses to women and occupational ill-health are explored in the second section of this book. Here I consider the extent to which the strategies outlined above were perceived to work in practice in relation to 'dangerous' work and what were the consequences of such actions. In the case of lead industries and in match-making it was argued that poisoning continued despite constant enquiry and increasing regulation. Ultimately, in these industries at least, the failure to consider prohibition of the single source of poisoning was fundamental.

Throughout the period there was considerable opposition to the State's failure to prohibit. This came from many quarters. The press were often vociferous campaigners in favour of the principles of the Factory Acts and gave publicity to investigations and inspectors' annual reports on working conditions. Newspapers constantly bemoaned the failure of legislation to bring improvements and looked for reasons for that failure in employers, enforcement and in the content and extent of the legislative remedy. Reformers in the House of Commons, many of whom were also supporters of women's causes, constantly used the floor to demand changes in approach. Sir Charles Dilke, in the 1899 Committee on Supply, pleaded: 'I hope we shall not again be put off with mere dentistry, because we had that last year at full length': a reference to the approach taken on necrosis.[109] Feminist activists, at least those who by this time had accepted that factory legislation was necessary to improve conditions for women workers, were adamant that in this case the 'protection' of women was not necessary as there was an alternative. This was particularly important for those who continued to pursue class as well as gender interests, since prohibition would have benefited all workers. As with other critics, they continued to be sceptical about the extent to which 'special rules' could be effective. As the women's periodical *Shafts* put it with respect to phosphorous:

> The insistence on the providing of hot and cold water, nail brushes and towels is all very well in its way . . . but as a prevention against necrosis they are in the nature of a dip out of the Atlantic with a teacup . . . It is hoped that he [*Mr Asquith, Home Secretary*] will see the wisdom of promptly supplementing the present regulations by prohibiting the use of phosphorous in its dangerous forms altogether.[110]

Such views were also shared by the State's own officials responsible for the enforcement of regulation, as Miss Vines informed the 1909–1910 Committee on the Potteries:

> Unless you go to the source of the evil and stop the material itself from being unhealthy, and make it innocuous you cannot really deal with the difficulty. While the use of lead continues, I do not believe that you will, as it were, even sufficiently strengthen the fence at the top of the cliff, so as to prevent the need of an ambulance at the bottom.[111]

Interestingly, similar metaphoric analyses have been offered recently in relation to the failure to divert resources from health services to prevention targeted at the social causes of ill-health.[112]

For women inspectors and many labour women activists, the calls for more effective measures were rooted in their own observations of the failure of 'special rules' on the ground. It was not just that employers failed to comply, it was that their attempts to do so were frequently based on a lack of knowledge about the techniques and mechanics involved (as in ventilation) or that what was provided gave little consideration to the workers who had to use them. Inspectors' reports reveal many instances of inadequate washing facilities; washing troughs which had to be shared by women; the requisite number of basins without the requisite number of taps and a lack of towels to name but a few. It was not surprising, they concluded, that women and girls would not want to use them.

There were similar problems with respirators. As one report noted: 'I found them to be of such a shape that they could not be worn over the face without flattening the nose, and were so old and dirty that no self-respecting woman could put her face into one, nor could she see if she did.'[113] Yet, despite doubts about their effectiveness, the importance of respirators continued to be emphasized and workers blamed for not wearing them. One medical witness, who had commented that women did not wear them 'because they do not like to disfigure their beauty' was further questioned by Gertrude Tuckwell as to whether he had 'ever seen a respirator which you think would be comfortable to wear', to which he replied: 'No, I have not, I am sorry to say they are very nasty things at the best of times.'[114] This is not to argue that workers were not sometimes guilty of not observing regulations or that 'thoughtless[ly] young persons bring to their work cakes or apples and eat them when at machines',[115] but to emphasize that these actions were more often those which seemed reasonable to workers, given the conditions under which they laboured.

This point is also valid in relation to observations that a 'fatalistic' attitude prevailed toward the 'dangers' of work. It was not just those unsympathetic to women workers who observed this tendency. Gertrude Tuckwell, following a trip to the Potteries in 1898, wrote: 'Apathy is one of the first things an outsider notes. Accustomed to the prospect of suffering, they duly accept it when it overcomes them, treating it as inevitable fate.'[116] Hilda Martindale, observed that:

> Amongst the poor there is a marked tendency to live merely in the present and an inability, perhaps in some ways fortunate for themselves, to consider the future; so in order to earn the weekly wage they refuse to acknowledge any signs of coming illness and poverty which must follow them in the future.[117]

Without any other form of material support and where increased surveillance could result in suspension or permanent exclusion, it was hardly surprising that illness was concealed. Such 'fatalism' was rooted in the often continual suffering and illness of working-class women, whether they worked or not. This aspect of their lives continued at least until the setting-up of the National Health Service in 1948.[118] And, given the combination of their social and working conditions, it is not difficult to imagine how the long hours of domestic labour and the lack of power that many experienced contributed to the women appearing apathetic or, more often, just plain exhausted.

Working women themselves also shared some of the preventive beliefs the experts considered important. Witnesses in lead work, for example, would often point to personal responsibility and individual characteristics as implicated in good or bad health. These lay explanations present a view that it was not so much the work that was dangerous, but how women responded to that danger. Mary Young put her not being ill as 'a great deal to do with the food you take'.[119] Mary Ann Ingram, a smelter, argued 'I do not think it affects any of them if they are very particular about keeping themselves clean'. The work was not dangerous, she said, 'it was women's fault that they were ill'.[120] Mary Killoran accounted for her good health because 'I take good care of myself and I get my food as I ought.'[121] Women's own perceptions about risk may have offered them some protection from poisoning, but ultimately it did not matter how clean or diligent workers were. It would not necessarily provide protection which was why women trade-unionists in particular argued so strongly for prohibition.

Finally the inability of an approach toward the 'dangerous trades' which focused on working conditions alone would have limited success. That women would continue to be employed in such industries was in part due to poverty and low wages in general. Women's disadvantage within the family in these circumstances would also impinge on their ability to withstand the rigours of such employment. It was frequently noted that women were 'ill-fed' and 'ill-clad'.[122] It was common practice in working-class households for whatever food that was available to be given to men first, then children and finally, if there was any left, women. Women told the Women's Cooperative Guild in 1914[123] of how they often pretended to have eaten first, so that their husbands would not be aware they had not food for themselves. Some recognition of this is found in recommendations that milk drinks and hot food should be provided in lead industries, but they were optional because of employers objections. Characteristics of working-class lives could also function ideologically. In the same way that gender susceptibility was a biological constitution of vulnerability to 'disease' and served to both direct attention to 'classes of worker' rather than industries themselves, so class could be viewed as a 'social' vulnerability (and often in combination with gender) could be used to account for why women and men continued to get poisoned. This was not just a problem of their material circumstances but attitudes and beliefs, a 'culture' which was accused of ignorance of both danger and the necessity for regulation.

What may have limited the extent to which exclusionary strategies were pursued in the 'dangerous trades' was marked sexual divisions in labour. There is little evidence that male trade-unionists in the potteries, for example, or in lead manufacturing supported exclusion, except as part of an accepted rhetoric. In general there was little competition between men and women for the jobs women did in the 'dangerous trades'. Sometimes this was because they were the 'worst in terms of skill required and conditions', and there is evidence that when women were excluded from white lead processes, one London firm resorted to importing Italian migrant labour.[124] In other cases the work was perceived as 'naturally' suited to women. As Thorpe and Oliver concluded in their 1899 report about majolica painting 'as a manual occupation it is particularly suited to females, but if they are permitted to pursue it, both the spirit and the letter of the law must be complied with'[125], and one male trade unionist in evidence to the 1910 Committee, favoured the exclusion of women from lead processes 'except majolica painting and other decorative work'.[126] In the Potteries at least there had been a long tradition of the interpenetration of home and work which enabled women to be considered part of the labour market.[127]

Agitation, intervention and regulation of the 'dangerous trades' marked a departure in concerns about the impact of working conditions on health and on the health of women. They fostered a development of medical knowledge and expertise in the identification of 'industrial disease'. The potential offered by a medical model of occupational ill-health to eliminate causes of pathology by the removal and substitution of poisons and other hazards was not, however, forthcoming. Rather, there seems to have been a continuance of earlier sanitary or 'public health' traditions of using legislation to ensure the cleanliness of bodies, air and workplaces and to expand the policing of the health of workers prior to and during work, consistent with developing traditions of observation and surveillance of the public in institutional settings and in the private domain of the home.[128] Thus the concept of 'dangerous trades' became subverted into a concern with 'dangerous' workers. For women it was not that their employment in such trades was a 'danger' to themselves, but that it posed the possibility of disorder in relation to the working-class family and ideals of separate spheres.

That such 'dangers' could not be confronted by exclusionary tactics was a measure of the extent to which this would have interfered with other cherished principles of the industrial system – and also the pervasiveness of the idea that women and thereby men could be 'protected'. Despite the considerable toll on health these scheduled industries took, they nevertheless represented at best only a partial recognition of the 'dangers' of work to health. At worst, attention was deflected away from all those broader aspects of working conditions that would continue to undermine the health of many more workers. The strategy pursued in relation to the 'dangerous trades' was, as with other areas of occupational ill-health, not preventive but protective. Suffering, sickness and deaths because of work continued as a consequence.

Notes

1   The reason for using inverted commas here and throughout the chapter is to indicate that this term was used in the discourse. Through legislation it defined only particular kinds of work in this way. It indicates that this also represented a problematic conception of danger.

2   See, for example, Hutchins and Harrison (1903) *A History of Factory Legislation.*

3   As indicated, the work of Sir John Simon and his colleagues at the Privy Council was particularly important. Wohl (1983) *Endangered Lives* Chapter 10 and Simon's *Annual Reports to the Privy Council* in the 1860s.

4   Reports by Redgrave on *White Lead Works*, PP XVIII 1882 and PP XVIII 1883.

5   Arlidge (1892) *The Hygiene, Diseases and Mortality of Occupations* p.4.

6   See, for example, Lee (1973) 'The emergence of occupational medicine in Victorian

Britain' and Harrison (1991) 'Women's health or social control? The role of the medical profession in relation to factory legislation in late nineteenth-century Britain'.

7   The text of the Schedule is in PRO HO45/9848/12393A.

8   *Hansard* (1895) Vol. 32, p.1408.

9   In the First Reading of the Factories and Workshops Bill, *Hansard* (1895) Vol. 31, p.178.

10   Frequent references to this can be found in the Home Office Files about the pottery industry in particular: PRO/HO45/9898/12393D.

11   See Harrison (1990) 'Suffer the Working Day: Women in the 'Dangerous Trades' 1880–1914'.

12   Oliver (Ed.) (1902) *The Dangerous Trades* p.14.

13   May Abraham resigned from the inspectorate after her 1896 marriage to Harold Tennant, because of 'family pressure' (see McFeeley (1986)) but she continued her work on the Committee.

14   The brief for the Departmental Committee to Inquire and Report upon Certain Miscellaneous Dangerous Trades is outlined in the First of their *Interim Reports* (1896) PP XXX.

15   Ibid., and (1897) PP XVII and *Third, Fourth and Fifth Reports* (1899) PP XII.

16   Committee Debate on Home Office Supply, *Hansard* (1900) Vol. 85.

17   Squire (1902) 'Rabbit down', in Oliver (Ed.) *The Dangerous Trades* Chapter LII, p.724.

18   Mr Walmsley, a Factory Inspector for Staffordshire, argued that higher wages for lead workers induced them to 'run all risks', by returning to work immediately after recovery. But it is equally likely that this was the main form of employment available and it was work with which they were already familiar. See *Annual Report for 1895*, PP XIX, p.144.

19   Squire (1902) 'Rabbit down', in Oliver (Ed.).

20   Cited by Henderson, Inspector of Factories for Newcastle, in a Memorandum to the Home Department, PRO/HO45/9848/B12393A.

21   As expressed in the *Report of the Interdepartmental Committee on Physical Deterioration* (1904) PP XXXVII, p.55.

22   Ibid., p.214, Minute 1464.

23   *Annual Report for 1897*, PP XIV, 1898.

24   *Committee on the Dangerous Trades, Reports*, PP XXX, 1896; PP XVII, 1897; PP XII, 1899.

25   *Annual Report for 1895*, PP XIX, 1896, p.129.

26   *Annual Report for 1910*, PP XXII, 1911, p.147.

27   Squire (1902) 'Women's labour in tin-plate works', in Oliver (Ed.) *The Dangerous Trades*.

28   Anderson (1922) *Women in the Factory* Chapter IV on the 'Dangerous and injurious trades'.

29   *Annual Report for 1906*, PP X, 1907, p.238.

30   Dry metallic bronze powders were used in letter-press printing and lithographic printing and for coating metal-sheeting.

31   Deane and Slocock, *Conditions of Work in Printing Works, Annual Report for 1906*.

32   See Harrison (1993a) 'Are accidents gender-neutral?' for a discussion of women inspectors' views of machine safety.

33   Both Rose Squire and Hilda Martindale received such complaints. See *Annual Report for 1906*.

34   *Report of the Chief Medical Inspector for Factories and Workshops for the year 1906*.

35   Ibid.

36   Cited in Anderson (1922) *Women in the Factory* Chapter IV.

37 The Anthrax Prevention Act required that all imported materials, a principal source of the problem, be disinfected on arrival in the country.

38 *Fifth and Final Report of the Departmental Committee* (1899) PP XII, p.231.

39 Collett (1893–4) *Report on Conditions of Work in London*, PP XXVII, p.643.

40 Harrison (1993a) 'Are accidents gender-neutral?'

41 Anderson (1922) *Women in the Factory* argues that records in 1920 showed men as 30 times more likely to have accidents than women.

42 Hilda Martindale also pointed out that this prevented the usual treatments for such injury being pursued: the scalp was too cold by the time it got to the infirmary. *Annual Report for 1906*, PP X, 1907, p.142.

43 Thursday, 15 December 1892, in PRO/HO45/98448/12393A/13.

44 Employment Returns in the *Annual Report for Factories and Workshops for 1895*, PP XIX, 1896.

45 There were many other occupations in which men were particularly at risk, but it was only well into the twentieth century that this raised concern. For example, notifications among house-painters and coach body-painters were high.

46 *Report of the Departmental Committee Appointed to Inquire into the Dangers Attendant on the Use of Lead, and the Danger or Injury to Health Arising from Dust and Other Causes in the Manufacture of Earthenware and China and the Processes Incidental Thereto in the Making of Lithographic Transfers* (1910) PP XXIX. (This will be referred to as the *Potteries Report of 1910*, from here on.)

47 Ibid., Minutes of Evidence, p.727.

48 Humphries (1981) 'Protective legislation, the capitalist state and working-class men: the case of the 1842 Mines Regulation Act'.

49 John (1984b) *By the Sweat of their Brow*.

50 *Report of Alexander Redgrave Esq. upon the Precautions which can be Enforced under the Factory Acts and as to the Need for Further Powers for the Protection of People Employed in White Lead Work* (1882) PP XVIII.

51 *Copy of Communications addressed to the Secretary of State for the Home Department on the Subject of White Lead Poisoning, and a Report by Alexander Redgrave, Her Majesty's Chief Inspector of Factories on the same Subject* (1883) PP XVIII.

52 Clippings in PRO/HO45/9848/B12393.

53 Bulley and Whitley (1894) *Women's Work* p.134.

54 *Report of the Departmental Committee on the Various Lead Industries 1893–4* PP XVII. Referred to as The White Lead Committee.

55 *Report of Her Majesty's Principal Secretary of State for the Home Department on Conditions of Labour in the Potteries, and the Injurious Effects upon the Health of the Workpeople and the Proposed Remedies 1893–4* PP XVII. (Referred to as The Potteries Committee of Inquiry.)

56 *Reports of the Assistant Lady Commissioners to the Royal Commission on Labour 1893–4*, PP XXXVII, pp.597 and 699.

57 The 'Dutch Process' involved the use of hand labour. It consisted of stacking crates of blue lead to be converted by the action of tan and acid into carbonate. Stacks were opened and the lead was stripped out. It was then crushed and subjected to processes that separated out the white lead. This was then put into pans and dried out in stoves. When dry, the lead was packed into casks or bins. Many of these processes were very dusty and involved direct contact with white lead.

58 See the *Annual Reports of the Medical Inspector for Factories* from 1898.

59 For example in the *Evidence to the Committee on the Various Lead Industries*, of

thirteen medical witnesses, eight agreed and five disagreed about a sex-susceptibility 1893–4 PP XVII. See also Harrison (1989) 'Some of them gets lead poisoned' for a discussion of medical evidence.

60 *Report of the Medical Inspector for 1899*, PP XI, 1900.
61 See Ehrenreich and English (1973) *Complaints and Disorders*; Jalland and Hooper (1986) *Women from Birth to Death*; and my own chapter on 'Women's health', in Purvis (Ed.) (1995) *Women's History, Britain: 1850–1945*.
62 1893–4, PP XVII. Witness Mr Bainbridge, Minutes of Evidence, 5770–3.
63 See the discussion of Dr Reid's studies in the *1910 Report*, PP XXIX.
64 *Annual Report of Chief Inspector for 1897*, PP XIV, 1898. This aspect is discussed at length by the Chief Inspector, pp.53–5.
65 *Report on the Employment of Compounds of Lead in the Manufacture of Pottery* (1899) PP XII, (Referred to as the *Thorpe/Oliver Report*.)
66 *Annual Report of the Medical Inspector for the Year 1898*, PP XII, 1899.
67 Oliver (Ed.) (1902) *The Dangerous Trades* p.296.
68 'Fritting' involved mixing lead oxide with silicates to achieve low solubility. Thorpe and Oliver claimed that a 'double measure of silicate would give equally good coverage' and that there were really no obstacles to its use in pottery manufacture. Employers contested this.
69 *Thorpe/Oliver Report* (1899) PP XII, 1899.
70 These figures are taken from the *Annual Reports of the Medical Inspector*.
71 *Report on the Regulations in the Potteries by Inspectors Pendock and Werner* (1914) PP LXXI.
72 *The 1910 Report on the Potteries*, PP XXIX, p.207.
73 Ibid., p.223.
74 Ibid., Witness Mary Fellowes, Minute 9788.
75 *Report*, PP XXVIII, Minutes of Evidence 11492–530.
76 Ibid., Minute 1554.
77 Ibid., Minute 9276.
78 Ibid., Minute 11 960.
79 Ibid., Minute 1518.
80 *Annual Report of the Medical Inspector for 1914*, PP XXI, 1914–16.
81 Arlidge (1892) *The Hygiene, Diseases and Mortality of Occupations* p.4.
82 In particular the *Children's Employment Commission Reports*, PP XVIII, 1863 and PP XX, 1883.
83 See Webb and Webb (1911) *A History of Trade Unionism*; and Beer, R. (n.d.) *The Match Girls Strike, 1888*.
84 See her letter to the Shareholders of Bryant and May, *The Link*, No. 24, 14 July 1888.
85 See Satre (1982) 'After the match-girls strike: Bryant and May in the 1890s'.
86 *Annual Report for 1898* (1900) Part II, PP II.
87 PRO/HO45/9849/B12393D contains these views.
88 *The Star*, 19–27 January, covered the issue. See Satre (1982).
89 PRO/HO45/9849/12393D contains a Memo from Sprague-Oram to this effect.
90 *Annual Report for 1892*, PP XVII, 1893–4.
91 Collett (1893–4), *Report on the Conditions of Work in London*, PP XXVII, p.544.
92 Ibid., p.643.
93 Squire (1927) *Thirty Years in the Public Service: An Industrial Retrospect* p.54.
94 Dilke (1895) *The Industrial Position of Women*. See also Black (1891) 'Matchbox making at home'.

95 *Report of the Chemical Works Committee of Inquiry into Lucifer Match Works* (1893–4) PP XVII.

96 Report is contained in the *Annual Report for 1898*, PP XII, 1899.

97 Ibid., p.168.

98 This newspaper coverage, including the report of Harold Tennant's speech, is in PRO/HO45/9849/12393D.

99 Lucy Deane makes this point in the special report, *Annual Report for 1898*, PP XII, 1899, p.168.

100 Evidence in PRO/HO45/9845/12393D.

101 Ibid. The Memo is on page 52.

102 *Reports to the Secretary of State for the Home Department on the Use of Phosphorous in the Manufacture of Lucifer Matches*. Each expert submitted an individual report as well as a joint report (1898) PP XIV.

103 See Harrison (1995a) 'The politics of occupational ill-health in late nineteenth-century Britain: The case of the match-making industry'.

104 *Thorpe/Oliver Report*, (1899) PP XII, p.553.

105 *Report of George Cunningham*, ibid., p.670.

106 Ibid., p.701.

107 Countries in Europe had banned white or yellow phosphorous much earlier, but by the early-twentieth century Bryant and May was experimenting with alternatives.

108 *Report to the Secretary of State*, (1907) PP X.

109 *Hansard* (1899) Vol. 66, p.225.

110 *Shafts*, 31 December 1892, p.138.

111 *1910 Report*, PP XXIX, Minutes of Evidence, p.501.

112 A much-quoted example comes from McKinley (1974) 'A case for refocusing upstream – the political economy of illness'.

113 *Annual Report for 1900* (1901) PP X, p.384.

114 *1910 Report*, PP XXIX, p.430.

115 *Report on Regulations in the Potteries* (1914) PP LXXI.

116 Tuckwell (1898) 'Commercial manslaughter'.

117 Martindale (1944a) *From One Generation to Another* p.88.

118 See Spring-Rice (1939) *Working-Class Wives:their Health and Condition* second edition 1981.

119 *1910 Report*, PP XXIX, Minutes of Evidence, p.80.

120 Ibid., p.78, Minute 2362.

121 Ibid., p.44.

122 This comes from the earlier quote (note 19) of Thomas Oliver, cited in a report by Henderson sent to Sprague-Oram, who forwarded it to the Secretary of State. In PRO/HO45/9849/B12393D.

123 Davies (1915) *Maternity: Letters from Working Women*. Several letters testify to this practice.

124 There is a reference to a firm in Millwall in the PRO/HO45 file.

125 *Thorpe/Oliver Report* (1899) PP XII, p.239.

126 *1910 Report*, PP XXIX, Minutes of Evidence, Mr B., p.192, Minute 6292.

127 See Whipp (1983) '*Pot bank and union: a study of work and trade unionism in the Potteries 1900–1925*', unpublished PhD Thesis, University of Warwick.

128 See Donzelot (1980) *The Policing of Families*; Foucault (1979) *Discipline and Punish*.

Chapter 3

Work, Maternity and Domestic Labours

Central to the political struggles which ensued around women in the labour market, the effects on their health of working conditions and the rationales for legislative protection, was the ideology of women's nature and place in society. It was the perception of women's role in relation to the nurture, care and responsibility for men and children within the domestic domain which ensured that women's work in the paid labour market would become a major 'social problem' of the late-nineteenth and early-twentieth centuries. The issue of occupational ill-health needs to be considered in this context because 'domestic ideology' both framed the discourse within which women's health in this and other respects was considered and it impinged directly on women's lives.

In order to explore some of the ways in which women's role within the domestic sphere framed occupational health problems identified in the paid and public domain of work, this chapter focuses on three issues. First, the extent to which it was argued that participation in the paid labour market affected the health of women as mothers and their children. Here the idea of work as directly impinging on the health of the domestic sphere is explored generally with reference to debates about the causes of infant mortality. Second, the case of possible reproductive damage from 'hazards' encountered in the workplace is examined, using the specific example of lead work. The final section is concerned with homework and domestic workshops as forms of paid work which were located in the domestic domain. Such work was considered to be a component of 'sweated labour' and a major factor in the identification of women as 'sweated' workers. This posed the paradox of women being where they were supposed to be, but not doing what they were supposed to do. It also raised issues about occupational ill-health.

Maternal Health and Infant Mortality

Although the sub-heading for this section indicates that a consideration of issues of maternal health might be important within any analysis of the possible health implications of paid employment for women, it will be evident that maternal health was not the central concern in the period discussed here, or indeed later in the twentieth century.[1] It was the damage to 'motherhood' rather than to mothers from paid work, particularly in factories, which was perceived to be the problem. The source of this 'social problem' as it came to be defined,[2] was the continuing high rates of infant mortality, 'a massacre of the innocents'[3] which persisted, although there was a decline in mortality for this group alongside that of other age groups.[4] Despite new social circumstances the debates about the consequences of factory employment on motherhood in this period were not new. As with other areas of occupationally related ill-health, there were continuities in the way problems were framed within medical and public health circles. In the 1830s and 1840s concern had been expressed that factory employment had a detrimental effect on domestic life and that infant care, alongside other responsibilities for their families, would suffer if women engaged in it.[5] Specific references to rates of infant mortality arose later, particularly because of developments in vital registration statistics. In the 1850s and 1860s, medical officers of health, and in particular those working under John Simon at the Privy Council and Simon himself, gave increasing emphasis to a possible relationship between the factory employment of mothers and high infant mortality. In the *Fourth Report* (1862) Simon argued that different infant death rates:

> are attributed to the varying prevalence of two local causes: first, to differences of degree in common sanitary defects of residence; and secondly, to occupational differences among the inhabitants.[6]

As with others who would take up this latter line of reasoning it was where 'women were greatly engaged in branches of industry away from home' that the consequences were 'the home was ill-kept, children ill looked after, being improperly fed and quietened by the use of opiates'. In his *Sixth Report* Simon concluded 'infants perish under the neglect and mismanagement that their mother's employment implies'.[7] It is evident from Simon's own reports that the relationship of mother's work to infant deaths was not because that work damaged her own health, or directly that of her child, but that it led to a dereliction of her duty to care. Greenhow, a colleague of Simon's at the Privy Council, reported that:

> on going to Sheffield we saw a haggard infant and asked what was the matter with it. A woman gave it a glance and said 't mother works', a disease with which I was sufficiently familiar, but for which the name was new.[8]

Disease metaphors were then, as now, powerful tools for representing perceived threats to the social order.[9] At the same time as considerable emphasis was given to the failure of factory mothers to adequately care for their infants, others contended that poor living conditions, inadequate sanitation, lack of food and other problems associated with material deprivation and the environment were implicated. Attempts to establish an evidential basis for particular causal relationships, were pursued with increasing vigour as the high rates of infant deaths continued.[10] By the late-nineteenth century the same factors remained in contention.

Dyhouse[11] suggests that by this time there were two factors around which there was some consensus: the consequences of high-density urban living and the associated problems of sewage disposal and artificial feeding, especially as safer supplies of milk became available. However, the differences in infant mortality rates between urban areas served to override what consensus there was and lent support to those factors which were still contested, such as environmental factors and the importance of maternal employment and the adequacy of working-class mothering, whether employed or not.

The medical profession assumed a high profile in these debates, both within the profession more generally as represented by the British Medical Association (BMA) and locally based medical officers of health, as well as those practitioners who held State office.[12] Many actively pursued the possibility of regulating the work of mothers. There was disagreement between practitioners, however, just as there was in the social and political domain over the possible 'causes' of infant deaths.

One early prominent figure in the 1890s was George Reid, a medical officer of health (MOH) in Staffordshire, who also undertook some of the enquiries on the impact of lead on women workers (see Chapters 2 and 6). In 1892 he read a paper at the annual meeting of the BMA in which he argued there were observable differences between the South Staffordshire mining towns with their relatively low infant-mortality ratio (IMR) and low employment of mothers and the towns of the Potteries with high IMR and employment of mothers. He further classified towns in terms of 'many women engaged in factory work'; those with 'fewer women engaged in factory work' and those with 'practically none'. He argued the difference between the rates of the first two and the third accounted for the annual loss of 300 infants. Further enquiry undertaken by the public medicine section of the BMA on a national basis confirmed that 'the practice of married women working did have an injurious influence on the lives of their children' although the differences were less pronounced over England as a whole.[13] However, the evidence was sufficient for the BMA to push for further regulation. A paper by Dr Jones to the Royal Statistical Society citing Dr Reid's work in support, concluded that there was an association between the employment of women and infant deaths.[14] But such assertions and the evidence for them did not go unchallenged.

In 1894 the BMA sent a deputation to the Home Department to 'bring notice that excessive infant mortality was due to the employment of married women in factories'. Dr Reid, a member of this deputation, continued his argument that infant mortality was linked to differential proportions of married women working. He also related this to artificial- as opposed to breast-feeding. Asquith, the Home Secretary, concluded:

> At the same time gentlemen I cannot say that it is as yet established to my satisfaction as a scientific conclusion that the increase in infant mortality which has undoubtedly taken place and is taking place . . . [that] the chief cause is the increase in the employment of women in factories early after the period of childbirth.[15]

The BMA were demanding that the regulation introduced in 1892 requiring women to take a compulsory period of four weeks' leave after childbirth should be extended, although it had largely proved unenforceable and ineffective. This was also contrary to some of its own members' concerns about the possible harmful consequences of depriving women of the material resources of paid employment. While Asquith responded that their views would 'receive careful and respectful consideration' he pointed out that employers, inspectors and female operatives had concerns about legislating for any longer period. The minutes of the meeting also reveal that the Home Secretary was at pains to reinforce the accepted view that 'we may see the time when the employment of women in factories will be entirely discontinued'.[16]

The acceptance of this ideal of the non-working married woman was evident elsewhere, even by those who doubted the quality of the data and the conclusions drawn from it. Among the women who disputed the Reid and Jones papers was Clara Collet. Following her period with the Royal Commission on Labour, she carried out a number of investigations on statistical questions connected with female labour.[17] She considered their evidence to be imprecise and impressionistic – 'bad science'. The proportion of middle-class households in towns and cities, she argued, had obscured the relationship. The relative rates of maternal working and infant deaths in relatively homogeneous working-class communities she concluded, demonstrated no particular pattern. Dyhouse[18] claimed that Collet was not interested in the question as part of any feminist agenda, as she also believed that maternal employment was 'inadvisable'. Similar contentions were made in relation to the crisis over the 'national health', when other women with a more explicit feminist agenda were among the debaters.[19] Like Collet, however, few fundamentally eschewed the ideal of the undesirability of women 'having to work' although seeking their right to do so. I return to the issue of feminist attitudes to the family in Chapter 8.

There were sections of the medical profession who refused to recognize the economic basis for married women's work. This was evident in their belief that extending post-confinement leave to three months would not be 'a great hardship'. In addition to maternity leave they advocated legislation to enable local authorities to set up crèches in those districts where working mothers were 'common practice'. This suggests they believed that although women did not necessarily require the economic returns from work, they would probably continue to work nevertheless. In these terms:

> it is surely not unreasonable to expect mothers who disregard maternal responsibilities in order to supplement the already in many instances, ample earnings of their husbands, by engaging in work away from home, should part with a portion of the money they receive to provide for their proper care which their children are thus deprived of.[20]

There were difficulties around proposals for the provision of crèches. On the one hand these could be seen to make it 'easier' for women to work and would thus defeat the object of ensuring that ideally mothers should provide infant and child care themselves. Advocates, early in the next century, emphasized that crèches should not be seen as a 'service' to working mothers. Some observations were made that one result was also that women could be seen rushing to factories with their children half-dressed.[21] On the other hand it seems that crèches would not have been a popular choice in any case for many working-class women. They were perceived to be a kind of 'institution' and institutions carried stigma. There were already in existence established patterns and preferences for local family or neighbourhood patterns of childcare.[22] While their quality no doubt varied, especially in terms of the environment, we certainly need to treat middle-class assumptions about such care critically.[23] Contemporary commentators themselves noted the differences in breast-feeding patterns among women workers. In Preston, for example, factory workers nursed their babies at mealtimes and before and after work at the mills.[24] Hilda Martindale pointed to local values in the potteries which emphasized a woman's responsibility to contribute to the family income and 'that men and boys appear to willingly do their part in the domestic work of the house'.[25]

The debates about working mothers and infant mortality continued both inside and outside the medical profession. By the early-1900s the evidence of infant mortality and the poor health that recruitment for the Boer War revealed led to a perceived crisis in the state of the national health. New discourses fuelled fears about the possibility of physical deterioration and national degeneration. Particularly important in this respect was Social Darwinism and its associated 'science' of eugenics, with concerns that the high birth rate among the physically weaker working-classes would lead to an increasing pool of unfit individuals.[26] The Inter-Departmental Committee on Physical Deterioration (1903–4) was set up to investigate the 'reality' and possible explanations for poor health. High infant-mortality rates were inevitably a major topic of concern for the Committee. Witnesses to the Committee continued to stress 'married women's labour is the root of all mischief'.[27] Women inspectors also noted a 'striking degree and amount of ignorance especially of feeding and cleanliness'. They drew attention to the stresses and strains of general life and the conditions of industrial work, which left little energy for the family washing and house-cleaning that had to be done on a late Saturday afternoon. As a result 'dirt and discomfort abounded'.[28]

Women factory inspectors considered that not only was the case against maternal employment not proven, but their own experience led them to conclude that factory work might also bring some benefits to women's health, especially those of the poorer classes, as long as they worked in hygienic surroundings and for limited hours. In her evidence to the Inter-Departmental Committee, Adelaide Anderson observed 'that despite some improvements in the conditions in factories there had not been a similar improvement in the physical condition of women, which suggested the external conditions outside factory life might be responsible'.[29] The weight of her evidence was against the view that 'factories in themselves did harm'[30] except for specific injuries. Hilda Martindale found it was hardly surprising that women prefered factory life, given the lack of healthy recreations and amusements and the prevailing squalor and gloom of the towns. Girls would need to be taught, she argued, 'to find pleasure in domestic work'.[31]

The Inter-Departmental Committee took up the question of extending the four-week post-confinement leave, as agitation continued. The problem was, as Adelaide Anderson told the Committee, the wording of the legislation. It included the phrase 'shall knowingly' which led to general evasion and failure of prosecution because in these terms it was difficult to prove that employers had full knowledge of the facts.[32] She noted that no case had been brought for six years. Inspectors also appreciated that the women themselves evaded the legal restriction by shifting the date of the birth or by seeking work elsewhere. As another inspector reported, women in Dundee who had returned early 'asked helplessly "what could they do?"'[33] The Chief Medical Inspector of Factories told the Committee that he opposed any extension of the four-week period because he 'did not see how they are to be supported'.[34]

In her retrospective account of the women's inspectorate, Anderson credits women inspectors with raising questions about some form of State support for maternity.[35] There was, she argued:

> no notion (publicly expressed) that national responsibility for the release
> of the child-bearing woman from wage paid employment should be recog-
> nised by some form of maintenance at the time of their greatest need.[36]

Despite the plethora of opinions and evidence, which the Committee agreed was inconclusive, and a certain sympathy with the view that women's social and economic position should be considered alongside the question of employment, the Report concluded that it 'was in no doubt that the employment of mothers in factories is attended by evil consequences both to themselves and their children'.[37] Equally legislative prohibition of work would cause practical difficulties. It would have consequences for those unmarried mothers for whom work currently saved from degradation, as well as the high proportion of women in some districts who were the breadwinners. Hilda Martindale's evidence from one such investigation in the Potteries showed that of 62 women sampled, only 24 had husbands in regular work and of these, 14 brought in insufficient income. The remaining group included women with husbands in irregular work or out-of-work, or in poor health, and those deserted and widowed.[38]

Following the Report of the Inter-departmental Committee, the first National Conference on Infant Mortality was held in 1906. In his address, the President, John Burns, laid most of the blame on mothers, but there was only one paper specifically on women's employment.[39] The Home Office initiated further enquiry through its medical officers of health in industrial centres. Direction was given in terms of whether extension to the period of post-confinement leave was necessary and also 'whether such restrictions might a) lead to a further fall in the birthrate or b) through increasing poverty in homes previously dependent on maternal income, actually diminish the chances of infant survival'. However, this enquiry did not result in any collation of national information, nor were there any further considerations on national policy initiatives.

Thus in the period up to the First World War, competing claims around possible environmental causes and whether the factory work of women was implicated in infant mortality continued. There was also evidence of a concerted attack on working-class mothers, whether or not they worked, which focused on their knowledge and infant-care practices. These arguments were most clearly made by Sir George Newman. He emphasized that high infant mortality did 'denote a prevalence of those causes and conditions which in the long run, bring about the degeneration of race'.[40] It was an 'index of *social* evil' (his emphasis) and although he acknowledged antenatal influences such as infections and prematurity, it rested 'most of all upon the absence of the mother from the home'.[41]

> The deaths of infants is not a problem of sanitation alone, or housing, or even of poverty as such, but it is mainly a question of motherhood.[42]

Simon's accusations levelled at factory mothers in the 1860s were still evidently part of early twentieth-century perceptions. They formed an important basis for both voluntary and official interventions in the development of infant welfare. Many of these initiatives[43] pursued improvements in infant-feeding and care through forms of home-visiting and education. Thus they constituted what Donzelot has called 'the policing of families'.[44]

The developing science of social statistics, which itself owed much to its direct links with public-health activists,[45] was constrained by 'official' limitations in collection and classification, but this did not prevent officials from entering into the infant-mortality debates. Both Sir George Newman at the Board of Education and Arthur Newsholme at the Local Government Board ignored 'alternative' sources of evidence, although they were in general careful statisticians.[46] As a result, despite differences between them on the relative importance they put on aspects of motherhood, it confirmed the importance of pursuing this line of investigation and intervention. Women activists continued to be concerned about the quality of data. In her evidence to the Inter-Departmental Committee[47] Adelaide Anderson laid great emphasis on the inadequacy of the statistical evidence. The Committee took these criticisms seriously. They included the absence of localized infant-mortality rates, especially in industrial towns, a general infant-mortality ratio for individuals nationally and the occupation of all mothers to be shown on the Registrar General's records. (It was nearly 100 years before women's own occupation was recorded on their death certificates.) Barbara Hutchins accepted that 'industrial employment was in some degree responsible for high infant mortality', but she also pointed to the lack of conclusive evidence.[48] Diarrhoeal deaths which were often linked to improper feeding as a result of a mother's employment were far fewer than those caused by respiratory disease.

Discussion following the presentation of her paper to the Royal Statistical Society in 1909 revealed that statistical evidence and its interpretation were as contentious as they had been 10 years earlier. Furthermore, the use of infant mortality rates as an indicator of health ultimately obscured the importance of viable infant lives and the overall improvements in survival of about 8 per cent between 1901 and 1911 – although by this time the gap between countryside and town and between the classes had widened considerably.[49] Indeed, it is argued that historians and demographers have missed the significant contribution which the decline in infant deaths made to reductions in overall mortality.[50]

If neither the science of statistics nor the clinical knowledge of medicine could resolve the problem of causation, it was not surprising that the discourse on infant mortality remained essentially within the social domain. In these terms some kind of consensus could emerge. By the early-twentieth century, Armstrong argues,[51] infant mortality provided an analytical framework that enabled a particular discursive articulation of social well-being linked to infant mortality rates to emerge. In this way mothering and domestic life acquired a new status within the public domain and in turn would be subject to increasing surveillance.

The debates about infant mortality thus rested on available and widely accepted ideas about the morality of women's work in factories, in particular wives and mothers. A 'scientific' discourse failed to establish countervailing evidence that would challenge the increasing strength of what Davin[52] has called the 'ideology of motherhood'. These new meanings of motherhood and a 'separate infant life'[53] were also constitutive of what could be considered as evidence.

As with other aspects of maternal and reproductive health in the period up to the First World War, there was little recognition that the health of infants might have something to do with the health of their mothers and not just the fact that they worked or had inadequate 'mothering skills'. This was spotted by women activists. Countering arguments that women were 'poor managers', Anna Martin exclaimed:

> it was easier to attack the problem of infant mortality by founding Babies Institutes, and by endeavouring to screw up to a still higher level the self-sacrifice and devotion of the normal working-class woman, than to incur the wrath of vested interests by insisting on healthy conditions for mothers and infants alike.[54]

These opportunities could also be seized on to oppose legislative interference and reiterate suffragist demands. Those who sought to prohibit women from work would 'leave untouched the causes which drive them onto the labour market (and) seems to them about as wise as proceeding to cure a broken leg by removing the splints'.[55] Other less-militant women investigators had noted the 'incapacity of a mother to deal with her existence however she may struggle' mainly because of her own failing health, because of poor diet and unhealthy surroundings.[56] One detailed study of Birmingham women concluded that there was little discrepancy in the homes of women who did or did not work; evidence, according to the authors, 'shows how many women keep up the intense apathetic drudgery entailed by doing two kinds of work'.[57] In the introduction to *Maternity*, the letters collected by the Women's Cooperative Guild, Margaret Lewellyn Davies argued:

> Writers on infant mortality and the decline of the birth-rate never tire of justly pointing to the evils which come from the strain of manual labour in factories for expectant mothers. Very little is ever said about the same evils which come from the incessant drudgery of domestic labour. People forget that the unpaid work of the working-woman at the stove, at scrubbing and cleaning, at the washtub, in lifting and carrying heavy weights, is just as severe manual labour as many industrial operations in factories.

She went on to point out that this work will be carried out until the day the child is born.[58]

As Davin argues, it was a case of where the ideology and rhetoric of motherhood obscured poverty and maternal ill-health. 'It was easier to blame them and to organise a few classes than to expand social and medical services, and it avoided the political problem of provoking rate and tax payers.'[59] It was the cultivation of the maternal instinct rather than the health of mothers that was central to developing policy and intervention. As in other areas of developing State intervention, there were practical as well as political constraints that necessitated targeting the 'failures' of individuals rather than a restructuring of the economic and social order.

Lead and Reproductive Damage

In Chapter 2 I argued that the idea of female susceptibility to lead-poisoning had been important in the way in which the 'dangerous trades' were viewed as posing particular problems for women workers. Poisoning attack rates showed disproportionate rates of female sufferers overall and some medical practitioners were also of the view that women suffered more severely. Thomas Oliver, for example, argued 'that females contract lead poisoning more readily, the symptoms are usually more acute, they suffer more severely and they succumb to it more quickly . . .'[60] A second view of female susceptibility was a sufficient, but not necessary, precondition for overall female susceptibility; the belief that lead exercised a pernicious affect on women's reproductive biology. In this case lead resulted in disordered menstruation, both excessive and amenorrhoea, and impinged on fertility, as well as causing miscarriages and stillbirths. It was thought to be implicated in high infant-mortality and in the deaths of infants from convulsions. Reproductive biology was a possible 'cause' of high attack rates overall, and there were consequences for reproductive health in particular of exposure to lead.

The possible effects of lead on women's reproductive system brought to the fore the issue of whether the prosecution of State regulation with respect to women would include *all* women or whether it should be married women in particular. Here the essentially biological arguments about the threat of lead work became confused with the social arguments about the responsibilities of motherhood and the causes of high infant-mortality. If women's biological characteristics made them vulnerable then, logically, all women were at risk, yet the most vociferous demands were for the exclusion of married women. If lead impinged on women's reproductive systems, then it would probably do so from puberty. So there would be little difference in terms of the potential for damage between the employment of a young girl or a woman. These dimensions were debated at the time, but 'women' and 'mothers' were terms that were conflated or used interchangeably.

In the 1899 *Thorpe/Oliver Report* into the Potteries, the authors expressed the view that:

the medical history of the pottery industry led us, in the interests of women themselves, and to avoid the disasters which plumbism entails upon the progeny of the mother, to urge that women should no longer be employed in the dipping house and as ware cleaners.[61]

Lead, they concluded, exercised a 'pernicious influence upon her reproductive functions', based on their observations that time after time for women in the Potteries 'maternity was all but an impossibility, for pregnancy after pregnancy ended in abortion or the child was born dead or died soon after birth'.[62]

By the time the 1910 Committee of Inquiry into the Potteries had reported,[63] the case for female susceptibility in general and the possibility of reproductive damage had been set. Women workers were questioned about their menstrual cycles in the context of other possible symptoms of lead-poisoning. This discussion was conducted with some 'delicacy'. Euphemisms for 'periods' were commonly used and the evidence indicated that both excess flow and lower-than-normal flows, as well as irregularity, were possible signs of disorder. Mary Fellows was asked 'I understand that at your time for *being unwell* you still lose far too much, do you not?' and she indicated that it was more than usual. Mary Woodall was asked whether 'her female life was quite regular'; Sarah Cooper whether 'she lost a good deal when (she) was unwell' and Mary Ann Ford if she 'was quite regular at her monthly times'.[64] Women's replies to these questions did not help to settle the question: while some reported their periods were not normal, others indicated they had experienced no change in them whatsoever.

Inevitably the controversy surrounding the issue of maternal disorders also surfaced in the 1910 enquiry, since there were still strong calls for prohibition or further restrictions on women's employment. One member of the Committee was Dr Reid, the MOH for Staffordshire who, as the discussion of infant-mortality revealed, was concerned with the consequences of work on maternity. He had conducted an enquiry following the 1907 Home Office circular. This had been sent to all MOH's in industrial districts to 'ascertain whether the employment of women in factories and workshops has effect prejudicial to either mothers or children'. Comparing mothers who had worked in the lead industry before marriage, and those who worked in there after marriage with the wives of artisans, he concluded that there was an excess of miscarriges in lead workers of three times and four times respectively. However, he argued it seemed to have no effect on fertility or on infant health.

In view of this 'alarming tendency to miscarry' and the paucity of data,[65] the Committee asked Reid to conduct a second study among mothers currently working with lead. This produced a different conclusion: almost an indication that lead work might protect against miscarriage. Sensibly, it was concluded that little reliance could be placed on this investigation, as Dr Reid himself was also to conclude that women probably underestimated the number of miscarriages they had, knowing that the purpose of the enquiry might affect their employment opportunities.[66]

Local practitioners did not help in reaching a consensus. Mr G.P. Johnson had enquired into 300 infant deaths and 'could not decide if the lead work of the mother or father had anything to do with it'.[67] Mr Dawes, the MOH for Longton, noted that lead-poisoning had diminished but infant mortality had not.[68] Mr Moody, a physician and surgeon from Hanley, thought both married and unmarried women should be excluded because 'An unmarried women's health is of great value to her, even apart from the question of the reproduction of the race.'[69] Mr Faulds, a surgeon, favoured exclusion, but it might 'cut the other way. If you cut down the living of a family you get dirt and poverty.'[70]

As with the general debates about infant mortality and the employment of mothers, the specific issue of possible reproductive damage reiterated arguments as the proposed remedy in both cases was the same: to exclude women from work. It was not only medical witnesses to the committee who favoured exclusion and they thought there were practical difficulties and external circumstances to be considered. This view was also held by some members of the women's factory inspectorate.[71] Adelaide Anderson argued:

> It is clear, if administratively possible, that it would be right on public grounds, apart from the welfare of women themselves, to exclude mothers from lead processes during pregnancy and the nursing of their infants, but there is a practical difficulty of achieving this by legal prohibition . . . the absolute prohibition of so large a number of adult workers cannot now be considered apart from their own wishes.[72]

It was perhaps not surprising that the Committee was cautious in its approach. They argued that existing precautions provided within regulation might reduce the liability of miscarriage and that the statistical evidence to support such action as exclusion was too limited. They concluded that seeing how grave the miscarriage rate was in women who had worked before marriage 'the exclusion of married women would not itself serve as an effectual preventive'.[73]

The Chief Medical Inspector told the Committee he thought lead did cause miscarriage. Dr Prendergast pointed to women with a tendency to miscarry whether they worked in lead or not: it might aggravate the possibility.[74] In some respects it was understandable that this particular result of lead work could be more readily accepted. Lead was commonly used as a abortifacient and there seems to have been a common perception of its qualities. But this also raises another difficulty for establishing the validity or extent of the possible risks of lead work. High rates of miscarriage were in any case commonplace for working-class women. In the 'Maternity Letters' collected by the Women's Cooperative Guild,[75] maternal or pregnancy biographies similar to those presented in the context of factory work were commonplace. Given that abortion was the principle means of family limitation among working-class families[76] and there were particular reasons why working women might pursue this line of action, it might be difficult to argue that the incidence of miscarriage and indeed stillbirths and infant deaths in factory women, including lead workers, were a direct result of the work itself. McLaren[77] has argued that increasing middle-class opposition to abortion utilized factory work as the 'immoral' root of the abortion problem.

There was a perception of reproductive damage from lead beyond that of the 'experts' – medical practitioners and factory inspectors. Male workers also expressed such beliefs. Union officials and organizers in the Potteries were in favour of restriction in the form of prohibiting women from working in lead processes. They drew heavily on the threats to women's health in doing so. Representatives from the National Amalgamated Society of Male and Female Pottery Workers observed that women had stillborn children 'because they worked up to their confinement': they supported the idea of greater female susceptibility. 'They are not so likely to be able to withstand the inroads that lead makes on them', was couched in terms of children who suffer because their mothers worked in lead.[78] There were contradictions in male unionists' positions, however, as they did not think women should be prohibited from the 'decorative processes which seem to be more suitable for women',[79] yet these involved exposure to lead. They claimed that their interest in restricting women was only motivated by health and that their objection would be removed if safe glazes were available. Yet Mr C. argued:

> they ought not to work in a lead process. I think that their husbands should support them without that. If he studies the health of his wife at all, I should think a man would grieve very much to see his wife doing such work.[80]

Recognizing that women did sometimes provide the sole support for a household by their lead work, he recommended that married women with husbands should be prevented, then single girls and widows not at all. In this context, the health of women was not essentially the issue; it was the position of men as the 'breadwinners' and the protection of an established gendered division of labour within the Potteries and the family.

Not all medical opinion considered that it was only damage to reproduction in women that occurred from lead work. From the evidence given at an earlier enquiry there were one or two examples of medical practitioners who raised the possibility that it might also have an effect on men,[81] or expressed the opinion that there was no difference in 'susceptibility'. Susceptibility remained closely linked to reproduction all the same. One medical witness argued that periods actually functioned to get rid of lead from women's bodies. Another said that the offspring of fathers who worked in lead were more likely to have epilepsy.[82]

It was not surprising that in 1893 such arguments were ignored, as this Committee was less concerned with the reproductive issue even though the question of female susceptibility itself was pursued to some extent. But the question of effects on male reproduction continued to be raised. The *British Medical Journal*, commenting on lead-poisoning in the Potteries in 1898, thought a lowered birth-rate among lead workers was common 'even if the father alone worked in lead'. In the 1910 Report, Mr Moody presented the case of one of his caretakers who had worked in lead for many years while his three wives had not, yet out of 22 children only one had lived. While he favoured the exclusion of women, he considered there might be a contribution by men.[83] Thomas Oliver,[84] in his text on lead-poisoning, pointed out that other researchers had raised the possibility that the influence on the progeny of men in lead might be greater than on the expectant mother. This was contrary to his experience, he argued, but lead 'was a racial poison; it destroys the foetus in utero directly or it cuts short its stay in the womb by its action upon uterine muscular fibres'.[85] Oliver strongly believed that the menstrual cycle and women's reproductive organs were connected to women's predisposition to poisoning and hence had consequences for pregnancy. He would probably not have been swayed by research or arguments about toxicity in relation to men.[86] In any case, to have accepted such a possibility would have raised serious practical problems for a preventive strategy that was recommending that it should only be men who worked in some processes and the non-acceptability of interference in men's work.

'Sweated' Work and the Home as a Place of Paid Work

Before the late-nineteenth century there had been a long tradition of domestically based industry in Britain. In some areas of manufacture or production of raw materials, the transfer of domestic productive relations persisted in new factory-based production, notably cotton manufacture.[87] Other forms of hand production occurred in domestic workshops often adjacent to dwellings, such as nail- and chain-making, file-cutting and laundries.[88] In general, whether or not the home constituted the workshop, it was usually only members of the family who were employed in them. However, by the end of the nineteenth century home-based production came to be seen as typical of 'sweated work', characterized by low wages, long hours and very poor working conditions. As such, in this period, there was an increasing association of 'homework' with 'sweated work'.[89] There were evidently 'sweated' conditions to be found in some factories and workshops and it also encompassed forms of 'outwork' which included women whose working day consisted of both factory-based employment and work which they brought home to complete.

> Sometimes a woman is found who works in a factory during the day, cards buttons and hooks and eyes before and after going to the factory, and in addition attends to her house and children as best she may. One such woman's working day was from three or four in the morning to eleven or twelve at night.[90]

Estimating the number of women who might have been engaged in such work is difficult for several reasons: the sometimes casual nature of the employment; the lack of registration at all or only in specific cases and, especially before 1901, the failure to comply with such requirements; the problems of categorization within local authority and census returns;[91] and the hiddenness of homework when it was associated with other full-time employment. In the *Annual Report of the Factory Department for 1901*, when outworkers were required to be registered by employers for the UK as a whole, there were 2370 lists accounting for 50 549 outworkers, of which 21 642 were in London. This would have been a small proportion of all homeworkers.

Whether or not 'sweated' work was confined to outwork, or whether 'sweating' was a result or an effect of the changing nature of late nineteenth-century capitalism and associated with particular characteristics of certain funds of work or a central structural feature was a matter of discussion and dispute at the time and has continued to be so in later analyses. Feltes, for example, has argued that the difficulties of defining sweating, most evidently seen in the context of the House of Lords Select Committee Inquiry – and the production of its Report in 1890 – revealed the extent to which the contested meaning itself 'marked an important moment in the ideological history of capital'.[92] He suggests that historians have tended to accept a dominant view that emphasized characteristics (such as long hours, low wages and insanitary conditions) to the exclusion of a consideration of 'sweating' as a 'system', an endemic and central feature of a particular form of economic organization.

In this context the problem of 'sweated work' became closely aligned to attacks not only on the organization and results of late nineteenth-century capitalism, but also more particularly with forms of industrial work associated with women's labour as outworkers or homeworkers. Recent analysts of the causes of 'sweated' production emphasize different aspects of late nineteenth-century industrial development and how these impinged on homework. Some consider 'sweating' to have been a kind of 'residuum'[93] of earlier industrial production. Others have considered it a direct outcome of industrial expansion. Schmeichen,[94] for example, placed considerable emphasis on industrial growth and development and its association with technological development. That encouraged an increasing subdivision of labour, the dilution of skills and therefore the possibility of very low-paid, unskilled work. Jenny Morris agreed that these features of the industrial system were important but that the availability of female labour was essential. According to Morris the subdivision of labour occurred along gender lines: women provided a necessary pool of unorganized, unskilled labour who could also be paid below subsistence wages.[95] Moreover, she argues, this had the result of forcing down wages generally.

In addition to the dilution of skills associated with the employment of women in the contracting-out system, there was also evidence that some of these trades were subject to fluctuations of demand for the product and, therefore, for labour. Seasonality created a demand for employment through resultant poverty, enabling employers to utilize a mainly female secondary labour market as required.[96] Thus, although there was an association between persistent poverty and 'sweated' labour, there was a difference between the late nineteenth-century phenomena and the large pool of male casual labour that characterized the mid-to-late nineteenth century.[97] Reports of conditions among the poor, particularly in London,[98] were still important, however, to agitation around 'sweating', but the focus was increasingly on the fact that the majority of 'sweated' workers were women.

Tailoring, which is often held to exemplify a 'sweated trade', consisted of a mixture of mechanized and hand processes. In large cities, especially, where rents were high and larger and larger teams of workers were needed, systems of contracting out and sub-contracting developed. This led to a more complex division of labour with individual workers allocated particular tasks. Thus, in order to avoid any expansion of factory or workshop-based production, some systems of contracting and sub-contracting took the form of homework. Miss Vines describes a typical homeworker in the industry who worked on 'finishing trousers': 'She had to supply her own trimmings, thread, cotton, soap and heat (for irons). She was paid 2s $\frac{1}{2}$d for each pair which took her two hours, and a further half hour per day was spent in collecting and delivering work.'[99] Morris describes the London tailoring trade at the turn of the century as an 'anarchy of competition' encouraged by easy entry into production of small units, high rents and the seasonal nature of demand, all of which mitigated against investment.[100] Many contemporary commentators also saw the continued existence of 'sweated' labour' as a direct result of capitalist interests in profit, secured by saving on capital investment and costs at the expense of humane working conditions. Fabian socialists, in particular, saw a considerable similarity between the reasons employers' opposed factory legislation and their use of home-work to extend production.[101]

As in other areas of 'sweated' industry, in tailoring there were accusations that foreign immigration was responsible for sweating. Enquiries had noted, for example, that employment conditions in many foreign-owned businesses (this largely referred to Jewish-owned firms) were particularly bad and also that cheap foreign labour was 'flooding' some trades, a convenient use of racism to avoid acceptance of 'sweat-ing' as widespread through out the industry generally.[102] As a result there were calls for immigration controls in the 1890s,[103] although this aspect of agitation was less evident in the early twentieth-century demands for reform.

Despite the considerable problems that were evident in the production of a consensus from the enquiry of the House of Lords Select Committee (1890), it was probably right to give emphasis to the wages paid to homeworkers as a primary characteristic of 'sweating' and for this to dominate not only subsequent analyses but also proposed remedies. Levels of pay provided clear evidence that everyone could see. Examples abounded in reports of what were evidently below-subsistence wages and the amount of work needed to earn them. Cadbury and Shann high-lighted the continuing problem by using Seebohn Rowntree's standard of the min-imum weekly expenditure required for an average family man, wife and children to have the bare necessities: 21s 8d a week.[104] Women working at carding hooks and eyes were paid 9d to 1s 4d per pack (i.e. two dozen gross of completed cards). Each card required stitching 384 hooks and eyes together and out of the 9d they also provided their own cotton and needles. In this 'scandalous trade', they pointed out, it would take two women working together to make 3s a week each.[105] Clementina Black reports on a:

> most worn out girl I remember ever to have seen . . . She may have been eighteen or nineteen; she was absolutely colourless, and although there was no sign about her of any specific illness, seemed exhausted literally almost to death! She sat day after day pouring powdered cocoa into ready made paper packets which she then folded down the tops and pasted on

the wrappers. She received a halfpenny for every gross. In the week previous . . . she earned 7s. Each shilling represented 24 gross of packets: she had therefore filled, folded and pasted in the week 188 gross or 21 792 packets.[106]

Low wages led to excessive hours of work and contributed to poor working conditions because of the nature of the work that could be undertaken in the home or domestic workshop. Low wages were not directly responsible for the unsanitary state of most domestic working conditions, as most working-class homes in any case were already typically overcrowded, unventilated and inadequately heated and lit.[107] But low wages and carrying out work in the home would have exacerbated the conditions in many cases. Another investigator emphasized the 'strain and wear and tear of working in a crowded space, in the midst of cross tiresome children, leaving off constantly to mind a fretful baby', as well as the time lost in fetching and carrying work and standing for two to three hours to get it examined.[108] As far as unsanitary and poor working conditions were concerned there seemed to have been more interest in the possible threats these posed to the consumers of the products than in the dangers to the workers who made them. A 'public health' dimension identified by the outbreaks of scarlet fever, small pox and typhus linked to such conditions led to some medical interest in 'sweating' in the late 1880s. One such outbreak in Leeds was investigated in 1888 by *The Lancet*. It confirmed the existence of conditions of 'sweating', called for an enquiry and demanded that homework and domestic workshops should come within factory law. The dangers were real enough, as the trade-union activist Mary MacArthur discovered when she caught diphtheria from a woman lacemaker.[109]

Following the Inquiry by the House of Lords Select Committee and the Report, which bypassed the whole question of the conditions and relations of production, denying that there was 'a system of manufacturing which produces misery', remedy was seen to lie in alleviating miserable conditions.[110] In the event any legislative regulation was minimal, with only limited interventions under the Public Health Acts. A minority report of the House of Lords Select Committee had advocated the prohibition of homework outside the umbrella of factory legislation but this was not implemented. This was not surprising given that, as far as factory legislation was concerned, there had always been a distinction between factories and workshops on the basis of whether mechanical power was used. Workshops could also be distinguished from domestic workshops or homework, in that in the former, employer and employees engaged in manual labour on a similar basis to the factory. Yet even here, workshops which employed adult labour were in the main excluded from legislation[111] and in these circumstances it was clearly difficult to countenance the need to regulate domestic workshops.

The 1891 Act gave factory inspectors limited powers of access.[112] Although the Royal Commission of Labour excluded domestic workshops from their main recommendations, a minority report called for them to be under the same regulations as factories, supporting both Beatrice Potter's and Charles Booth's suggestion of making landlords liable for compliance. There was no further regulation until the

1895 Factories Act sought to prevent the evasion of hours-of-work legislation by prohibiting the sending of work home after the end of the day: a practice which had turned day-workers into night-shift homeworkers. However, this kind of outwork was distinct from a division of labour in which certain tasks were undertaken entirely by outworkers or by homeworkers.[113] For the proponents of legislation, the neglect of homework within the regulatory framework was detrimental in its own right. It also provided employers with a means of evading the restrictions of existing legislation. In this way, as some feminist activists argued,[114] it was probably the case that factory legislation itself contributed to a growth of homework and 'sweated' conditions.[115]

Given the widespread view that it was not desirable for women to enter the public domain of paid work, there were some supporters of homework for women on the grounds that if, as it seemed, it was economically necessary for them to have work, then it was preferable that they did this in the home. Homework, it was argued, did not expose women to the moral risks associated with performing hard physical labour in male company and it would let a woman care for her children while she worked. Those women activists who defended women's right to homework unfettered by legislative regulation had also argued this for other employments. But in this case it was particularly evident that a defence of such rights could utilize in support the discourse of separate spheres. As one exponent argued:

> Women with invalid or disabled husbands, widows with young children, women who are not strong enough for the long hours and exhausting conditions of factory life – are they to be deprived of the power of earning a livelihood at home? Is it not moreover probable that if a mother can be at home children will be better looked after than if she is absent all day?[116]

In reality there were problems with this conception, since the wages paid did little to ameliorate general impoverishment and to earn a meagre wage women worked so many hours that they were left with little time for domestic duties. The overwhelming concern of factory legislation throughout the nineteenth century had been with limiting children's employment in factories and workshops, it was in homework that child labour continued to flourish. Opponents of legislative regulation also considered it unthinkable for the State and its official representatives to intrude into the private domain of 'respectable women who practise honest industry' as one male factory inspector described it.[117]

The 'sanctity of the home' argument was also used by those who sought legislative reforms. They emphasized that the extremely low wages, the likely transmission of infectious diseases and the consequent neglect of children from the long hours of work were all detrimental to domestic life. Here again such arguments increasingly drew on the prominence of maternal neglect as a factor in the perceived 'deterioration' of the national health.[118] For those reformers who favoured legislation, it was once again the fact that it was women workers who bore the brunt of 'sweated' conditions that necessitated regulation. Feminist activists argued that this lack of legislation left the homeworker in the unskilled trades having to protect their own conditions, when they were the ones least able to do so.[119]

The interest of pro-legislative feminists in homework led to their involvement in drafting Bills for presentation to Parliament in 1899 and 1902 under the auspices of the Women's Industrial Council (WIC).[120] This followed an extensive investigation by the Council into the conditions of 400 homeworkers in London in 1897. The report singled out fur-pulling and matchbox-making as the 'most wretched forms of homework', an opinion that concurred with those of others who had witnessed these trades.[121] Out of 384 women workers the investigators ascertained that about one-third earned 1s a day or less, 127 between 1s and 1s 6d; 66 between 1s 6d and 2s and only 67 2s. However, the most 'striking fact' was that the highest pay was received by the wives of men in work and the lowest by those who most needed it. The report suggested this might be because of age, health and infirmity and thence the efficiency of the worker who was dependent on piece rates. Equally, they argued this evidence disputed the assertion that women's 'supplementary' earnings drove down male wages.[122]

The WIC Bill proposed that premises used for homework should be inspected and licensed as 'fit for work', although this raised the interesting possibility that if homes were not fit to work in they were probably not fit to live in either. The idea of licensing was not a new one: it had been advocated by the Royal Commission on Labour in 1893 and by women factory inspectors. The Bill also sought to give powers to factory as opposed to sanitary authorities, especially as the Council had been unhappy that workshops were viewed mainly as a local authority responsibility on the grounds that there was a potential conflict between rigorous enforcement and conflict with local ratepayers.[123]

Outside of women's organizations, however, little attention was paid to homework in the 1890s. The issue returned to prominence mainly as the result of an exhibition organized by the *Daily News* in 1906 to publicize sweated conditions, under the auspices of the Anti-Sweating League (ASL), the campaign which became one for 'the minimum wage'. Women's organizations and other middle-class labour reformers were in its forefront.[124] While it may seem logical that an attack on low pay was fundamental to any anti-sweating campaign, a distinct gender dimension underlined the political struggle for a minimum wage. Where there was a high proportion of young, unskilled women, employers assumed lower subsistence needs and thence paid the lowest possible wage. Any idea of homeworking wages as an additional supplement to that of a male breadwinner was far from the reality. However, male trade-union attitudes toward 'sweating' reflected their broader concern that women threatened wage levels in general. They sought measures to prohibit women from working or to restrict their employment altogether rather than reform this pattern of industrial production itself. Clementina Black had called for 'a living wage', recognizing that a minimum wage did not necessarily guarantee subsistence. The ASL rejected this because it might be too ambitious and lose them support.[125]

Social feminists remained divided over the proposed remedies for homeworking in the early decades of the twentieth century. WIC and its principal spokesperson Margaret MacDonald continued to argue for the licensing system. Clementina Black, who had taken a leading role earlier in WIC, now put her energies into the ASL; she was adamant that minimum-wage legislation was the answer. Margaret

Figure 3.1 *Sweated industries exhibition reproduced by permission of Mary Evans/ Fawcett Library.*

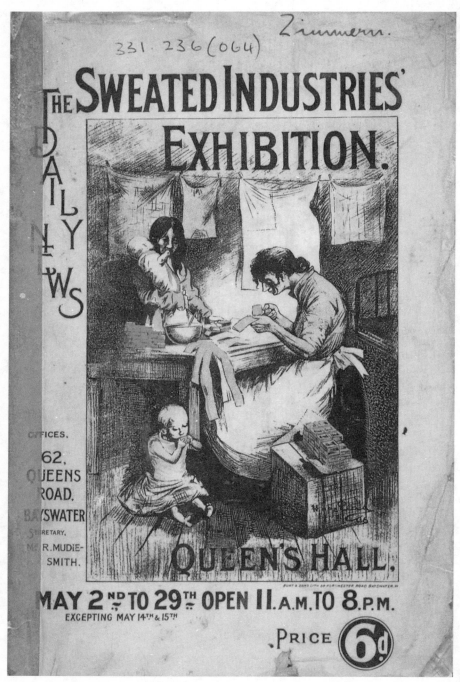

MacDonald's husband, J. Ramsay MacDonald, continued to present legislative proposals in the House of Commons which would introduce a system of licensing, although Margaret MacDonald admitted this would not touch the hours of labour.[126] Ideally, it seemed, both the Macdonalds would have preferred women not to work in the home at all. As with other pro-legislative activists at this time, they saw the State as having a duty to protect mothers on behalf of the wider community.

Views about the desirability of State intervention and what remedy it should recommend if it did intervene appeared again in the context of the further enquiry in 1906, the Select Committee on Homework (1907).[127] This considered and reported on conditions in trades in which homework was prevalent and the proposals to establish Trade Wages Boards and licensing as remedies. Two competing claims were presented by women activists to the Committee. Both marshalled the voices of some women homeworkers in support, their evidence reflecting the now-familiar differences of view about regulating women's work. Mary MacArthur of WTUL brought representatives whose evidence was heard both anonymously and as a group. Others were brought by representatives of the National Homeworking League, who opposed intervention and indeed the whole idea of homework as 'sweated' labour. It is difficult to assess the extent to which these women were typical homeworkers. Miss Vynne of the National Homeworking League admitted that her witnesses were all skilled, although 'not above the average': despite the fact 'they lost their heads in giving evidence', they generally gave a positive view of homework. In doing so they frequently contrasted homework with factory work, emphasizing the benefits to their health of the former. Mrs King of Clerkenwell, who had previously worked at flower-mounting in a factory, told the committee:

> I found my child neglected. When I had the second child I stayed at home and looked after it and had my work at home. I found an improvement in my health, in my home, in my children and in every way.[128]

Miss Bamford of Leicester echoed that she 'enjoyed better health since I have been at home and I have been at home for 15 years'.[129] Despite protestations to the contrary, the Committee asserted that two of the League's seven witnesses provided evidence of 'sweating' in the form of 'gross underpayment'. One of the WTUL witnesses, identified only as Mrs F., had worked in shirt-making for 16 years, earning on average 10s a week for a 15-hour day. She did not have time for household duties, her husband did them for her.[130] This group said that proper rates of pay should be made compulsory. The Committee itself would seem to have concurred:

> A very large number of people are unable to, or at any rate do not earn more than a mere pittance, and consequently live under conditions which are conducive to anything but social, material and moral well-being.[131]

Thus the demand for minimum-wage legislation, by setting rates for particular trades, can be seen as a response to the revival of interest in 'sweating'. The continued scandal of working conditions in homework was a direct result of the fact that women were the workers. Reform had, at this time, a broader social and political context which stemmed from the health of the physical and social body of the nation. Metaphors of disease were again evident in the campaigns to establish the Trade Boards. As Harold Tennant told the House of Commons on the occasion of the Bill's introduction, it was intended:

> to be applied exclusively to the exceptionally unhealthy patches of the body politic, where the development has been arrested in spite of growth in the rest of the organism. It is to the morbid diseased places – to the industrial diphtheria spots – that we should apply the antitoxins of the trade boards.[132]

According to Morris,[133] arguments that health and stability were threatened by 'sweated' work, work done by women who should not have been at work at all, contributed to an atmosphere that made intervention in the form of the 1909 Trade Boards Act possible. The primary motive was 'the harm that sweated trades were doing to the quality of labour' and thereby the existing social order. No society, Clementina Black argued, 'can be sound in health which has this undrained morass of wretchedness'.[134] Some improvements that would maintain existing class and gender relations would thus be in the interests of both employers and the State. Feminist activists agreed with other reformers that although waged work did not always have a detrimental effect on children and family life, it was desirable for married women not to work. Middle-class, male assumptions about women's primary domain of work were thus reinforced. The spectre of physical deterioration was never far away and it was difficult for women's opposition to prohibition and restriction in the working domain to escape from the debate about the social problems of infant mortality, motherhood and work. Less-than-subsistence wages, Gertrude Tuckwell argued, perpetuated a system:

> by which sickly anaemic workers are rearing a feebler generation, whose fight for work must be appreciably weaker, who soon swell the ranks of the unemployable and disappear into the abyss.[135]

Once again, however, legislation did not deliver what it promised. Following the Act, women workers, impatient at delays in establishing minimum rates, went on strike in several industries. Paradoxically, it had been the difficulty in organizing women to secure improvements by collective means which had provided the impetus for a legislative alternative, which in turn was a failure and led to a period of militancy and a growth in trade-union organization among women workers. Neither the Trade Boards nor strike action, however, would achieve any alteration in the inequalities of pay or in the acceptance of women's right to work.

Overwhelmingly, there was a construction of the problem of women's work in the industrial sector as having consequences either for the health of others, for whom they had primary responsibility, or for the physical and social health of wider society. It was not that women were not fit to enter paid work, it was that work was not fitting for them. A view of women's physical constitution as ill suited to the rigours of employment was but one example of where the idea of biological susceptibility in relation to reproductive functioning was utilized to deny women participation in the public domain.[136] As such, health itself had a constituting role in gendered social relations.

Notes

1 This was particularly evident in the continued high rates of maternal mortality, as well as the focus of growing intervention in infant welfare. For a fuller discussion of this see Harrison (1995b) 'Women's health', in Purvis (Ed.) *Women's History, Britain: 1850–1945*, Chapter 7.

2 This is indicated by the title of Newman's influential 1906 monograph, *Infant Mortality: A Social Problem*.

3 Wohl (1983) *Endangered Lives: Public Health in Victorian England*, calls his chapter on infant mortality in these terms.

4 See Woods, Watterson and Woodward (1988) *The Causes of Rapid Infant Mortality Decline in England and Wales, 1862–1921*.

5 See Mockett (1988) '"A danger to the State"'; and Gray (1991) 'Medical men, industrial labour and the State in Britain 1830–1850'.

6 *Fourth Report of the Medical Officer to the Privy Council* (1862) PP XXVII, 1863.

7 *Sixth Report of the Medical Officer of Health to the Privy Council* (1864) PP XXVIII, 1864. Appendix 14 addressed 'The excessive mortality of infants'.

8 Cited in Wohl *Endangered Lives* p.27.

9 See Sontag (1977) *Illness as Metaphor* and Sontag (1990) *AIDS and its Metaphors*. This relationship is evident in Verbrugge's analysis of women's health in relation to social change in nineteenth-century Boston: (1988) *Able-bodied Womanhood*.

10 These arguments are summarized in Smith (1979) *The People's Health*.

11 Dyhouse (1978) 'Working-class mothers and infant mortality 1895–1914' p.251.

12 In the 1890s George Reid was most prominent and into the twentieth century such views were promulgated, in particular by Sir George Newman as Chief Medical Officer to the Board of Education and by Arthur Newsholme, Medical Officer to the Local Government Board 1908–18.

13 PRO file HO45/9884/B16701.

14 Dyhouse (1978) p.252. For the full essay, see Jones (1894) 'The perils and protection of infant life', *Journal of the Royal Statistical Society* LVII, pp.1–98.

15 PRO file HO45/9884/B16701, transcription of the Deputation. Asquith's response is on p.34.

16 PRO file HO45/9884/B16701, pp.39–40.

17 These were largely carried out as part of her job as Labour Correspondent for the Board of Trade.

18 Dyhouse (1978) p.253.

19 Members of the Fabian Women's Group, such as Barbara Hutchins, also used their statistical expertise to challenge evidence about working women.

20 PRO/HO45/9884/B16701, Public Medicine Section of the Parliamentary Bills Committee of the BMA to the Home Department.

21 May Tennant makes this point against crèches in her chapter 'Infant mortality', in Oliver (Ed.) (1902) *The Dangerous Trades* pp.73–84.

22 Hewitt (1958) *Wives and Mothers in Victorian Industry* Chapter 9.

23 Dyhouse (1978) p.262.

24 Medical witnesses to the Committee on Physical Deterioration drew attention to such differences (1904) PP XXXII.

25 Cited in Anderson's *Memorandum on the Employment of Married Women, Report of the Select Committee on Physical Deterioration* (1904) PP XXXII, p.127.

26 See Porter (1991) '"Enemies of the race": biologism, environmentalism and public health in Edwardian England'; and in relation to infant mortality Davin (1978) 'Imperialism and motherhood'; Smith (1979) *The People's Health* pp.119–22; and Lewis (1980b) 'The social history of social policy'.

27 Garrett (1904) *Report of the Interdepartmental Committee on Physical Deterioration*, PP XXXII, p.53, *Minutes of Evidence*, 9015–65.

28 Anderson in her *Memorandum on The Effects of Employment on the Employment of Mothers in Factories and Workshops*, cites such evidence from other women inspectors to this effect. Ibid., See p.124. She also pointed out that practices varied widely.

29 Ibid., *Minutes of Evidence*, p.214, Minute 1464.

30 Ibid., p.217.

31 Ibid., *Report*, p.49.

32 Ibid., Appendix V, p.123.

33 Evidence from Miss Paterson cited in Anderson's *Memorandum*, Appendix 5, Ibid., p.124.

34 *Minutes of Evidence*, Dr Legge, Ibid., p.235.

35 There were already some calls for the endowment of motherhood in socialist and feminist circles elsewhere, although campaigns for a family allowance did not really begin until after the First World War.

36 Anderson (1922) *Women in the Factory* p.151.

37 *Report of the Interdepartmental Committee on Physical Detorioration*, PP XXXII, 1904, p.49.

38 Cited in Anderson's *Memorandum*, p.126.

39 Davin (1978) 'Imperialism and motherhood' p.28.

40 Newman (1907) *The Health of the State* p.110.

41 Ibid., p.118.

42 Ibid., p.124.

43 See Lewis (1980a) *The Politics of Motherhood*; Lewis (1980b) 'The social history of social policy: infant welfare in Edwardian England'; and an examination of a specific intervention Marland (1993) 'A pioneer in infant welfare: the Huddersfield Scheme'.

44 Donzelot (1980) *The Policing of Families*.

45 See Szreter (1991) 'The GRO and the public health movement in Britain 1837–1914'.

46 See Woods, Watterson and Woodward (1989) 'The causes of rapid infant mortality decline in England and Wales 1862–1921'. For example, they continued to examine the variation in rates, rather than the overall decline.

47 *Report of the Interdepartmental Committee on Physical Deterioration* (1904) PP XXXII. See her *Minutes of Evidence*, p.213. Anderson also submitted a separate *Report on the Employment of Mothers in Factories and Workshops*, see Appendix 5.

48 Hutchins (1909) 'Statistics of women's life and employment'.

49 Smith (1979) *The People's Health* pp.122–3.

50 See Woods, Watterson and Woodward (1988) 'The causes of rapid infant mortality decline in England and Wales 1861–1921' Parts I and II.

51 Armstrong (1986) 'The invention of infant mortality' pp.213–14.
52 Davin (1978) 'Imperialism and motherhood' pp.12–14.
53 Armstrong (1986) for example makes the argument for the significance of this conceptualization and notes the increasing age differentiation in mortality statistics from here on.
54 Martin (1911) *The Married Working Woman* p.4.
55 Martin, ibid., p.41.
56 Bell (1907) *At the Works*. This study of Middlesborough did not find a high proportion of women workers (814 out of 44 420 in 1901) but a high infant mortality.
57 Cadbury, Mathieson and Shann (1906) *Women's Work and Wages* p.222.
58 Davies (1915) *Maternity*, Introduction, pp.5–6.
59 Davin (1978) 'Imperialism and motherhood' p.26.
60 Oliver (Ed.) (1902) 'Lead and its compounds', in his *The Dangerous Trades* p.298.
61 *Thorpe/Oliver Report* (1899) PP XII, p.287.
62 Ibid., p.291.
63 *Report* (1910) PP XXIX.
64 Ibid., *Minutes of Evidence*: Mary Woodall 11 069–130; Sarah Cooper 9681–734 and Mary Ann Ford 4900–5019.
65 *Report* (1910) PP XXIX, pp.205–6.
66 *Report* (1910) pp.205–6.
67 *Report* (1910) *Minutes of Evidence*, p.513.
68 Ibid., p.528.
69 Ibid., p.536.
70 Ibid., p.538.
71 See the evidence of Miss Vines and Miss Anderson to the 1910 Committee PP XXIX, 1910.
72 *Report* (1910) *Minutes of Evidence*, pp.730–1.
73 *Report*, ibid., p.205.
74 Ibid., pp.423 and 456.
75 Davies (1915) *Maternity: Letters from Working Women*.
76 See Brookes (1986) 'Women and reproduction *c.* 1860–1920', in Lewis (Ed.) (1986b) *Labour and Love.*
77 McLaren (1977) 'Women's work and the regulation of family size'.
78 *Report* (1910) See evidence of Joseph Lovatt, PP XXIX, pp.168–216, especially Minute 5567; and of Samuel Clowes, p.185.
79 Ibid., Mr B. employee and society representative, p.192.
80 Ibid., pp.196–8. See especially Minute 6465.
81 *The Committee of Inquiry into the Various Lead Industries* (1893–4) PP XVII. See Evidence of Drs Debenham and Johnson. One employer, a Mr Webster, also suggested that men were just as susceptible.
82 Ibid., Mr Webster and Dr Johnson's evidence.
83 *Report* (1910) *Minutes of Evidence*, PP XXIX, p.531.
84 Oliver (1914) *Lead Poisoning* pp.183–4.
85 Ibid., p.184.
86 The fact that this research evidence was from abroad may also have made it difficult to accept.
87 See Mark-Lawson and Witz (1988) 'From family labour to "family wage": the case of women in nineteenth-century coal mining'; Rose (1992) *Limited Livelihoods*.
88 See Malcolmson (1981) 'Victorian laundresses and the laundry trade', *Victorian Studies*.

89 See Pennington and Westover (1989) *A Hidden Workforce: Homeworkers in England, 1880–1985*.
90 Cadbury and Shann (1907) *Sweating* p.37.
91 There was not only a problem related to how women defined homework i.e. often as housework, but also in registers one woman might appear several times, since she took in work from several employers.
92 Feltes (1992) 'Misery or the production of misery: defining sweated labour in 1890' p.441.
93 See Stedman-Jones (1984) *Outcaste London: A Study of the Relationship between the Classes in Victorian Society*.
94 Schmeichen (1984) *Sweated Trades and Sweated Labour*.
95 See Morris (1986a) 'The characteristics of sweating: the late nineteenth-century London and Leeds tailoring trade', in John (Ed.) pp.95–124. Also Morris, *Women Workers and the Sweated Trades* (1986).
96 This analysis of women's role within the labour market of late nineteenth-century capitalism is similar to the original Marxian concept of 'the reserve army of labour'. This thesis was later developed with reference to gender divisions in labour markets more generally; see Beechey (1983) 'What's so special about women's employment?' and the use of a dualism between primary and secondary labour markets: see Barron and Norris (1976) 'Sexual divisions and the dual labour market', in Barker and Allen (Eds).
97 See Stedman-Jones (1984). He identifies this casual labour market with dock-work, construction and other typically male areas of employment.
98 See White (1885) 'The nomad poor of London' pp.714–26 and Booth (1888) 'Conditions and occupations of the people of East London and Hackney'.
99 Miss Vines in evidence to *The Select Committee on Homework* (1908) Minutes of Evidence, PP VIII, Cmd. 246, 1133.
100 Morris (1986a) 'The characteristics of sweating' pp.46–7.
101 See Hutchins (1907) 'Homework and sweating: the causes and the remedies'.
102 Poor foreign labour occupied a similar position to women in relation to this kind of work and were equally viewed as a part of the 'residuum' mentioned above.
103 It is suggested that immigration control was the primary motivation of Lord Dunraven and the House of Lords Select Committee.
104 Based on Rowntree's classic study of York, which provided an empirically established baseline for estimating proportions of populations in poverty.
105 Cadbury and Shann (1907) *Sweated Industry* p.36.
106 Black (1907) *Sweated Industry and the Minimum Wage* p.26.
107 See Wohl (1983) *Endangered Lives* Chapter 11.
108 March-Phillips (1902) 'The evils of homework for women' pp.4–5.
109 See Solden (1978) *Women in British Trade Unions* p.65.
110 For a fuller discussion of what I would call the 'backroom politics' of the report's production, including the role played by Beatrice Potter (later Webb) especially around the issue of whether sweating was a system or a symptom, see Feltes (1992).
111 There were some restrictions on hours for children and young people employed in workshops from 1867.
112 Anderson (1900) *Legislation Affecting the Conditions of Employment in Homework and Domestic Industries*, although MacDonald (1906) pointed out that because many exclusions operated the Royal Commission saw little evidence of change in conditions.
113 Morris (1986a) 'Characteristics of sweating' p.96. She emphasizes the need to distinguish homework and outwork and argues that a conflation of the two has resulted in an

association of outwork with 'the backward sections' of the tailoring and clothing trades. In fact not all outworkers were homeworkers, nor were they necessarily unregulated.

114 For an example of this argument, see Tuckwell (1902) 'The more obvious defects of our factory code', in Webb (Ed.) p.141.

115 Both pro- and anti-legislative camps acknowledged this. The *English Women's Review* 16 January 1899, p.11, noted that while it was right to draw attention to the misery, after the 1895 Act 'employers . . . now gave out work to be done at home in preference to taking women into the Factories'.

116 Knightley (1901) 'Women as homeworkers', *Nineteenth Century* p.288.

117 Cited in Knightley (1901) ibid., p.289.

118 Hutchins (1907) 'Homework and sweating'.

119 See Tuckwell (1902) 'The more obvious defects of our factory code', in Webb and Webb (Eds) *The Case for the Factory Acts* p.141.

120 Mappen (1985) *Helping Women at Work: The Women's Industrial Council 1889–1914* pp.88–98.

121 See Squire (1902) 'Fur-pulling', in Oliver (Ed.) *The Dangerous Trades*; Black (1891) 'Matchbox making in the home', *English Illustrated Magazine* August, p.629. The novelists Charles Dickens and John Galsworthy had also noted the conditions of matchbox makers. (For a summary of the latter, see Beer (n.d.) *The Match Girls Strike, 1888.*

122 Mappen (1985) *Helping Women at Work* p.94.

123 This issue was discussed in Chapter 1, where it was noted that a failure to effect improvements in sanitary conditions was considered to be partly due to political influences on local authorities.

124 Notably Edward Cadbury, whose own investigations with co-workers Mathieson and Shann into women's working conditions fuelled an appreciation of the problem of achieving improvement. Mallon of Toynbee Hall was also involved.

125 See Morris (1986b) p.199.

126 MacDonald (1906) p.35.

127 *Report of the Select Committee on Homework* (1907) PP VI, p.55.

128 *Select Committee on Homework* (1908) PP VI, Minutes of Evidence, p.125, response 2879.

129 Ibid., p.124, Minute 2841.

130 Ibid., p.1786, Minute, 2050–52.

131 *Report*, PP VI, 1908, p.14.

132 *Hansard* (1909) p.344.

133 Morris (1986b) *Women Workers and the Sweated Trades*.

134 Black (1907) p.*xxiv*.

135 *International Morning Post*, 10 December 1907 cited in Morris (1986b) *Women Workers and the Sweated Trades* p.151.

136 See Harrison (1995b) 'Women's health', in Purvis (Ed.) *Women in Britain 1850–1945*.

Chapter 4

Out of the Factory: Health and Work in Non-industrial Occupations

In reviewing the problem of women's occupational ill-health in this period, it has been suggested that because factory legislation was the major form of intervention to limit the worst effects of working conditions, this resulted in a narrow perspective on the possible problems women workers confronted. Factory legislation as applied to industrial work and women workers did not encompass all areas of factory work: its applicability addressed only a few specific issues. Thus some aspects, such as heavy lifting or the provision of appropriate lighting, remained outside regulation until very late in the period. Similarly, there was no regulation of workshops until 1895. The control of conditions in domestic outwork or homework happened even later. The omission of certain categories of industrial employment, however, is relatively minor compared with other areas of working and middle-class women's employment that were excluded, in particular domestic service and service industries such as shop-work, bars and catering although the latter two were subject to some enquiry and intervention.

The other major exclusion affected by a focus on 'protective' legislation and an association with the 'hazards' of industrial work was the growth of some new employment opportunities for women: in office work as clerks and typists and in 'professional' work. Although the occupations themselves were subject to examination, it seems that middle-class women's work in particular was rarely considered to pose occupational health problems or to require intervention. For many contemporary women activists, an interest in widening the employment opportunities for women was paramount and white collar and 'professional' occupations were particularly important. This resulted in many historical accounts neglecting the topic of work-related health.[1] These work arenas sometimes provided better pay and working conditions – but because they also had the potential to damage health, they need to be considered. Poor working conditions were not the prerogative of the factory or the workshop. Both working and middle-class working women often recognized how their health was undermined by their work in other contexts.

Domestic Service

In 1881, one in every three young women between the ages of 15 and 20 worked in domestic service.[2] In the period considered here it was the largest single source of employment for women. The 1911 census showed that 1 359 559 women and girls were employed in 'indoor domestic service'.[3] In this period, too, the sexual division of labour in domestic service changed to the extent that it was only in very wealthy homes that men retained such positions. Representations of domestic service often presented an ideal of the beneficial and improving potential of the occupation; manuals such as the one by Mrs Beeton (1863) reinforced an image of household management based on the model of the large country house. As contemporary commentators[4] and more recent historical analyses[5] have shown, the reality was different.

Typically, domestic servants were scattered across the country, working alone in middle-class households. Most middle-class families had average annual incomes of around £300 which was not enough to pay more than one servant. Higgs'[6] study of late nineteenth-century Rochdale found that 64 per cent of servant-employing households were 'middle-class'. In many such households, daughters or other women in the family performed unpaid domestic duties for their kin (this factor caused some difficulties in census enumeration and classification).[7]

In 61 per cent of Rochdale households there was only one servant, a 'maid-of-all-work', which led to many domestic servants being overworked. There were concentrations of domestic servants, however, especially in London. Booth's[8] survey found 399 178 domestic servants in London, of whom 205 500 were indoor servants. The percentage in one-servant households was not so high – 65 000 – with a further 52 000 in two-servant households. However, Booth's classification of service was quite wide. It included a number of male occupations such as grooms, as well as the specific aspects of London households. By 1916, when the Butler Report for the Women's Industrial Council (WIC) appeared[9] there seems to have been little departure from nineteenth-century patterns of employment, but there was a widespread view that there was a 'servant problem'. Considerable discussion occurred on the difficulties employers encountered in getting 'satisfactory' servants and from servants in getting 'good places to work'. Some contentment was expressed by both employers and servants to the enquiry, but it was a minority. For servants, in particular, the problems lay not just in their working conditions but in the social relations and social status that accompanied the work itself.

Thomas Oliver devoted some attention to domestic servants in his work on the 'dangerous trades' published in 1902.[10] While it was only two pages of a massive text, it indicates he did consider there to be some health consequences in the work – arguably important ones, given the large numbers of women in such positions. He noted there were considerable variations in the conditions under which domestic servants laboured and lived. They shared problems with many shop-workers and other service-workers: they were expected to live in, which increased the likelihood that they could be called on to work excessive hours. The accommodation itself often offered little respite from the working conditions. Servants rooms were often in attics or basements; they were small, badly lit, without heat and poorly ventilated.

These aspects were noted in evidence given to the Royal Commission of Labour in 1893,[11] when Mr Greenman of the London Domestic Servants Union contended that conditions were by 'no means satisfactory'. Commenting on the report in *Shafts*, Jane Clapperton argued 'It was trying to be run off one's feet all day long in obedience to the requirements of other people, or the demands of a capricious mistress.'[12] This was only one of a number of commentaries noting the diversity in conditions which depended on the type of house worked in. According to the *Shafts* article, the worst were in London middle-class households, while in 'the mansions of the aristocracy the servants suffer from enforced idleness than overwork ... in the main their sufferings are social rather than physical'.[13] According to Oliver, domestic servants in small houses with large families and in lodging houses suffered the most:

> Their hours of toil are long, and the demands made upon domestic servants are numerous, often exacting and frequently protracted well into the evening. Small wonder that, owing to their deprivation of fresh air, the monotony of their work and in many instances the conflict of tempers and the imperfect food obtainable in many poorer families or lodging houses many young women break down in health.[14]

In addition to physical illness such as anaemia, headaches, 'derangement of the digestive and pelvic organs' and stomach ulcers, Oliver noted that a large number of females admitted to asylums were domestic servants. In Northumberland between 1886 and 1890, of 415 admissions, 48 or 11.3 per cent were domestic servants and a further 15 were housekeepers. Interestingly, 189 were housewives. The further 101 with 'no occupation', Oliver suggests, were young women who were probably engaged all day on 'housework'.[15] Such figures raise the possibility that being confined to domestic work, paid as well as unpaid, may be implicated in wellbeing. The health differentials in both physical and mental health to this day have continued to show the relatively poorer health status of women without paid work outside the home.[16] Studies have suggested a link between health status and the extent to which both paid and unpaid work provide women with sources of social esteem and a sense of control over their own lives. The thesis also has relevance in the historical context.

Lack of self-esteem and control over their lives was particularly evident in domestic service. It was not just the hazards of the occupation which Oliver highlighted: many young women experienced a lack of personal liberty both within the work itself and in terms of available alternative employment. As with many women confined to unpaid domestic labour, they felt trapped. Studies that have used the oral testimony of women workers show that domestic service, although becoming unpopular among women themselves, was often the only alternative to one other dominant trade in a town. In Bornat's study in the Colne Valley, one respondent gives an example of where someone had commented that her employment:

> in the mill 'was common' to which I says 'well I think skivvies are common'. She says 'what do you call skivvies?' I says 'we're not servants, we can please ourselves when we come and go. Skivies can't ... we consider that the girls in Barnsley that have to go into service are very unlucky'.[17]

In Colchester, according to Westover's respondents, tailoring and domestic service were the only two possible kinds of work. Often the girls' mothers pushed their daughters into domestic service, seeing it as 'more respectable', while their daughters preferred tailoring: 'No I could not bear to bow and scrape' and 'when I started I either got to go into the factory or service . . . No fear I didn't want to go into service.'[18] Servants interviewed for the WIC enquiry repeatedly referred to the tie of service: the perception of being restricted involved a number of interrelated dimensions. It included the feeling of always 'being under orders', of 'never being off-duty' and the limitations imposed by living-in, in its impact on workloads, free time and social contact. For some 'service is like a prison'.[19] A parlour-maid who survived only seven days in the job described it as:

> too monotonous to endure day after day without being able either to have friends perhaps to see you, or being able to go and see them; and naturally one loses all interest in life, and it is not worth living.[20]

This absence of free time was a constant complaint made by those in service, regardless of whether they were happy or not. It was the one aspect they most desired to see reformed:

> Speaking of myself, I am very often shut right indoors from one week to another, Tuesday to Tuesday. I never have a day out . . . I consider all maids should have two hours each day to call their own . . . Domestic service would not be nearly such a monotonous occupation if a little variation were included. A good home and good food *is not all* that is required by servants.[21]

This lack of free time, either indoors or to go out, was closely linked to the problem of long hours. Domestic servants themselves complained at their exclusion from the Factory Acts: 'I wish with all my heart the Factory Acts limiting the hours of labour could be applied to domestic service'[22] and a cook/general servant commented favourably on the WIC enquiry that 'I am very glad something is being done for domestics, as I think the factory girls are studied far more than we are. I think there ought to be laws for us as well as them.'[23] Among the report's recommendations were that domestic servants should be given an average of two hours off-duty each day, excluding mealtimes, and a half-day-a-week holiday as well as Sundays.

As arduous as other forms of work may have been, women themselves increasingly turned against domestic service as an avenue of employment. Higgs'[24] study noted that rural migrants were an important source of recruits, while their urban counterparts regarded it as not only personally restricting but degrading. The Butler Report for WIC describes this as the 'loss of caste'.[25] Witnesses highlighted two aspects in their investigation: first, the deliberate rudeness from employers which encompassed a view that employers tended to treat them as 'machines rather than human beings'.[26] Then there was the stigma of social inferiority. One servant described it as 'I consider servants are a despised race. Not by the ladies, by the girls of their own class who are in business'. Another echoes 'once a servant, you are treated as belonging to an inferior race to all other workers: it is as if the low-est point has been reached'.[27] Such perceptions varied from place to place, often depending on whether there were other employment opportunities, but the stigma was also noted by both employers and servants who were positive about service and felt it to be undeserved. Although I came across no discussion of possible sexual harassment in relation to domestic servants, they must have been subject to this both in single- and multiple-servant households. Perhaps the silence is because it would have been impossible for domestic servants themselves to mention it to anyone, both because of their reliance on references and because discussion of such matters would have been improper.

Those with a specific interest in the regulation of factory conditions did not see domestic service as a better alternative either. In 1893, Clementina Black con-sidered the conditions of domestic service 'are still those of an earlier industrial and social system'.[28] In particular, she noted employer/employee relations were differ-ent to other employments in that when the hours of labour were over the relation-ship continued: the 'servant has no life of her own'. The reality for most working women was that there was little time or energy left for such a life in other kinds of work either! In the same article, Black argued that if she personally were the mother of girls who had to choose between factory work and service, 'I would give my voice unhesitatingly to the factory'.[29] The Women's Industrial Council, with which she was associated, confirmed in their report that 'girls are apt to prefer lower wages, less material comfort and much less security of employment in shop, office or factory work, to the oft-quoted advantages of domestic service'.[30] There were then important differences between domestic service and other forms of wage-earning for working-class women. Not only was the work not carried on for profit, it was conducted on the employers' premises, making any bargain for wages and conditions essentially an individual and private matter. These material differences had consequences for the variability in work experience of domestic servants and evaluations of it as an occupation. In turn, these differences impacted on physical health and psychological wellbeing.

Women factory inspectors often commented that one of the consequences of any restrictions on factory work might be to drive women to domestic work and in particular to 'charing' which was equally damaging to their health. From time to time, trade unionists also raised the issue of the plight of domestic servants. Mary McArthur, Secretary of the WTUL in 1909, pointed to the 'hard life' of the single servant; she reiterated the problems of long hours, lack of solitude, little freedom and isolation from others of their social class. She told the TUC that she would welcome legislation to restrict the hours of work of any woman.[31] There were pro-posals to organize domestic servants, but such a task posed particular problems given the conditions of the work.

In considering ways to reform domestic service it was evident that it shared a similar obstacle to the control of conditions for homework: it was not considered appropriate for there to be any regulation of work that intruded on the private sphere.

Just as, for much of the nineteenth century, it was difficult to countenance intervention in family life, the domestic domain was considered inappropriate for the kind of surveillance carried out by factory inspectors. There was already some erosion of these ideas in the case of working-class families, as the development of early health-visiting indicates.[32] With the 'crisis' over 'physical deterioration' into the new century, such surveillance was to expand considerably.[33]

But it was a different matter when it came to middle-class households. In 1909, when Horatio Bottomley introduced a Bill to limit the hours of work to eight hours a day, the question of including domestic servants was raised. In opposition, one inspector had said: 'It was intolerable and unthinkable that inspectors should visit, good mistresses know much better how to conduct their houses, look after their servants and regulate the work.'[34] In any case, some argued, it was social rather than physical conditions that were the problem in relation to domestic service and 'the State cannot possibly curb social suffering'.[35] In the event, domestic servants had to bargain for themselves, helped by the competition provided by widening employment opportunities.

Serving Others in the Public Domain: Shop Assistants, Barmaids and Waitresses

The growth of shop-work for women and the problems that arose in connection with its conditions were a product of changes at this time in the retail trade. As with clerical work, the pool of cheap labour that women provided was welcomed in an expanding and increasingly competitive market for the sale of mass-produced goods. By 1901, 243 000 women were engaged in the retail trade, the majority as shop assistants. As a result, both the division of labour and its gender composition changed. At the same time, it is difficult to generalize about shops and shop-work as size, geographical location, goods retailed and the use of 'living-in' were variable and these differences impacted on recruitment and the conditions shop assistants experienced. Despite this, the general picture was of deteriorating working conditions. Holcombe[36] suggests these may have been a direct result of the increasing number of women employees and rising public agitation for shops to be included within factory legislation.

The 1876 Factory Commission had noted that long hours were a feature: as many as 84 hours a week were reported.[37] These also occurred within traditional retail outlets, where certain goods were both made and sold on the premises. This gave rise to considerable problems in enforcing hours-of-work legislation, as women could be switched from shop-work to manufacturing. The Commission concluded that shop-work 'could hardly be considered fatiguing, much less unwholesome'. Thus feminist organizations such as the Society for the Employment of Women (SPEW), who campaigned for women's work opportunities and to provide some training for them, were not alone in considering that commercial work such as retailing was 'ideal'. There were advantages in women being able to serve women customers and, paradoxically, the occupation retained a middle-class image of respectability while being publicly condemned for conditions no better than either domestic service or factory work. But investigators such as Booth[38] noted how shop assistants 'preferred' this hardship, 'rather than lose caste', a term also used by WIC in reference to urban women's concerns about domestic service, revealing once again the salience of class distinctions in employment. Shop assistants were drawn from a wide social spectrum: by 1914 they were the largest group of middle-class women workers, numbering almost half a million.[39]

Clara Collet concluded in one of her reports to the Royal Commission of Labour that the 'idea that a shop assistant's work is less arduous than that of persons in a factory seems to be erroneous'.[40] Her investigations for the Commission gave credence to the need to look beyond factories and workshops to other areas of women's work. Hours of work were also a particular problem for shop assistants and the effects were often exacerbated because they were spent standing, with few proper mealbreaks. They often experienced differential pressure due to demand for goods and some of Collet's informants 'got worn out' in the summer, reporting painful swollen legs.

In her report on shop assistants in London, Collet referred to one witness who had worked a 72-hour week to find herself dismissed because of absences caused by headaches and illness.[41] Such hours were typical of East End shops, while in the West End the average was 54 to 64 hours per week. Other investigators also noted very long hours: Bulley and Whitley cited 84–85 hours from the *1888 Select Committee Report on Shop Hours*, noting that the worst excesses were to be found in the suburbs.[42] Later still, Margaret Irwin drew attention to the fact that country shops were probably the worst of all because the assistant was often the sole employee.[43]

As with other 'service' occupations, particular aspects of the work added to the strain experienced by shop assistants. Collet perceived the patience and politeness shown to the most trying customers; being subject to constant supervision and the liability to instant dismissal as features that 'render the occupation of shop assistants most trying to the nerves and injurious to health'. 'It is a significant fact', she concluded:

> that whereas large numbers of factory girls cannot be prevailed upon to give
> up factory work after marriage, the majority of shop assistants look upon
> marriage as their one hope of release, and would as one girl expressed it
> 'marry anybody to get out of the drapery business'.[44]

One of the factors that may also have contributed to such a negative view was that 'living-in' was common in shop-work. Over and above the difficulties to which these often 'barrack-like', overcrowded, ill-ventilated accommodations gave rise, the system was viewed as depriving young women of the normal companionship of men in their leisure time, as well as making it less likely that leisure could be claimed.[45] Holcombe cites the case of a girl in Baker Street, London, who lasted two days in a situation where 22 girls shared three bedrooms and she had to share a bed with two others. In another example, an apprenticed draper's assistant reported that the sheets on her bed were changed once every three months.[46]

The living-in system contributed to a considerable amount of illegal overtime in shop-work. Even if they did not live-in, assistants were often required to take part of their pay in meals, further depressing their already low wages. Some of these wages had to be spent on their own 'presentable' clothing. The poor conditions of living-in were also characteristic of 'eating rooms' which were often damp basements, poorly ventilated, overcrowded and infested with vermin. Clementina Black found examples of 'houses of good repute' which still provided nothing but a basin in which to wash.[47]

Food quality also varied widely, but at its worst it was poor, badly cooked and insufficient; shop assistants often got just bread and butter. Collet reported that shop assistants were often interrupted during their meals. They had acquired a habit of 'bolting' their food, so it was not surprising that they suffered from indigestion and craved 'unwholesome food': 'sweet stuff and pastry'.[48] Margaret Bondfield an early active member of the National Union of Shop Assistants (NAUSA), found cases of shop assistants who would spend 2s to 3s a week of their own money on food.[49] The combination of such factors led investigators to conclude that it was not surprising that ill-health was commonly found among shop assistants. One WIC investigator who spent 15 weeks in a shop reported that:

> out of 16 assistants I worked with, one was anaemic, one had varicose veins, one chronic indigestion, all suffered from lassitude and headaches, and four frequently lost their voices through weakness. One who left broke down from extreme weakness and had to give up altogether.[50]

The Royal Commission of Labour led to an enquiry into the possible health consequences for women who worked in hotels, public houses and 'other places of refreshment'. Eliza Orme, who conducted the enquiry,[51] found that views about this work were tainted by notions of respectability. Issues of morality were at stake, not least because of the presence of drink and examples of sexual harassment. In one case she describes, the woman 'left her third situation after two days in consequence of the attempted familiarity on the part of her employer. She then took a place in the City where the customers were of a low class using bad language and subjecting her to insults.'[52] Such problems, she suggested, contributed to a high absenteeism. Again, as with all occupations, hours of work were a major problem, but Eliza Orme's report is interesting for the emphasis it gave to the provision of seating, noting that this alone does not benefit the worker: 'a girl may be far more tired by being in a bar for many hours, even if there are seats in it, than by standing for a few hours with the prospect of a complete rest at a fixed time'.[53] A WIC enquiry found a teashop worker whose hours were 9.00 am to 9.00 pm for five days and 9.00 am until 11.30 pm on Saturdays, with no breaks for meals as she was in sole charge. Evidence to the Select Committee of the House of Lords on Early Closing of Shops suggested that hours of 70 to 96 hours per week were common in restaurants. One waitress commented, 'When I get home I just sit down and cry with fatigue.'[54] In 1913 barmaids' hours were restricted to 63 per week, but many reported still having to work a 17-hour day. In his study of Victorian barmaids,

Bailey[55] describes the physical regime as 'punishing', but also notes that conditions varied considerably with the best to be found in large establishments. However, it was the moral dimension of barmaids' work that most exercised reformers' attentions, not the hard work. As Bailey puts it, pubs managed both the flow of drink and the flow of sexuality, despite the controls of pub protocols that provided some protection for women.[56]

Long hours of standing was also an issue returned to again and again in shop-work. Some time before the Royal Commission on Labour, the *Englishwoman's Review* (ER) had reported on a survey conducted in Edinburgh shops in 1880. It found that only 28 out of 126 had seats: the girls were not actually forbidden to sit on them, although there was often little provision for them to do so.[57] ER suggested that seats were more often found in shops which were owned or managed by women. With increasing competitiveness, shop-owners did not want their assistants to sit down in case it looked like slackness. Over and above the long hours of standing, enforced civility, as noted by Collet, and the problems associated with the 'living-in' system, shop-work was also characterized by insecurity and unemployment. Margaret Bondfield remembers having to trudge the streets of London to join long queues of young women applicants for a job that offered 25s plus live-in for a 65-hour week. Instant dismissal was not uncommon and older women, especially if their health broke down,[58] could find themselves replaced by younger ones. Poor as they often were, this could mean they also lost their homes.

As with other areas of work, shop assistants were frequently fined for being late, giving the wrong change, breakages and 'bad manners'. Two commentators on shop work in the 1890s described such deductions as 'capricious'.[59] Examples included fines of 6d for standing on a chair or sending a bad coin to the cashier. They concluded: 'one wonders how human ingenuity could devise so many punishable offences'.[60] Fines extended to house rules associated with living-in. Margaret Bondfield[61] gave examples of loitering in passages, no flowers in rooms and no visiting each other's rooms. She found one firm where there were 159 rules, 'the most objectionable being that all employees are liable to be searched any or every time of leaving the premises, the door-keeper having the authority to do so'. An analysis of these kinds of problems with shop-work suggests that activists had developed a sensitivity to the ways in which work could damage health. Clementina Black noted:

> that in many, indeed most shops, the space behind the counter is too narrow, and the assistant is jostled every time another passes her. To a tired woman with aching back and feet, the repetition of this discomfort grows, and toward the end of the day, becomes intolerable.[62]

The combination of all these circumstances may have been just as damaging to shop-workers' health as those that confronted factory workers. In fact despite some level of inactivity, this, alongside anxiety, may have been more tiring. At least one informant told Margaret Bondfield that her sister who had worked as a shop assistant in a small country town, 'at the end of the time was carried home in blankets, having broken down completely at the hard conditions of her life'.[63]

By the 1890s there was noticeable concern about shop-workers' conditions. There were early attempts at organization. In addition to NAUSA, formed in 1891, a union of cooperative employees was formed in 1895, although a number of the factors discussed above, such as a 'middle-class' image and job insecurity, mitigated against it. Although women were admitted to the union, men took little interest in women's concerns, but by the early-twentieth century leading women activists, such as Margaret Bondfield, gained more senior places in the union and worked to increase women's interests.[64] This was especially evident in campaigns for a minimum wage. Both unions continued to argue for differential rates for men and women, using the well-worn arguments about 'pin money', physical strength and the worth of women's labour. However, in some instances unions were able to reach voluntary agreements over pay and conditions.

The second major front for trying to achieve change was through legislation. This mainly concentrated on hours and The Shop Hours Act 1886 restricted them to 74 per week including mealtimes, but there was no provision for enforcement. The unions continued to press for a 50-hour week, with fixed closing times, and a half-day holiday for both men and women. They also wanted to regulate against Sunday trading. Despite the presentation of a number of Bills to Parliament over the first decade of the twentieth century – and some sympathy in government circles for regulation –[65] these attempts largely failed. Churchill introduced one in 1911 but it was 'pulled to shreds and patched together' in debate, so he conceded many of the provisions that were being sought by unions and shop-workers' supporters.[66]

Legislative intervention was considered desirable in other areas too. In 1899 it was a requirement to provide one seat for every three workers, although there was no system of either inspection or prosecution. There were attempts to have shop assistants included within the Truck Acts in order to control the use of accommodation and meals in lieu of wages. The 1908 Departmental Committee on the Truck Acts included shop assistants in its remit. Lucy Deane reported that assistants could live better out than in, in terms of employers estimates of 'cost'. She refuted claims that living-in provided a 'moral safeguard'.[67] The committee were not convinced and recommended that fines or deductions should not exceed 5 per cent of wages. In the event any legislation on these areas was slow and was eventually hampered by the onset of the First World War. Little in the way of legal limitation had been achieved in the two decades of activism.

Into the Office: Clerks and Typists

Office work expanded rapidly in the late-nineteenth and early decades of the twentieth century. Although men were still predominant, some authors have called it 'a white blouse revolution'.[68] The 1901 census revealed 307 889 men and 55 784 women in commercial and business occupations. There were also 42 475 men and 14 312 women in the civil service: of the women, the majority were in clerical grades, in particular within the Post Office. In 1892, *Shafts*[69] argued that typewriting

Figure 4.1 *Post office clerks, reproduced by permission of Mary Evans Picture Library.*

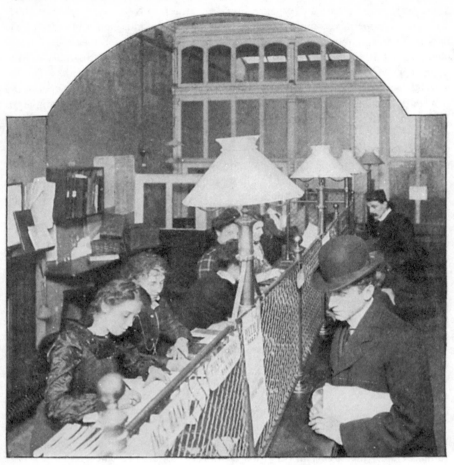

was an 'ideal' occupation for women. In the context of a demographic surplus of women, offices provided another alternative to becoming a governess for the middle-class woman. There was enthusiasm for a form of daily work, conducted in offices that were run by women, which was 'often very interesting' in contrast to the 'dry routine' of many employments. The popularity of office work also owed something to a perception of the work as 'light' compared with manual labour.

Zimmeck and Lewis[70] suggest that clerical work was also seen to have considerable advantages over other possible employment for women, in terms of Victorian ideas of 'suitability' which were closely linked to notions of moral respectability. Clerical work did not involve contact with social inferiors, as teaching or nursing did, nor did it involve living-in, as shop-work did, which might present moral dangers. Zimmeck suggests that clerical work, was seen as clean, 'dainty' and where appropriate feminine dress could be worn. Women themselves certainly saw the work as without 'danger'. In a 1907 survey for the Board of Trade [71] Clara Collet found that those conditions which were positively rated by clerical workers in the civil service were 'safety', protection from sexual harassment, permanency, liberal sick-leave and pensions. However, the survey was conducted in the context of a perceived crisis in the retention of clerical workers in the civil service, where wages were lower than in many private businesses. It was the latter that began to offer incentives to those women with ambition and a desire for career advancement.[72]

Particularly in the early years of expansion, there were those who thought that typewriting offices had all the characteristics of a sweated industry: long hours, low pay and poor environmental conditions. On the whole, however, it does seem that hours were not excessive, and that outside of a tendency that seemed to be present in all occupations of asking workers to meet externally instigated pressures of work, conditions were considerably better than those in many other forms of work. No doubt there were many exceptions to this and long hours, unprotected breaks and low pay were to be found. There were also offices which were dirty, over-crowded, lacking in ventilation and natural light and where the noise caused by telephones and typewriters would have been considerable. The Association of Clerks and Secretaries, founded in 1903, pointed out to the 1912 TUC[73] that thousands of girl clerks worked in smaller spaces than factory workers with poor sanitary provision.

An earlier enquiry in 1906 by the Association of Shorthand Writers and Typists revealed that the majority of women worked from 9.00 am until 6.00 pm with an hour for lunch.[74] There could also be demanding workloads. Dohrn describes clerks working at one insurance company in 1910 as having to fill in 60 policies per minute, for which they received a annual salary of £22.[75] In 1914 a study of women in the professions conducted for the Fabian Women's Group described the 'whole profession to be in a chaotic condition'.[76] They found some women being paid as little as 5s per week, while there were some firms who paid annual salaries of £100 to £150 per year. However, 'well-paid posts' were 'exceptional' and had remained static since the 1890s.[77] A manager in Manchester, told the enquiry that 'it is impossible for girls to live on their salaries unless they are at home with their parents', when in fact many clerks and typists were the chief breadwinners. There were also examples of low pay combined with long hours and social isolation, especially in the case of the individual employment of a private secretary. One described:

> my two years in the house of Sir – the most hopelessly isolated and uninteresting existence within the four walls of his study. A secretary should certainly stick out for a free weekend once in a month when living in. Isolation is horribly bad for one.[78]

An Edinburgh woman said that 'in her first post . . . my time was never my own . . . my work began at 9.00 am and often did not end at midnight. Sunday work was quite common.'

An enquiry conducted in 1910 by Adelaide Anderson and Mr Robinson[79] for the Factory Department to consider whether the Factory Acts should be extended to typewriting offices found that outside public employment, it was difficult to estimate the number of people employed. Their report noted there were different classes of women in such employment. At the top were those with education, often with foreign languages and proficiency in shorthand and typewriting who were mainly employed in business houses. Conditions here were very good: pay was £3 to £4 a week for a 10.00 am to 5.00 pm or 9.00 am to 6.00 pm day. In the middle group were those 'intelligent and capable in typewriting and copying'. They worked in better-class offices, usually as bookkeepers and clerks, earning about £1 to 30s a week in generally satisfactory conditions. Finally, at the lower end, were women who may have had some training from large commercial schools, who chose office work in preference to domestic service, but 'who will never become very proficient'. For this group hours were not considered to be excessive, although overtime was sometimes worked and wages were generally low. Overall the report concluded that generally conditions were fairly good, although in some smaller firms suitable and separate sanitary accommodation was an issue. Equally, given the rapid development of the employment, some regulation might be required in the future. Inspectors were alert to the fact that materials and new technology such as stencilling, copying and the addressograph might need to be monitored.

Bills were introduced with respect to underground workrooms – some of which would have been offices – and to control the sanitary conditions in offices and railway offices each year from 1911 until the First World War but none received a second reading.[80] Unionization was to prove problematic. As with many other new areas of employment, a combination of competition-based insecurities, notions of middle-class respectability which often led to an identification with employers' interests and a positive view of conditions and opportunities resulted in little perceived need for collective organization. After three years of operation, by 1900 the National Union of Clerks only had 82 members.[81] Lewis[82] suggests that women clerks shared gendered ideas of men employers and employees about their work, so it did not prevent them from having a sense of pride or satisfaction in it.

It is important to consider other aspects of clerical work beyond the immediate working environment and conditions that might have had an impact on health and well-being even if they did not present the same 'dangers' as factory work. Statistical information about the health of clerks and typists is hard to find. Common ailments seem to have been neuritis, anaemia and nervous breakdown, with strain on both eyesight and hearing particularly for typists.[83] In the case of the rapidly growing class of clerical employees within the Post Office, many of whom worked as telegraphists, the work was seen as 'exacting and exhausting to the nervous system' so that special attention was called for in terms of both the equipment provided and the need for rest-rooms.[84]

Clerical work did not escape the constraints of either 'separate sphere' ideology or patriarchal attitudes about women's abilities and their eligibility for paid employment. As elsewhere, what was deemed suitable work for women and a sexual division of labour was rigidly enforced: thus women's self-esteem was potentially undermined. Women obviously experienced overt discrimination and their wages were much less than for male clerks on the grounds of lesser eligibility.

Women were not envisaged to be self-supporting and the opportunities to move beyond a small increase in pay were rare. While they earned more than the average industrial wage, this was still not a great deal. Telegraphists and counter-clerks in the Post Office had the minimum rate, set at £65 in 1881, actually reduced to £55 in 1897 'as a concession to male staff'.[85] They were on a incremental scale to £100 but the majority remained at the lower end.

Poor pay and unequal pay remained important grievances. While women were prepared to work for lower pay than men, men perceived this as a threat to the male wage. This acted as a further block to collective organization.[86] As the Parliamentary Secretary to the Royal Commission on the Civil Service (1912) argued, lower pay for women was justified because they 'ought to be got as cheaply as possible, and if they can be got for less they ought not to be paid the same as men'.[87] For those women employed in the Civil Service, a marriage bar also operated. Typically, women were physically segregated from men to the extent, as Zimmeck describes it, 'this took on a surreal importance' to justify the non-employment of women.[88] This undoubtedly contributed to the lack of sexual harassment Clara Collet noted and to some advantages that many contemporary activists considered accrued to having women managers or supervisors. But it was also an 'unnatural isolation from men that reinforced the boundaries of women's work in the mechanical sphere and closed off opportunities for mobility except in supervising women'. It was 'endless snakes and no ladders'.[89] The effect of this work organization around sexual segregation of both the spheres of work and the physical environment was to make much of the work done by women routine and devalued. Women worked with women, under women and in women's jobs and processes. Women's abilities were considered suited to the monotony and drudgery that sometimes ensued.

There was some ambivalence toward clerical occupations where women experienced the restrictions of 'lesser eligibility', but where there were also new opportunities for work. Many women voted with their feet, seeking betterment through job change. Many of them also enjoyed working and gained considerable satisfaction from their skills and the work they produced. Generally, although clerical work altered in complexity and intensity there is little doubt that for many women it was a popular option. The increase of women from 1851 to 1911 was 83-fold, compared to a seven-fold increase in men and the demand for posts exceeded the supply.

Professional Work

The late-nineteenth and early-twentieth century was also a period of forging new 'professional'[90] occupations for women. In some cases, as in medicine or factory inspection, this required challenging a male monopoly, in particular the 'credentialist' tactics that men used to define women as ineligible and thereby exclude them, or for women to develop a form of occupational closure – a separate women's profession – as in nursing.[91] Other areas which were popular with many middle-class women, such as forms of philanthropic work, offered opportunities to 'break out' of the confines of a stultifying domestic existence without challenging the legitimacy of it by claims to paid employment.[92] In time, some areas of 'voluntary' work were transformed into a salaried profession. This applied to early settlement work prior to the origins of social work, in voluntary health or sanitary societies and for 'bible' women as the forerunners of locally employed health visitors.[93] There were also traditional women's occupations that were to undergo processes of transformation, for example, relatively untrained but 'genteel' women who moved from isolated, paid duties in the private domain to the public arena, as in teaching; and occupations that had been traditionally unskilled and mainly working-class in recruitment to ones suitable for middle-class women, such as nursing.

There were also broader social influences in the move of middle-class women into the professions. What avenues were possible reflected the extent to which there were differences in women's education and training. From the 1890s an increasing number of middle-class women had been through high school and further or higher education and wanted professional work. Women themselves entered into the debate about the 'proper' sphere of their professional work, eligibility and the limitations imposed on entry, emphasizing the lack of information about them.[94] Advocates and analysts alike accepted that there were distinct masculine and feminine aptitudes and character but that this was an argument *for* women's employment, not a limitation. As Clara Collet put it: 'I do not urge women to compete with men because they can do what men can, but because I believe that they can do what men cannot.'[95] Phoebe Sheavyn similarly argued: 'We must lay stress upon woman's positive capacities not upon her limitations' and 'the woman's special characteristics are needed in many occupations outside the boundaries of the family, the schoolroom and the sick-room'.[96] Lady Jeune also suggested that what was important was 'that their health has stood the strain of the pressure of work in an unexpected manner. The false prophets who foretold the complete destruction of the female constitution from overwork have been confounded.'[97] From the 1880s an increasing number of texts pointed out the advantages and pitfalls (less evident) of alternative forms of professional work for women.[98]

A further important context was the serious demographic obstacle to the possibility that middle-class women could look forward to marriage and family life. Clara Collet's analysis of census data showed that in many districts the ratio of women to men was often double and in London these were mainly middle-class districts. (In the East End the ratio was better.) Thus it was also a material necessity that propelled many middle-class women into work.[99] These general features of the increasing employment of women in professional life can be illustrated by a closer examination of three examples: teaching, nursing and factory inspection (civil service). They reveal the different ways in which work and working conditions impinged on women's lives and health – and the response.

Teaching

Teaching underwent considerable development in this period, reflecting the changes toward compulsory schooling and educational provision and opportunities. It had been an occupation for women before the 1870s when they had mainly been single governesses in private homes. While domestic service was sometimes viewed as an occupation of last resort for women, middle-class women considered being a governess in exactly the same way. This was how Charlotte Brontë characterized it:

> many a time when her charge turns unruly in her hands, when the responsibility which she would discharge faithfully and perfectly becomes unmanageable to her, she will wish herself a housemaid or kitchen girl rather than a baited, trampled, desolate, distracted governess.[100]

While Brontë's vision was earlier in the century (1848), the traditional governess persisted in some households. In 1850 there were 21 000 but after the 1870 Education Act, which brought compulsory elementary education, other forms of teaching opened up. Those who were already governesses suffered similar conditions to those of domestic servants: long hours, low pay and having to perform domestic duties for their charges. Many governesses were little more than glorified 'babysitters'. Their social position was more complicated: they were tapped between the family above them and the servants below. The result was often confinement either to the nursery or the schoolroom. Being a governess was rarely seen as an occupation of 'choice' but rather of necessity – and they were observed to be one of the most common categories among women asylum inmates.[101] Although conditions probably improved for private governesses, residential posts became less attractive. Schools, 'where the work though fatiguing, is kept with fixed hours, and where time out of school is (nominally at any rate) at the teacher's own disposal',[102] seemed more appealing.

By the end of the century the increased numbers of trained, certified teachers who could claim higher pay freed the occupation from its old association with domestic service. In the 1881 census there were 123 000 women teachers. By 1911, the census revealed 183 298 women teachers, the majority of whom were unmarried (171 480).[103] There were marked differences in the nature of the work and working environments in teaching, from those involved in local elementary education through to those communities of women, described by Vincinus, in boarding schools and women's university colleges.[104] For the latter, Vincinus highlights the importance of 'discipline' as a cornerstone not only of how these communities operated but also of empowerment. This was a profession, she argues, which allowed women to discipline others and required in its turn considerable self-discipline. On both counts it enabled women to have legitimate occupancy of public space. For other teachers there was neither empowerment nor companionship. Teachers in rural areas, for example, had to contend with social and intellectual isolation over and above the usual teacher's lot of 'extraneous duties' and the 'number and many-sidedness of the responsibilities'.[105]

While hours were relatively short – in high schools, for example, from 9.00 am to 1.00 pm and 2.30 pm to 4.00 pm and the pay was better, ranging from £85 for a trained assistant to £150 in 1893,[106] both were considered to be unsatisfactory. Bulley and Whitley[107] pointed out that with high school work, the worst part 'is the correction of homework, which in many cases takes up most of the evenings

Figure 4.2 Gordon Memorial School, Cambridge Road, Kilburn. Nature study class in an elementary school, reproduced by permission of Hulton Deutsch Collection Limited.

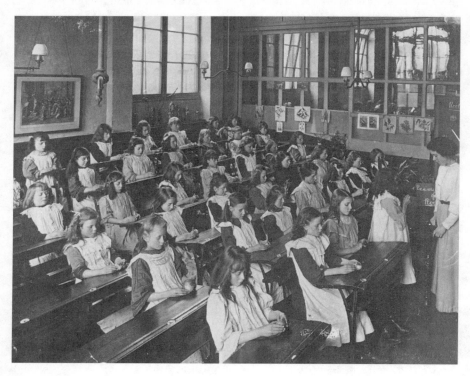

of the week. Such expenditure of energy is almost pure waste, and the mistress comes to school most mornings tired and dull.' On salaries, they pointed to the years of experience required before teachers earned anywhere near £160. Classroom teaching in many social settings was not easy: classes were often large and could be intimidating. Maintaining control, let alone the interest of the students, was often difficult. One London School Board elementary teacher in the 1880s recalled 'classes taught in one large room were noisy and nerve-racking, and large classes with rigid discipline tended to crush out anyone with refined manners or soul'.[108] Some teachers admitted that they sometimes found the routine 'deadly'.

Although there were Board of Education building regulations, many school buildings were badly built, presenting problems of ventilation, temperature and dirt. Thomas Oliver observed that the quality of air in schools was 'often anything but satisfactory' and 'usually worse than factories'.[109] The teaching of certain subjects presented teachers with particular hazards, including the nature of classrooms. This was especially so in practical subjects, where teachers were often not provided with specialized accommodation.

In the case of domestic-subjects' teachers, Annmarie Turnbull[110] found primary-source examples of accidents, exposure to noxious fumes, explosions caused by gas ovens and defective piping, crushed fingers and scalds. These teachers also experienced an inferior status, a downgrading of their skills, the struggle to claim the value of their subject and conflicts with colleagues and parents. All this contributed towards feelings of isolation and low self-esteem. Citing a report in a 1914 *The Times Educational Supplement* that noted 'a high proportion afflicted with nerves' among those teaching domestic economy, Turnbull concludes:

> Certainly for the period 1870–1914, the domestic subjects' teacher, as a result of poor training, class antagonisms, difficult working conditions, and what many considered to be a dubious role in the classroom, was isolated from the general life of the elementary school. In retrospect her susceptibility to 'nerves' is perhaps understandable.[111]

For teachers generally there seemed to be such a susceptibility. Despite a medical inspection of fitness for work at the end of their training, there were 'an alarming number of cases of consumption reported to the Benevolent Fund of the National Union of Teachers (NUT)' and the strain of a teacher's life resulted in an increasing number of nervous breakdowns.[112] The impact of teaching on health went beyond the environmental aspects of working conditions.

A source of frustration for teachers may have been that this profession was one of only a few limited opportunities for work. Collet summarizes this ambivalence:

> all they see is teaching. For those who have to earn their living, the only brain work offered them, and badly paid as it is, it is better paid than any other work done by women. The result . . . after a few years, growing weary and sick of it, tired of training intellects, and doubtful about the practical value of the training . . . discontented with a life for which they are naturally unsuited, and seeing no other career before them.[113]

In her own early career as an assistant mistress at a girls' school in Leicester, Collet expressed those same frustrations. In her diary[114] she records: 'I have been indulging in a fit of hysterical crying tonight. I feel so perfectly wretched and miserable and hopeless and worthless and tired. The worry of school and the feeling of impotence makes me feel miserable.' She goes on to express a wish to go to Girton or University College and to give up teaching or to emigrate. While there were undoubtedly aspects of teaching that women experienced as 'tiring', monotonous and a strain on their health, equally, attributions of 'nerves' were part of a wider discourse that sought to emphasize the negative consequences of women's attempts to participate in a professional, working and often urban life. The results of doing so in a climate hostile to women's attempts in this direction may have also taken a 'real' toll on their nerves. One teacher, who described her health as 'excellent usually', said her 'nerves seem the only vulnerable point . . . a term in X – brought me to the brink of a regular nervous breakdown.'[115]

Despite such perceived disadvantages, Holcombe argues that by the turn of the century working conditions and the professional status of elementary and secondary school teachers had greatly improved. At the same time, despite growing union-ization, issues relating to salaries, equal pay, security of tenure and opportunities for promotion remained in the forefront of the political struggle within the pro-fession.[116] Problems of teachers' health and wellbeing were subsumed in both these 'equal opportunities' areas and in the perception of a comparatively healthy occupation for women. In one of the last issues of the ER in 1909, Dora Jones wrote that of all the women's professions, 'teaching offers the best prospect', with shorter hours, long holidays and good salaries.[117] Although it took its toll on health in terms of the 'double-day' which, like many women workers, women teachers also worked, there was, at least until the early-twentieth century, evidence of a greater acceptance of married women in teaching. In a study of London's women teachers, Copelman shows that four weeks' leave for childbirth was the most common and that many stuck by their decision to combine marriage with a career.[118]

Nursing

Nursing exemplifies a particular approach to two important issues surrounding the politics of women's employment. First, here was an occupational struggle that remained largely outside contemporary feminist politics which, whatever its vari-ants and class interests, recognized the centrality of gender in the problems of working women and work opportunities. Second, it demonstrates how the politics of professionalizing an occupation left many aspects of the work itself, including occupational health issues, marginal or invisible. There have also been influences of this contemporary emphasis on the subsequent construction of nursing's occu-pational and professional history. In particular, although not unique to studies of women's occupations at this time, historians have focused on a 'single standard bearer' – Florence Nightingale, who had considerable political and social influence in her own time. Although her own biography and role in professional politics have been constantly reassessed,[119] this has failed to move nursing history away from its leading players and their own ideological construction of it as a field of women's work.

Before the late-nineteenth century there had been attempts to 'reform' hospital nursing. Vincinus has described this in terms of a transformation of conditions, recruits and the nature of the work.[120] It was an unskilled occupation drawn sub-stantially from older women, who earned 1s a day and 'some food and beer'. The hours were long, with little time off, although different staff were employed at night. But 'they were no worse off than . . . a maid of all work, who toiled similarly long hours and slept on a pallet in the kitchen'. Hospitals, however, harboured disease and dirt; and in transforming the occupation into one suitable for single middle-class women, nursing reformers had to confront the working environment and the hard work entailed in hospital nursing. The emphasis on cleansing until the 1880s was both on conditions and 'old style' nurses. Subsequently the metaphoric 'battle' against dirt and disease shifted in favour of a more 'maternal' vision of the requirements of the occupation: of women's attributes as ideally suited to nursing and of nursing as a 'feminine' occupation with a particular place within a healthcare division of labour. Central to reformed hospital nursing was its hierarchy of work and discipline involving women with control over women – and the purifying influence of hard work.

Nightingale's idea of a probationer, the new recruit to be trained in the discipline of the 'new' nursing, was that she would have her time filled with work, exercise and study. The result was a gruelling day. Vincinus cites an early probationer's day at St Thomas's in London: a 15-hour day with short breaks, seven days a week, which began at 6.00 am and ended with supper at 8.30 pm prayers at 9.00 pm and lights out at 10.30 pm.[121] In evidence to the Select Committee of the House of Lords on Metropolitan Hospitals[122] in the early 1890s the long hours were complained of most of all, with poor pay close behind. Booth also noted that 'It can hardly be doubted that the long hours exacted during training are injurious to the vigour of body and mind.'[123]

Long hours were partly a result of hospital governors' reluctance to increase staffing levels; but while many senior nurses and defenders of nursing admitted to long hours, they also maintained that these were not always arduous. In some hospitals, nurses, including probationers, did get two hours off-duty daily and three hours on Sundays (so they could go to church).[124] One matron and superintendent of nursing admitted she could 'not altogether defend' a 14-hour day, but said there were mitigating circumstances, in particular that there were times in the day when the work was not hard. However, there were also 'times when they work hard all day, and have hardly a moment to sit down; but I know also there are times when they do not have so much to do'.[125] Comparisons were made with earlier times with the argument that 'nurses are not nearly so hard worked nowadays as they were formerly',[126] although again despite an ideal of daily time-off, it was admitted this was not universal. There were similar issues with respect to pay: some considered £30 per year with food and lodging was 'reasonable' compared to other women. Probationers were paid considerably less (perhaps £12 in their second year). Matrons, the most senior rank, could earn up to £150.

Thus, by the late 1880s, nursing began to take on the 'classic contours of a women's occupation, overcrowding, stagnating wages, uncontrolled entry and varying standards of training'.[127] By the 1890s, pay was lower than for teachers or social workers. Much of the work done by probationers was hard physical work and domestic duties were onerous if not unpleasant (even though there were maids to do most of the scrubbing and heavy carrying). The early days of a probationer 'through long hours of duty entails constant strain on the mind and body . . . on the memory as well . . . [she] finds herself face to face with disease of every kind, loathsome sights, foul smells and death in all its pathetic sad variety'.[128] There was monotony too. Prudence Herbert wrote to her sisters:

The monotony of life is dreadful. Day by day and night by night we do exactly the same thing at the same time. It is deadly. I sometimes long even for an earthquake to break the monotony. New cases become part and parcel of the monotony. One man goes out and another comes in. He is simply a 'case' – an arm, a leg, or whatever else it may be. The bed is there and someone is in it. That is all.[129]

The dehumanizing consequences for nurses and, importantly, for the care delivered are all too apparent, yet a 'military type' discipline and regimented work practices were never questioned as the appropriate basis for nursing.

In addition to the demanding nature of the work itself, probationers were often left hungry after gulping down their meals, or not eating them at all, under the eyes of the waiting nurses who had been served first. Life in nurses' homes 'sound like a combination of boot-camp and boarding school'.[130] At all levels nurses experienced the tiredness of overwork and the constant rotation of duty. An emphasis on class divisions, exacerbated by an hierarchical work organization and often accompanied by the arbitrary exercise of authority served to undermine any feelings of solidarity or corporate/community loyalties. Vincinus describes the extent to which the world of nursing became a rule-bound, hierarchical and severely disciplined arena within a 'family' ideology that in fact bespoke the opposite.[131] These features were a way of covering-up mistakes and getting the work done. The drop-out rate was high at 30 per cent and it remained so until the beginning of the First World War.

It was difficult for hospitals to shake the legacy of their environment and for nursing to be seen as suitable for middle-class women. In the 1880s there were still recruitment problems: even the respectable domestic servant whom Nightingale thought might be suitable failed to offer her services. But even if demand was not met it did grow: by 50.8 per cent in the decade 1881–1891 and by 1911 there were 77 060 women nurses.[132] Inevitably, even for some middle-class women, hospital work was one escape from a useless life or an unhappy home. However, the age at entry of 23 to 25 as well as the low salary once trained probably acted as a deterrent.[133] Even private nursing, which was bettter paid, was a world of working-class workloads and ladylike manners.

Working conditions were probably at the root of both recruitment problems, and poor nursing care.[134] Protests about nursing's working conditions emerged mainly from outside nursing itself – or if it did not, this accusation was often made of those who raised such issues. In 1888 *The Westminster Review* warned that 'a sentimental glamour has been thrown over the services rendered to the sick' and called for better conditions for nurses, improved pay and pensions.[135] An investigation conducted from 1890 to 1892 in one London hospital revealed a pattern of overwork, poor food and insufficient attention to nurses' health. Reports such as these usually led to accusations and counter-accusations.[136] In fact, discontented voices raised from within reformed nursing about its conditions were often looked on as a lack of commitment. In writing about nursing in the mid-1890s, Bulley and Whitley argued that:

> Nurses were supposed to take it up in a missionary spirit . . . without regard to their own comfort and health. Unfortunately the more 'noble' a profession is considered, the greater is the tendency to neglect the material wellbeing of those concerned in it; and nurses have reason to feel the full force of this misplaced sentiment.[137]

Essentially, however, both the nursing and the medical establishment considered that such problems would disappear with recruitment from the 'right' social class, more training and rigorous regulation and discipline. One hospital matron,[138] for example, while accepting that 'conditions surrounding life of a hospital are trying in the extreme', argued that 'the mixed class in the nursing profession is, to a large extent, responsible for the bad qualities'. She said that 'the public send us inferior types to train' and they will accept bad conditions. This particular writer did consider that conditions should be improved and discipline lessened, although her class snobbery was noticeable.

Women's self-sacrificing nature was a desirable attribute in nursing and demands about conditions of work were viewed as a contravention of it; it was as if these concerns were not those of nursing. The *Nursing Record,* for example, opposed recommendations for a reduction in working hours on the grounds: 'I can imagine nothing more trying than an eight-hour shift. At the end of the twelve hours one hardly knows how to go and leave the worst cases, the interest and anxiety over them is so great.'[139] The acrimonious struggle between the various factions of nursing over political strategies for achieving professional status, particularly around the issue of registration, only served to obscure the difficulties of these conditions for nurses even further.[140] These professionalizing projects served the class interests of a few higher-status women, leaving the mass of hard-working nurses with the results of a collusion with medical men that defined nursing as a subordinate women's occupation and ensured their 'stranglehold' of power at the top.

Other issues emerged from time to time indicating that despite the nursing leadership's preoccupation with its professionalizing project, working nurses cared considerably about their 'lives on the treadmill' as one probationer described it.[141] One of these issues was the lack of pensions, especially as nurses were expected to retire when they were 50. Given that the majority of women who remained in nursing were single, this left them without any means of support for the rest of their lives. As a result, many went into private nursing. A second issue concerned 'living-in' which also resulted in poor living environments. Increasingly, however, voices were raised about the 'requirement' to live-in. They argued it restricted opportunities for recreation and cultural activities and indicated more general frustrations with confined lifestyles. In the early-twentieth century, when these concerns were increasingly raised, one critic of the demand argued: 'If a woman can't live in, work in, eat in and even think in, she should choose different work with fewer demands.'[142]

Nursing work did expand in this period, as hospitals themselves grew, although problems with the census categories makes precise numbers difficult to estimate.[143] There was no legal definition until the Registration Act 1919. Maggs suggests there were 12 500 nurses by the end of the century, with only a quarter of them properly trained and qualified.[144]

Hospital or private nursing were not the only arena for women's nursing work. A relative lack of historical knowledge about women's work in asylums and poor-law infirmaries, for example, is another result of preoccupations with 'reformed' hospital nursing. (District-nursing and health-visiting have fared better, although they are not discussed here.) Asylum nurses suffered from the general negative conception of asylums and asylum patients. Asylum nurses, according to Carpenter,[145] were paid less than hospital nurses and engaged in equally incessant labour for long days. Pay of £19 per year for a working day from 6.00 am to 8.00 pm with a two-hour break for meals and one day's leave a week could actually be longer because of staff shortages.[146] The private nursing of such patients was even more unremitting as nurses often had to sleep with their 'disturbed' clients.[147] Even towards the end of the period, a study conducted by the National Association of Asylum Workers Union as part of a campaign to reduce hours found that in 1912 in all but two out of 31 hospitals, men and women worked more than 70 hours a week.

In a House of Commons Select Committee in 1911, witnesses justified the long hours on the grounds that 'duties were light' and that they were required to ensure continuity of patient care. One superintendent defended the practice of one day off a month: 'I think the effect of too much leave, too much freedom, too many hours off duty, would be distinctly demoralising, especially to female staff.'[148] It was argued that some of the hours on duty were 'pleasant, with walks, drives, tea outdoors and entertainments'.[149]

Such a view did not seem to be shared by asylum nurses. The low esteem in which asylum nursing was held was demoralizing, too, not just publicly but also by those who entered the occupation as 'a last resort'. Despite expressed wishes that it could mirror general nursing it remained an inferior order, especially for women, although many asylum nurses shared similar vocational ideas to the general nurse. Probably more important than the dangerous and trying characteristics of the work as attendants saw it, was the social isolation engendered by its physical separation, its institutional containment and contamination by ideas of 'insanity'. Long hours and living-in contributed to an institutionalization of both staff and patients: an 'occupational hazard' not recognized until much later in the twentieth century.[150]

For those who nursed in poor-law infirmaries, conditions were even more 'deplorable'. 'Of anything that could really be called nursing there was not a trace, nor was there any order, cleanliness or the most elementary comfort.'[151] The patients themselves were seen as unattractive: 'The average patient is an aged, worn-out being upon whom no nursing miracle can be performed.'[152] An indication that it was largely working-class women, usually 'the dregs of the population who could not obtain work even in hospitals' who were recruited to this work was the provision of £3 10s per year beer money. For patients there was little care, rather 'fear and terror'.[153] Some sought to reform poor-law infirmaries and women's role in relation to them, notably Louisa Twining, herself a Poor Law Guardian, but the debates about nursing work and nursing conditions were dominated by the 'reform' of hospital nursing.

Women Factory Inspectors

The particular role of women factory inspectors in relation to the health consequences of work for women generally is discussed in Chapter 7. Here we consider their working lives and conditions. 'Pioneering' a new occupation for women imposed its own stresses as well as its rewards. Women entrants experienced day-to-day sexism from male colleagues and constant threats to any autonomy they were able to achieve for their work. The work of women factory inspectors, however, was far from the regular hours experienced by women clerks or other professionals in the civil service. The peripatetic nature of their brief meant they were constantly travelling and not always in comfort, including travel by 'jaunting car' in Ireland.[154] In Ireland in 1897, Lucy Deane had shipped her bicycle. She describes how she walked or rode in inclement weather, 'long lonely walks undertaken (often by special request after dark) in wet and stormy weather'.[155] Hilda Martindale describes her time in Ireland as 'strenuous', moving from hotel to hotel, without office or clerk, having to send typing to London and undertaking long journeys.[156] These problems were not peculiar to a posting to this part of the country. It was not just travelling that was difficult for a woman alone, but also the fact that their work often took them out at night. There are many examples of how they would rise before 4.00 am to catch illegal overtime. Rose Squire reports that in all these kinds of night-time detection visits, she was never once molested in 15 years.[157] However, Violet Markham recounts that May Abraham was 'often frightened'. In one incident she was on the back stairs of a sweat-shop when the owner 'sprang out on them from the landing with a knife and the words, "if you come back here it will be the worse for you"'.[158] Such intimidating situations were probably not uncommon. Travelling alone and staying in accommodation alone, they were constantly 'out of place'; the frequent assumption of a 'pretence' role[159] must have been difficult and isolating. Rose Squire also described conditions in one of her hotels 'which could scarcely be called waterproof. When gales blew the peat fire in the sitting-room and bedroom smoked, the carpet rose in billows from the floor, rain penetrated the walls – even the bed was damp.'[160]

The sheer scale of inspectors' work in trying to meet the demands of inspection and special enquiry with a small staff meant that, like many of the women for whom they had responsibility, they were overworked and exhausted as a result. Rose Squire[161] remembered the impact on their health of being 'unable to meet anything like the demand made upon us. I do wonder if official supervisor at headquarters ever gave a thought to the strain on the workman [*sic*] in the task of cutting a coat out of insufficient cloth.' These shortcomings were compounded by the fact that they felt unrewarded and frustrated at the lack of support for the bureaucratic aspects of their work. As Adelaide Anderson put it in her 1900 Report:

> without clerical help and travelling as they never have done before, the able workers become steadily more over-strained as their years of service increase, and since no promotion is provided, no material encouragement lightens or rewards strenuous work.[162]

A perennial problem for the Principal Lady Inspector and her staff was the high incidence of sickness absence, often for prolonged periods. In 1896, Lucy Deane had typhoid and finally left the service in 1908 because of ill-health. The causes of these absences might not have been due to their occupations and women's health did not show any marked class differential, so sickness was a common experience.[163] But strenuous work in poor conditions can add to the risk of other infections and, as with working-class women, professional women were also exposed to a combination of factors that impinged upon their health and general wellbeing.

It is evident from this chapter that even when the conditions of work were materially or environmentally different, that all shared a relative devaluation of the skills and aptitudes women required *vis-à-vis* men, rewards which mirrored this devaluation and confirmed the lower social worth of women in general, as well as their lesser eligibility to enter and work in the public domain. There were few occupations that escaped these demeaning consequences, even when women did create communities that offered some opportunity for the exercise of power and control over the work and others. All too often such advantages accrued to a few, resulting in some women being party to the continued exploitation of other women. It was difficult for there to be a sense of 'sisterhood' that could overcome the rigidity of Victorian class structure, and class snobbery persisted within and between women's occupations. Equally, as Levine[164] argues, despite the divisions within feminism over work and working conditions, there was also a commonality in an identification of shared experiences of being working women that sometimes overrode those of class, and to this extent 'first wave feminism' did foster gender politics. For some occupational arenas the absence from 'first wave' feminist politics, in particular nursing, may have contributed to their inability to move outside of 'family' and class-based ideologies of appropriate work for women, and prevented the formation of an occupation that created good working conditions and opportunities for all entrants.

For some new occupations, eventual unionization would enable conditions to be addressed to a greater extent, while others would live with a legacy that 'dangerous' working conditions belonged elsewhere – to the factory. There certainly were not the 'dangers' we have seen in Chapters 1 and 2, but conditions were not good, and the organization of work and the social relations of a gender based division of labour and patriarchal control in the workplace were omnipresent.

Notes

1   I do not want to imply here that studies of middle-class women's employment did not discuss such issues. Rather, I emphasize that many incorporate it with other issues and that in most the relationship of the conditions they discuss to health remain relatively under-explored. I have also omitted agriculture for consideration in this book.
2   Murray (1984) *Strong-Minded Women,* p.328.
3   Butler (1916) *Domestic Service: An Enquiry by the Women's Industrial Council* p.1.
4   Ibid.
5   Higgs (1986) 'Domestic service and household production', in John (Ed.).
6   Ibid., p.133.
7   See Hakim (1979 and 1980).
8   Booth (1905) *Life and Labour of the People of London* Series 2, Vol. 4.
9   Butler (1916) *Domestic Service: An Enquiry.*

10 Oliver (1902) *The Dangerous Trades* Chapter LIX on the miscellaneous trades contains a section on domestic servants pp.799–800.
11 *Royal Commission on Labour*, PP XXXVII, 1893–4.
12 *Shafts*, April 1893, in an article called 'Reform in domestic life as required by scientific sociology', p.26.
13 Ibid.
14 Oliver (1902) *The Dangerous Trades* pp.799–800.
15 This is also confirmed by an analysis of the occupations of patients in Scottish asylums in the mid-nineteenth century. In Glasgow, domestic occupations accounted for 37.11 per cent of which 13.9 per cent were domestic servants and 8.12 per cent domestics. See Rice (1981) 'Madness and industrial society' pp.214–16.
16 There are too many relevant studies to list all of them, but see Verbrugge (1985) 'Gender and health: an update on hypotheses and evidence'. The connection between paid work and health remains an important part of contemporary research and debates on health inequalities. See Arber (1991) 'Class: paid employment and family roles' and Bartley, Popay and Plewis (1992) 'Domestic conditions, paid employment and women's experience of ill-health'.
17 Bornat (1986) 'What about that lass of yours being in the union?' in Davidoff and Westover (Eds) (1986) p.80.
18 Westover (1986) 'To fill the kids tummies', in Davidoff and Westover (Eds) p.64.
19 Butler (1916) p.73.
20 Ibid., p.28.
21 Ibid., p.16, emphasis in the original.
22 Ibid., p.51.
23 Ibid., p.54.
24 Higgs (1986) 'Domestic service and household production' pp.139 and 142.
25 Butler (1916) p.36.
26 Ibid., p.35.
27 Ibid. These examples are taken from testimony on pp.37–9 of the report.
28 Originally published in *Nineteenth Century* in 1893. An excerpt was reprinted in Murray *Strong-minded Women* (1984).
29 Black, ibid., p.339.
30 Butler (1916) p.11.
31 Report of the TUC Congress in 1909, in the files of the Gertrude Tuckwell Collection.
32 See Dingwall (1977) 'Collectivism, regionalism and feminism: health visiting and British social policy 1850–1975; Davies (1988) 'The health visitor as mother's friend: a woman's place in public health 1900–1914'.
33 See especially Davin (1978) 'Imperialism and motherhood', which documents the wide range of interventions considered to regulate working-class family life and conditions with respect to infant health.
34 See the report of the TUC Congress 1909 in the Gertrude Tuckwell Collection.
35 *Shafts*, April 1893, p.26.
36 Holcombe (1973) *Victorian Ladies at Work* Chapter V, p.108.
37 *Commissioners' Reports on Working of Factory and Workshops Act 1876*, PP XXIX 1 and XXX I.
38 Booth (1905) *Conditions of Work in London*.
39 Holcombe (1973) p.101.
40 *Report of Conditions of Employment of Shop Assistants, Milliners, Dressmakers and Mantle Makers in Provincial Towns 1893–4*, PP XXXVII.

41 Collet (1892–3) *Report on Conditions of Work in London, 1892–3* PP XXXVII, p.550.
42 Bulley and Whitley (1894) *Women's Work*, section on shop assistants.
43 Evidence before the Select Committee of the House of Lords on the early closing of shops, PP VI, 1901.
44 Collet (1893–4) *Report on Conditions in Provincial Towns 1893–4*, PP XXXVII, pp.635–6.
45 This was argued by Margaret Bondfield in an excerpt from her autobiography, in Murray (1984) p.359.
46 Holcombe (1973) p.113.
47 Black (1907) *Sweated Industry and the Minimum Wage* Chapter 3, p.59.
48 Collet (1893–4) *Report on Conditions of Work in London, 1893–4,* PP XXXVII, p.551.
49 Bondfield (1899) 'The conditions under which shop assistants work' p.278.
50 Black (1907) cites this example, p.56.
51 Orme *Conditions of Work of Barmaids, Waitresses and Bookkeepers Employed in Hotels, Restaurants, Public Houses and Places of Refreshment 1893–4*, PP XXXVII.
52 Ibid.
53 Ibid., p.703.
54 Miss Irwin's *Evidence to the Select Committee on the Early Closing of Shops* pp.5–6.
55 Bailey (1990) 'Parasexuality and glamour' p.160.
56 Bailey (1990) ibid., p.162.
57 *English Woman's Review* July 1880.
58 Described in an excerpt from her autobiography reproduced in Murray (1984) p.359.
59 Bulley and Whitley (1894) *Women's Work* p.51.
60 Ibid.
61 Bondfield (1899) 'Conditions under which shop assistants work' p.58.
62 Black (1907) p.50.
63 Bondfield (1899) p.58.
64 Holcombe (1973) pp.117–22: reference to the importance of Margaret Bondfield, p.120.
65 A prominent campaigner was Sir Charles Dilke, who also took up other causes on behalf of employment and women. He tried to introduce Bills on the number of occasions in the 1890s and early 1900s.
66 Holcombe (1973).
67 Departmental Committee on the Truck Acts 1908, PP LIX, Vols 1–3. Deane's *Evidence*, Vol. 1, p.70. Holcombe (1973) details the struggle around the minimum wage, 'truck' and living-in, pp.132–8.
68 Anderson (1988) *The White Blouse Revolution* is the title of his collected essays on the increasing 'feminization' of clerical and office work.
69 *Shafts*, 12 November 1892, p.31.
70 Zimmeck (1986) 'Jobs for the girls: the expansion of clerical work for women', in John (Ed.) (1986) and Lewis (1988) 'Women Clerical Workers in the late Nineteenth and Early Twentieth Century', in Anderson (Ed.) (1988).
71 Ibid., p.166.
72 Ibid., p.167.
73 *TUC, Annual Report of Congress 1912*.
74 Cited in Holcombe (1973) p.149.
75 Dohrn (1988) 'Pioneers in a dead-end profession', in Anderson (Ed.) p.57.
76 Morley (Ed.) (1914) *Women Workers in Seven Professions* Section VI, p.282.
77 Ibid., p.281.
78 Ibid., p.284.

79 *Special Report on Hours and Conditions of Work in Typewriting Offices, Annual Report of HM Chief Inspector of Factories 1910*, PP XXII.

80 Holcombe (1973) pp.157–61.

81 Ibid., p.155.

82 Lewis (1988) 'Women clerical workers'.

83 Morley (Ed.) (1914) pp.286–7.

84 Ibid., Section V, p.273.

85 Ibid., p.263.

86 Holcombe (1973) p.152.

87 Cited in Morley p.260.

88 Zimmeck (1986) p.160.

89 Ibid., p.160.

90 The concept of 'profession' is a theoretically contested one. Which occupations may be called 'professions' or how they come to claim 'professional' status is a subject in its own right. Here I use 'profession' to include mainly middle-class occupations which it was claimed opened up professional work for women in this period.

91 Witz (1992) *Professions and Patriarchy* discusses the role of gender in the professionalizing tactics of the healthcare professions in the late-nineteenth century in these terms.

92 Hollis (1987) *Ladies Elect* suggests this was also important in women's involvement in aspects of local government.

93 Vincinus (1985) *Independent Women*. Chapter 6 is about settlement work and health-visiting. See Dingwall, Rafferty and Webster (1988) *An Introduction to the Social History of Nursing* Chapter 9. A whole issue of the *Health Visitor* (1987) Vol. 60, 5, is devoted to historical aspects of health-visiting.

94 See Sheavyn (1911) *Professional Women* p.83 and Collet (1902) *Educated Working Women.*

95 Collet (1902) ibid., p.16.

96 Sheavyn (1911) pp.88–90.

97 Jeune (1893) *Paid Employment for Women* p.11.

98 See Bateson (1895) *Professional Women upon Their Professions* and O'Neill and Barnett (1888) *Our Nurses and the Work they Have to Do.*

99 Collet (1902) See especially the chapter on 'Prospects of marriage for women'.

100 Excerpt reprinted in Murray (1984) p.274.

101 Ibid., p.271 and in Rice (1981) the figures for the professional sector in Scottish asylums showed 14.8 per cent as teachers (although they were not categorized as governesses, the majority at this time probably were so).

102 Bulley and Whitley (1894) p.9.

103 Holcombe (1973) gives figures for the proportions of women in different professional groups in different census reports in her Appendix. These figures for teachers are on p.202.

104 Vincinus (1985) *Independent Women* Chapters 4 and 5.

105 Morley (1914) p.48.

106 Bulley and Whitley (1894) pp.10–11.

107 Ibid., pp.9–10.

108 Clara Grant, cited in Purvis (1989) *Hard Lessons* p.39.

109 Oliver (1906) *Maladies Caused by the Air we Breathe Inside and Outside the Home* p.19.

110 Turnbull (1994) "An isolated missionary" pp.89–96.

111 Ibid., p.95.
112 Morley (1914) p.48.
113 Collet (1902) pp.13–14.
114 Collet *Diary of a Young Assistant Mistress 1878–1885*. This entry is dated 2 March 1883.
115 This example is cited by Collet (1902) in her essay on 'The experience of middle-class working women' p.77.
116 Holcombe (1973) pp.31–8.
117 EWR, October 1909, reprinted in Murray (1984) pp.322– 4.
118 Copelman (1986) 'A new comradeship between men and women: family marriage and London's women teachers' 1870–1914.
119 See Smith (1982) *Florence Nightingale: Reputation and Power*; Maggs (1983) *The Origins of General Nursing* and Baly (1986) *Florence Nightingale and the Nursing Legacy* among many other examples.
120 Vincinus (1985) 'Reformed hospital nursing: discipline. and cleanliness', in *Independent Women* Chapter 3.
121 Ibid., p.91.
122 *Reports of the Select Committee of the House of Lords on the Metropolitan Hospitals, First Report* 1890, PP XVI and *Third Report* 1892, PP XIII.
123 Booth (1905) *Life and Labour of the People of London* second series, No. 5, p.198.
124 Gilpin (1923) *Scenes from Hospital Life*. This edited collection of letters from Prudence Herbert to her sisters reveals a number of aspects of a nurse's existence. Unfortunately we do not know when and where Prudence was based. She refers to this off-duty pattern on p.20.
125 Stewart (1890) *Murray's Magazine* p.168,
126 Burdett (1890) *Nurses Food, Work and Recreation* p.13.
127 Vincinus (1985) p.102.
128 Wilson and Wilson (1893) 'Hospital nursing', in Jeune *Paid Work for Women* p.98.
129 In Gilpin (Ed.) (1923) pp.85– 6.
130 Vincinus (1985) p.109. Prudence Herbert describes the problem of eating in terms of 'by the time the plate reached you everyone had finished . . . we reluctantly put down our knives and forks', in Gilpin (1923) p.21.
131 Vincinus (1985) ibid., pp.107–8, discusses these features.
132 For a detailed discussion of recruitment in this period see Maggs 'Nurse recruitment to four provincial hospitals 1881–1921', in Davies (Ed.) (1980a) *Rewriting Nursing History*.
133 Musson Matron of the General Hospital in Birmingham', in Morley (Ed.) (1914) p.178.
134 Johnston (1902a) 'The case against hospital nurses', *Nineteenth Century and After* Vol. 5, pp.595–603.
135 Cited in Vincinus p.112.
136 The Report mentioned here was on the London Hospital and was discussed in the *Nursing Record* in January 1891. There were also letters throughout the year. There had been a similar controversy earlier about Guys Hospital: see Lonsdale 'The present crisis at Guys Hospital', *The Nineteenth Century* Vol. 7 (1880) pp.677–84 and William Gull in the same issue pp.884–9.
137 Bulley and Whitley (1894) pp.28–9.
138 Rae (1902) 'Lady Superintendent of Coventry and Warwickshire Hospital', *Nineteenth Century and After* pp.972–4.

139   Cited in Vincinus (1985) p.119.
140   See Witz (1992); Maggs (1983) *The Origins of General Nursing* and Dingwall, Rafferty and Webster (1988) *An Introduction to a Social History of Nursing*, which give accounts of these struggles.
141   Stoney cited in Vincinus (1985) p.120. (This original document was reported lost by the British Library because of bomb damage.)
142   Vincinus discusses these two examples pp 117–18. The quote is from an article from *The Nursing Times* (1908) **4**, p.818.
143   Davies (1980b) 'Making sense of the census'.
144   Maggs (1983) pp.8–9.
145   Carpenter (1980) 'Asylum nursing before 1914', in Davies (Ed.) (1980a) *Rewriting Nursing History*.
146   Morley (Ed.) (1914) p.201.
147   Clifford (1893) 'Care of insane patients', in Jeune (Ed.) *Paid Employment for Women*.
148   Cited in Carpenter (1980) p.133.
149   Clifford (1893) in Jeune (Ed.).
150   This concept of 'institutionalization' was developed by Erving Goffman in his classic study *Asylums* (1961).
151   Seymer (1932) *A General History of Nursing*.
152   De Pledge (1895) in Bateson (Ed.) p.44.
153   Holcombe (1973) p.71.
154   Hilda Martindale describes such journeys in Ireland in *From One Generation to Another* (1944).
155   Deane *Business Diaries* 16 November 1897.
156   Martindale (1944) p.93.
157   Squire (1927) *Thirty Years in the Public Service: An Industrial Retrospect* p.67.
158   Markham (1949) *May Tennant: A Portrait* p.25.
159   For example Adelaide Anderson (1922) *Women in the Factory* describes assuming the role of a lady novelist in a hotel full of male guests lest her real purpose be discovered.
160   Ibid., p.83.
161   Ibid., p.132.
162   *Annual Report of Her Majesty's Women Inspectors for 1900*, PP X, 1901.
163   Johansson (1977) 'Sex and death in Victorian England', in Vincinus (Ed.) *A Widening Sphere: Changing Roles for Victorian Women*.
164   Levine (1990a) *Feminist Lives in Victorian England*.

Part II

Responses

Chapter 5

State Intervention: 'Protective' Legislation and Women's Health

It will now be evident from the data and discussion in Part I that there were conditions of labour and aspects of women's lives which threatened their health and wellbeing. Only some of these threats were attended to by lay activists, reformers, or by the State and its officials, who sought remedy for them. The selective focus on aspects of work and working conditions was directly related to gender divisions in the labour market, work and wider society. In terms of responses to perceived problems the State is an important starting point, because it was views of the State and its function in relation to the regulation of working conditions that in large measure conditioned the responses made by others.

Political struggles around working conditions increasingly incorporated a consideration of the role of the State. Some parties to the activities and debates about women's work were also inextricably part of a developing State apparatus. As such they had concerns about defining the parameters of what would be taken as 'the problem', and with the delivery of regulatory requirements and their enforcement. Important in this respect were the roles of the medical profession and the women's factory inspectorate which are examined in the next two chapters. Here, after some general points about the State and society as a locus for response by way of introduction, the analysis will be concerned with the relation of the State to a variety of political interests, but in particular to those of industrial capital – employers and manufacturers – and of men and women workers. However, an important focus for discussion will be an assessment of a regulatory strategy through 'protective' legislation for the prevention of occupational health problems in women.

By way of introduction the concept of the State itself requires discussion, recognizing that it is a contested theoretical area that also has empirical consequences. I am not going to engage in theoretical debate at this juncture, but some operational definition is clearly needed. It is axiomatic that whatever formulation is used it must provide for a consideration of the different positions of men and women in their relations with the State. I am defining the State 'as a complex conglomeration of agencies and institutions claiming some ultimate authority'.[1] However, it is neither a monolith or autonomous, so it does not act in unison, nor are its practices or authority immune from wider processes and interests including struggles within the State itself. For my purposes, the State will empirically include the apparatus, agencies and personnel of centralized national government, including the administrative systems that do the work of government, but also local government.

In the period considered here the latter is particularly important, since a characteristic of State formation and governance in nineteenth-century Britain was its local and limited character, including the institutions of social administration.[2] However, a focus on legislation does result in an emphasis on more centralized and bureaucratic forms of State action. There are also agencies who are more or less tied to the State, such as those who are established, and paid for, by government although these will not be a major focus in this instance. State intervention will encompass those activities initiated by the State, including policy-making and legislation, and the work of its own officials this necessitates.

This working definition will provide a basis for an examination of the political struggles around women, work and health that were occurring within the various and diverse interests within the State, as much as they were between the State and other interested parties. Thus although it is necessary to sometimes refer to 'the State', this is more often in reference to a final outcome of complex intentions, interests and negotiations. To this extent any piece of factory legislation is a product of the State, but it is equally important to appreciate the diversity of actors and the social processes that preceded it. Thus a final important aspect of the analysis to follow will be to examine the extent to which the broader concept of social interests can help to elucidate the idea that State action is motivated and intentional. Asking whose interests were served enables a consideration of the extent to which gender and class as key structural variables in any such analysis were important in respect of this particular aspect of late nineteenth and early twentieth-century British society. The focus for this analysis is factory legislation as 'protective' legislation.

State and Society 1880–1914

Some appreciation of the relation of State and society is a necessary context for what can only be an initial attempt to consider the complexities of State intervention in women's work in this period. The idea of the State and the role it should assume in public life – in social, economic and even private matters – was undergoing considerable change at this time. The political struggles around working conditions, and about women's work and issues of the nation's health, were important in the development and practical consequences of working out a new *modus operandi* for State action. The case of intervention in women's work is therefore a means of testing out interpretations of State action in different historical conditions. Hall and Schwartz[3] have argued that from the 1880s there was a 'profound crisis' in the British State, and that the period was marked by a discontinuity from the *laissez-faire* period which preceded it. In particular, it is argued, there was a qualitatively different form of State organization and social regulation which resulted in increasing intervention in social and economic life. At the same time, 'modern' forms of political representation made their appearance. The consolidation of monopoly capitalism, and the redefinition of the boundaries between State and civil society, had consequences for the nature of politics itself. It is suggested that forms of political representation and activism which had previously been class-based were transferred into interests that were both within and between class divisions, such as those arising from a fracturing of the working-class according to skill, and alignments such as those evidenced in the strong feminist movement that were no longer class-based.

> The effect of the feminist campaigns was to activate new sources of contention and antagonism, as well as new potentialities for alliances *across* popular movements of the day.[4]

These features of political representation and activism are visible in the responses examined in this chapter and the following chapters of the book. While there were working-class male interests in 'protective' legislation, they were not shared with working-class women; and there were middle-class and working-class women whose struggles with male trade unionists and with the State shared an experience of structurally based discrimination. There were also divisions between women, as will be evident in the discussion in Chapter 8, but these were as much within the middle-class as between the classes. The reconstruction of State boundaries and its role were thus in part necessitated by new political forces which were positioned against it. Out of this redefinition emerged the concept of a State which served 'collective' interests, a redrafting of citizenship where it could be seen to act on behalf of others. By assuming conciliation and arbitration powers, and in legislating for wages, the State assumed responsibilities which had traditionally been those of trade unions.

The demand for 'protective' legislation by some feminists was also a result of a failure of unionism. In this context, the problems of working conditions and women's factory labour became part of what was defined as the national interest. The economic decline relative to Germany and the USA, the crisis of Empire (posed acutely by the Home Rule for Ireland crisis) and the increasing evidence of poor standards of physical ill-health could all be linked to the industrial system. The stability of the social body necessitated State intervention for the collective good. 'Protection' of individuals was necessary to 'protect' all, as Clementina Black argued in relation to sweating:

> women cannot protect themselves, they are beyond the reach of organisation . . . It is the state alone which can take care of them, protect them against the rapacity of the oppressor and, in protecting them, protect itself also . . . No society can be sound in health which has this undrained morass of wretchedness.[5]

New categories or identities would become targets for intervention. As we saw in Chapter 3, the 'unfit mother' became such a category, requiring its own bureaucratic system, agencies and 'experts'. As Foucault has argued,[6] new 'social subjects' were a focus of 'proliferating discourses'.

Already existing discourses and ideologies were utilized, and in part provided a collectivist basis for the new 'problems'. In this period, it is evident that Eugenics and Social Darwinism served such as purpose, being visible in debates about factory legislation, education, sexuality, birth control, and the regulation of domestic and urban environments.

Another important aspect of the specific discourse around the State and reform was the imputation of moral and ethical responsibility. A number of different aspects of this moral dimension have been emphasized. For some, this responsibility represented the 'protection' of the weak, to promote moral conduct, largely by defining and then circumscribing the action and powers of others, as in the domain of sexuality.[7] In the context of factory reform, the idea of moral responsibility was closely aligned with a conception of progress, in which, it is argued, the law and State action reflect and sanction an already existing community-based normative framework.[8] Such needed constraints were underpinned by a rhetoric of factories and workers that distinguished between the 'good' and the 'bad', the 'deserving' and 'undeserving', extending to a characterization of many women workers as 'rough' or 'low' and their working conditions as 'inflicting injury on the moral character'.[9] Gray argues that the construction of moral responsibility was as important as the amelioration of conditions.[10] The defence of factory legislation by one contemporary commentator was that,

> The regulation of factories by law rests on the broad principle that it is the right and duty of the State to restrict the freedom of individual action in the interests of the community . . . Factory legislation is a history of conflict waged between humanitarian impulses and commercial interests.[11]

Thus, moral responsibility, industrial efficiency, and a new sense of collective interests, not least in the 'condition of England', resulted in a shift in thinking about the relationship of State and society.

However, despite considerable changes during this period, it is questionable whether they should be characterized as a major disjuncture: it was a change in degree and orientation. There had been factory legislation since the 1830s alongside forms of enquiry and intervention in respect of this and many other aspects of social life, especially in relation to conditions in towns and the relief of the poor.[12] There were also elements visible in the period where *laissez-faire* ideologies remained strong. As Hall and Schwartz argue, *laissez-faire* is not 'an absence of controls but a specific means by which market forces are politically regulated', and thus some intervention or regulation by the State might be necessary to preserve a 'free' market, such as the prevention of monopoly.[13] These authors, however, do consider the 1880s marked a profound discontinuity in social and political development.

There was an expansion of State institutions and practices, complemented and constituted by demands from below, which themselves represented new forms of politics. With a new concept of social instead of individual rights, and situations where traditional political mechanisms had failed to deliver reform, it was perhaps not surprising that the State might be viewed as an alternative. Equally, the State may itself have failed such interests, not least because those rights the State sought preserved the existing systems of class and gender relations.

The State and 'Protective' Factory Legislation: Precedents

Despite the idea that this period saw a transformation in ideas about, and practices of, the State, State involvement with problems of working conditions within the industrial system began much earlier in the century. But the idea of intervention had developed slowly and in a limited direction. In essence the orientation of that intervention was with the employment and hours of work of children and young persons (that is those up to eighteen years of age) and in a few industries – principally textiles and mining. A variety of Committees and Factory Commissions in the 1830s and 1840s, alongside articles and pamphlets – many produced under the auspices of local literary and statistical societies – had identified the possible harmful consequences of industrial work not only to children and young people, but also to women. At the outset, however, despite the inclusion of women in the debates, there did not seem to be any explicit intention to include women within the legislation.[14] In fact, it might be argued that outside the specific case of the exclusion of women from underground mine work in 1842, the inclusion of women within legislation as a 'special class' of worker, like children, in need of protection happened more by 'fiat' than design. In the case of the 1842 Mines Act, the major impetus for prohibition seemed to have been a construction of such hard physical labour in the presence of men as morally reprehensible.[15]

As noted above, such moral dimensions continued to feature in the demands for other forms of 'protective' legislation, although there does seem to have been some special attention to moral issues in this early prohibition that were not so evident elsewhere. The early debates were important, however, in that they undoubtedly served to create a climate of opinion in which such limitations were perceived to be 'natural' under the circumstances. In the debate around the 1844 Bill, Sir Robert Peel called for women to be included:

> read the account of lace manufacture which are not to be touched by the Bill, read the account of the hosiery trade, and above all read the account of the dressmakers and milliners employed in this very town. Is it right to leave these untouched?[16]

The possibility that work might be harmful to women's health and that there were social consequences arising from their employment were ideas that were already relatively entrenched by the 1860s – and thus so was the potential 'need' for legislation.

It has been suggested that this early approach of using factory legislation to remedy those 'special' wrongs identified and enabling regulation aimed at prevention to be targeted effectively also served to deflect attention from the need to control industry more generally. In making such an analysis, Barbara Hutchins, who took a special interest in factory legislation, saw the 1867 Factories Act as evidence of an important change in thinking:

> From this time we see the old concept of factory legislation as an exceptional remedy for troubles in exceptional industries abandoned and questions of regulation thenceforth hinges rather on the classes of persons employed.[17]

So while women had been included within the legislation of 1844 and 1847, it was the 1867 Factories Act that quite explicitly set out to regulate some conditions only in respect of women and young girls, notably in this case the first recognition of the 'dangerous trades', with the measure to prohibit them eating food in rooms where dangerous processes were carried out. To this extent, it is probably right to argue that the 'protective' principle of factory legislation as applying to classes of worker, and which treated women as if they were children, was established at this time. However, it is also the case that the older focus on 'troubles' in exceptional industries did not entirely disappear. Both investigation and factory legislation seemed to proceed by selecting problems that were industry specific, and specific industries, while considering only women, young persons and children within them.

By the 1870s there was widespread agitation around the 'protective' principle. There was opposition by feminist and labour activists, with support from politicians, who not only objected to the theoretical grounds for 'protection', but also to the potential practical impact of such legislation on women's work opportunities. From the outset, in the two decades prior to 1880s, the parameters of the political struggle around 'protective' legislation were set in terms of the right of the State to interfere in economic and labour matters, to interfere particularly in women's work, and in the approach that should be taken to ameliorate conditions.

The hostility of feminists and women union activists to the State at this time was not surprising given their lack of access as legitimate political agents to the political process. This view was often expressed as the ultimate injustice of a State that proposed to take action with respect to their work. It was perceived as men helping other men to preserve aspects of the public domain as rightly belonging to men, and perpetuating women's dependence. Josephine Butler, a feminist activist better known for her campaigns against State interference elsewhere (The Contagious Diseases Act), also drew attention to the fact that factory legislation was based on false principles, and against the interests of women.[18] Activists, pursuing such arguments, achieved some early successes in limiting the legislation. Henry Fawcett MP, a long-term supporter of 'equal rights' feminist demands, having failed to remove the category 'women' from the 1876 legislation, was able in 1878 to secure an amendment to remove domestic workshops – that is, private homes, if no children or young people were employed – from the legislation.

Despite arguments about whether or not the State should interfere at all, the development of legislation continued, in particular moving to consolidate that which had occurred to date in the 1860s and 1870s. It was, however, still on a small scale, and a tentative and essentially limited approach was taken. In an earlier paper, Helen Mockett and I[19] identified three main assumptions that established the case that women's employment required State intervention. First, that work threatened women's health in ways that was not the case for men; second, that there were particular social problems which resulted from their paid employment, expressed mainly through the neglect of domestic and maternal duty; and third, women were more susceptible to the adverse consequences of employment and therefore required special 'protection'. Opponents contested all these assumptions. We also emphasized that the idea of 'protection' encompassed 'needs' which arose from both a physiological predisposition in women to ill-health, and women's socially and politically dependent position. These features can be repeatedly discerned in the debates about whether or not State action with respect to women's work was desirable. Despite countervailing assertions, by the 1880s the idea of 'protection' was firmly established and the grounds for it widely accepted. In 1900, for example, Mr Talbot, MP for Oxford, told the House:

> much might be said for and against the protection of adult men, but what he was contending for was protection for a class whom everyone wished to see protected and who *could not protect themselves.*[20]

The development of State intervention in women's employment in the form of legislation is therefore only one dimension that needs to be considered. What these precedents established was the role of the 'protective' principle, the specific policies and forms of State action, and the political struggles that ensued around it as part of a wider social and political discourse that confirmed and reproduced gender relationships. The specific example of women's susceptibility to the consequences of factory employment on health drew on an existing set of ideas, including medical theories, that women's biological nature – in particular their unique menstrual cycle and reproductive organs – were the source of physical and mental instability and rendered them ill-suited to any kind of participation in the public domain. There was an available discourse that suggested women were 'unfit' for the world of work. What was prescribed and proscribed as the boundaries for women's own actions and opportunities in legislation was important, but more important may have been the constituting role legislation served within the discourse that it also drew on. The law as enshrined in 'protective' labour legislation demonstrates how political definitions of gender are incorporated into specific policies and, as Levine[21] has recently argued, enacted a system of discursive sexual differentiation in both the meaning of work and the separate spheres of home and work. The State, in this sense, defined normative patterns of behaviour for nineteenth-century factory life. The 'cautious and slow approach' of factory legislation aimed at specific classes of person – in this instance women, as Amy Harrison and Barbara Hutchins characterized it at the time[22] – can be seen to reinforce the idea that it was not factory work, but *women in the factory* that was the problem. For Levine, it was not so much work which 'protective' legislation regulated as the proper symbolic functioning of the separate spheres.[23]

State Intervention and Women's Work: The Response from 1880

State intervention in women's employment took three main forms during this period. By the 1890s there was already evidence, particularly from its own officials, that earlier legislation which had, for example, introduced regulations with respect to women in the 'dangerous trades' and had placed restrictions on hours of work in the textile and other industries, had failed to achieve any major improvements. In the early 1880s there was an enquiry into the white lead industry, and regulations were introduced aimed at improving cleanliness and ventilation to effect a reduction in lead-poisoning. But cases were still reported and deaths occurred, while factory inspectors found employers and workers less than diligent in their adherence to regulations.[24] Similarly, evasion of hours of work legislation was considerable.

The first response which was typical of this period was the use of enquiry and investigation – and these occurred in increasing numbers. The extent to which existing regulations were 'successful' formed one important remit for most enquiries. Another frame of reference were two related problems of women's employment: the impact of cheap female labour on male workers and wages primarily defined in terms of the possibility of displacement and a downward pull on earnings; and the possible damage that working mothers inflicted especially on their children.

The most evident indication of this was in the appointment of Assistant Lady Commissioners to conduct a special set of enquiries into women's work as a distinct element within the Royal Commission on Labour, 1892–3.[25] The investigative tradition was not confined to the *ad hoc* Committees or Commissions, but was also part of the administrative function of some departments. A number of writers[26] have identified the setting up of a Labour Committee at the Board of Trade in 1893 as a new initiative or function taken by the State.[27] The Committee collected statistical information on employment patterns, wages and hours of work; and one of its members, Clara Collet, was an important analyst of these questions in relation to women's work. Also, the particular brief given to the Women's Factory Inspectorate on its establishment in 1893 provided for it to have a role in special enquiry and investigation in addition to the usual statutory duties in 'policing' legislation. Feminist organizations and other reformers shared a commitment to the practice of investigation. They perceived it as having a function within their campaigns around State intervention. With positivist epistemology and its privileging of the empirical ascertainment of facts in ascendancy at this time, it was not surprising to find evidence of social investigation being used in relation to political strategies around intervention.

A second distinguishing characteristic of State intervention in the 1890s was a shift in the focus for regulation. It was not only that women were to feature prominently here, but, as argued above, it was still only certain problems about that work, or certain industries that were subject to scrutiny. The primary issue of the earlier Victorian period had been hours of work. It was in this period to shift to the 'dangerous trades'. There were Committees of Inquiry into the Lead Industries and Potteries in 1893 (two), 1898, and 1910, and two undertaken within the

Royal Commission of Labour and the Women's Factory Inspectorate in 1893 and 1897. The Chemical Works Committee of Inquiry examined Lucifer Match Making in 1893 and there was a separate enquiry in 1898 and again by women inspectors in 1898. Over and above this, a departmental committee was convened to examine the miscellaneous 'dangerous trades' in 1895: they met continuously until its final report in 1899, while Cotton Cloth Manufacture was investigated in 1897.

A final distinguishing characteristic of State intervention in this period was the increased use of expertise. This occurred in two ways. First, the employment of outside 'experts' for the purposes of special enquiry. While it is most common to see expertise as belonging to members of the scientific community and medical profession, the concept of expertise employed here was quite wide. In fact, the idea that expertise was located only among those with professional knowledge and training was actively contested in any case. There were trade unionists, women labour activists and ex-women factory inspectors who were also called on to serve on enquiries.[28] However, the use of medical expertise on questions relating to the health consequences of conditions did gain considerable ground at this time, as we see in the next chapter, and the State would seem to have affirmed a role for science and medicine within the development of social policy.

A second development of expertise was consistent with such an acceptance: salaried employees within the State's own service or administrative apparatus. Some commentators have noted the increasing professionalization of the factory inspectorate at this time, especially within the women's branch who tended to be middle-class and professionally trained,[29] in contrast to a tradition of working-class men with practical abilities. But new, professionally-based branches of the civil service were also established, such as a Medical Inspector within the Factory Department in 1898. Thomas Legge, who first occupied this post, is attributed with an important role in restoring the social and political dimensions of occupational medicine after the First World War.[30] Together, all three aspects of State intervention can be viewed as indicative of a new rationality, neutrality and bureaucratic form of organization that some sections of the new political spectrum claimed were a necessary basis for State welfare.[31] These claims of neutrality or objectivity, and the practical rationality inherent in jurisprudence, also led Catherine MacKinnon to argue more recently that the State exhibits and institutionalizes male power.[32]

Capital, Labour and the State: Employers

There were a number of groups whose interests could be viewed as potentially in conflict with State intervention in the labour market and world of work, but within the capitalist industrial system it would be expected that employers/manufacturers or industrialists would be to the forefront. The State–employer relationship is important to consider for two reasons. First, it seemed that the developing demand for State action with respect to the labour market and employment conditions was because of a perceived failure on the part of employers to attend to the needs of the human agents of production. As evidence of poor conditions, long hours and the evasion of existing regulations mounted, employers were targeted for their ruthless pursuit of profit and self-interest. Fabian socialists, who had been among the most vociferous in such demands, considered that the anarchy of the capitalist market, visible in the problems of working conditions, required an 'authoritarian' State to deliver the reforms necessary for 'national efficiency'.[33] Regulation was at the core of socially engineering the collective good. Some common set of standards imposed on employers seemed to be warranted. Beatrice Webb, for example, argued that the State 'must by one means or another enforce on all employers a minimum humane order as the inviolable starting point of competition'.[34] Even after the introduction of legislative measures, State officials frequently accused employers of negligence as well as of concerted attempts to defeat the processes of law, such as being involved in the intimidation of witnesses.[35]

A second reason for examining employers is that class interests have had considerable privilege in State theory,[36] with State action viewed as preserving class domination. We might expect, therefore, that if this was the case there would be both resistance to, and a lack of interference in, production or productive social relations. However, although women provided a cheap and flexible source of labour, as men, employers may have shared a belief that women should not be employed at all. Questions must be asked about the basis for the extensive gender and class divisions already established in the labour forces of most industries. At the outset this suggests there are some problems with a conflation of employers with either the male gender or bourgeois class interests. Employers had already colluded, with other men (workers and/or trade unionists) in the demarcation of women's work and skills in paid labour markets, which ensured male interests and power were preserved in the workplace, and this arguably suited employers in the management of their workforce. Equally, however, the 'naturalization' of some kinds of work as women's or men's both undermined the demands for restrictions on women's work, and the actual effects of legislation on employers' practices of hiring women. Gender divisions could thus be used by employers to secure their own economic interests.

Empirical evidence suggests that there were also women employers. Factory Inspectors received a letter from a 'Work Girl' complaining that 'our employer is one of the most unfeeling, unjust women you could meet'[37] and another letter asked if 'Mrs — could be compelled to give her work girls a fire?'[38] Equally, there were notable exceptions to either male or female ownership and management as associated with poor working conditions. The existence of a small number of women employers should not detract from either a class or gender analysis of employers' interests and their relations with the State. Both are relevant, and at various historical junctures these were in contradiction or coincidence to varying degrees. It is possible to view the State as leaving both class and gender relations intact while seeming to act otherwise. Gender divisions in the workplace simultaneously secured class and gender relations – both within production and within the context of reproduction – on women's responsibilities for motherhood. Motherhood and the 'breadwinner' were, as Rose argues, oppositional constructs, not just as ideological representation but because they were socially organized.[39] Despite the benefits of employing women, management practices did not make any concessions to the possibility that some of their workers had family responsibilities.

There is considerable evidence of employers' resistance to legislation on a number of grounds. They perceived regulation as limiting their supply of labour, including its cheapness and specialized skills; that it would affect the market for their goods and thereby their competitiveness; and because the 'reforms' required by regulation incurred costs. When employers were consulted on proposed amendments to the 1892 special rules for Lucifer Match Making there was a chorus of objections:[40] we would 'object to a medical man coming through our works once a month' and Collard Kendall of Liverpool claimed it 'would greatly interfere with our business – besides adding expense when there is no necessity for it'. (Interestingly, Inspector Richmond reported a case of necrosis from this firm in 1895).[41] One employer argued that if compulsory medical examinations were introduced this would frighten women off matchwork, doing them physical and mental injury. Pottery manufacturers frequently sent deputations and correspondence to the Home Office, including their objections to the discretionary powers of the Home Secretary to amend the special rules.

Although it seemed that employers were generally hostile to State intervention for the reasons outlined above, they were neither united organizationally nor ideologically. By the end of the nineteenth century, there is evidence that one of the strategies used by employers in their resistance to State-imposed regulation was their resort to a discursive distinction between 'good' and 'bad' employers. The argument mounted in several contexts was: why should a few 'bad apples' result in legislation that applied to all? The disease metaphor surfaced again here as 'cancers' within the industrial body. Fierce competition was part of a wider economic context that acted as a constraint on employers' motivations to make improvements. Interestingly, this kind of distinction was used by the State itself in order to achieve some measure of regulation in the Potteries. The 1895 Act had given employers the rights to arbitration in respect of proposed 'special rules' in their industry and, as indicated in Chapter 2, this was used by employers as a tactic to delay and defeat certain regulations. In the Potteries, arbitration occurred over a number of years over the use of 'fritted' lead in glazes.[42] Arbitration hearings continued to give some support to the employers' argument that the 'scientific case' was unproven. In the end the government resorted to exempting from regulation those firms who did use it.

There were also some arguments that because of the economic realities of competition, regulation put all employers in an industry on the same footing, and that 'responsible' employers would no longer be at a disadvantage. Fabian socialists had promoted this viewpoint. Other employers favoured regulation because it would also impose some discipline on the workforce. There were also firms who did not see business solely in terms of economics, but as opportunities for combining social and religious principles with business practice. Quaker firms such as Rowntree and Cadbury espoused broader interests in the welfare of the community and many prominent firms such as these, as well as Bryant and May, and Courtaulds, took on a paternalistic role with respect to their women employees in particular.[43]

Despite the fact that there could still be exploitation of workers in these firms, this resulted in welfare provisions and working conditions that were often considerably better than elsewhere.

However, it would be erroneous to leave the impression that there was some truth in employers' claims about the 'good' and the 'bad'. Based on many years experience the problem was, as one woman factory inspector put it:

> It is not the base manufacturer who needs prodding for his [*sic*] disregard, but those tender souled people [a reference to eminent potters] who talk about leadless glaze and then don't take the trouble to see that they get it . . . among certain manufacturers there is a 'sort of sanctified by time' feeling about glazes.[44]

Among the pottery manufacturers who showed themselves to be opposed to lead-free or low solubility lead glazes, were Doulton, Meakin, and Wedgewood. In fact by 1914 only 337 out of 481 employers had relinquished lead in glazes.[45] There was a visible change in the attitude of the State toward employers in the two decades either side of the turn of the century. Whereas the 1893–84 Committee on the Potteries recommended that lead substitution 'should be left to be settled by competition in the open market',[46] in 1910 the Committee concluded that lead-poisoning 'was largely due to defective conditions of labour'.[47] And despite offering employers some protection in their eventual recommendation, they concluded that they shared some responsibility for the disease: 'In the past many of the manufacturers do not have appeared to regard it as incumbent on them personally to insist upon it', (the observance of special rules).

A further strategy of resistance employers used in this competitive climate was to absolve themselves of responsibility either for the use of certain methods of production, or for the fact that, despite their best efforts, women still became ill. This had two components. In the first, the consumer was used as an excuse for why it was not possible to use lead-free glazes or non-dangerous forms of phosphorous in the case of the 'dangerous trades', or in the demand for their laundry at the end of the week, for fresh flowers on the table in the evenings, for printing and packaging, clothes and millinery, in the case of hours of work. The State seemed to give some credence to these claims, and exemptions were granted for seasonal and or unforseen demand – although in this context there were those officials who wanted to know why Ascot was regarded as 'unforseen'.[48] Sir Charles Dilke MP also asked why bottle-box-making could not occur\at any time of year, only to receive the response from manufacturers that the storage required 'was impossible' and 'they could not anticipate the variety required for next season'.[49] Consumer preferences in a competitive situation were also cited as reasons for not prohibiting either lead or phosphorous. This was also a potential weapon that could ensure compliance with regulations. The State, as a consumer in its own right, was frequently called on to buy only those goods produced under healthy conditions. For example, in reply to a memo from John Burns MP, the Chief Inspector denied the full extent of the danger from Lucifer Matches but conceded that future public sector contracts would give consideration to conditions under which matches were made.[50] From 1900 onwards, public service departments only bought leadless ware.

The second means adopted by employers to deflect attention away from their own unwillingness to seek improvements was to argue that it was the workers who were to blame for their ill-health, either through their own attributes, including attitudes and habits, or their failure to observe preventive measures or regulations. As one employer put it in a letter to the Home Office: 'When a man [*sic*] lays himself on the rails in front of an advancing train it is scarcely fair to put the whole blame upon the directors of the railway.'[51] Putting the 'blame' for the unhealthy consequences of work on the worker was not a view employers alone promoted. There was a degree of concordance on this issue expressed by State officials, particularly male factory inspectors and medical practitioners. Alexander Redgrave, Chief Factory Inspector in a report on the Cotton Industry (1890) commented that:

> her energetic industry is not infrequently an embarrassment to the inspector, for it makes her indifferent to the provisions of the Act of Parliament which has been passed for her own protection. She has practically *to be driven from her work*.[52] (my emphasis)

Thomas Arlidge suggested that the casting of blame 'more or less on the workpeople, unhappily is too frequently justified by the conduct of the latter', and he bemoaned those women who 'tossed aside' protective dresses 'because they hide the charms of the wearer'.[53] In the inquests into the deaths of Eliza Higgins, Lydia Cox and Ellen Pickering, all lead-workers, witnesses accused them all of 'neglecting themselves', yet the *Daily Post* argued in the case of Ellen Pickering that she 'was a careful girl and clean in her habits'.[54]

Because this was a pervasive view of the failure of prevention it was difficult to contest and, although women factory inspectors were not entirely immune from some tendency to see fault with women workers, they were much more inclined to resist such labelling and point to the structural basis for non-compliance with regulations, or for those ills which generally befell women at work. Clara Collet reported to the Royal Commission on Labour that she had been told that cases of severe injury in bottle-sighting were due to 'carelessness'. Employers bore the brunt of their counter-accusations, such as in 1896 when two inspectors reported that employers' ideas of unfitness were very different to their own, and 'the difficulty and often direct opposition, which has to be encountered in any attempt to obtain elementary conditions of decency'.[55] In the case of bottle-sighting, old fencing masks were provided in one factory and the coroner at the inquest into the death of the enameller, Harriet Walter, declared the respirators provided to be 'very objectionable'.[56] There was also in women factory inspectors' defence of workers' 'failure' an implicit critique of regulation itself. As Rose Squire argued:

> to prohibit taking meals in a factory or workplace without laying upon the occupier a legal obligation to provide a suitable place in which food may be eaten, is unfortunately merely to substitute one set of conditions injurious to health with another.[57]

Or, as Lucy Deane observed, such accusations that workers sit down at their workbenches the minute 'one's back is turned' seems plausible until one notes this is the only warm place available.[58]

This 'victim-blaming ideology'[59] extended from specific instances of occupational ill-health, to women in their capacity as mothers and homemakers responsible for the poor state of the national health. The importance of such an ideology should not be underestimated in this context. It served to deflect attention away from the underlying weakness in the State's preventive strategy of using legislative regulation; it obscured the origins of occupational ill-health and, moreover, the health of infants and children in material circumstances and environmental conditions; and, in the case of employers, it suggested that employment and production practices were not implicated. Workers were to blame, because women had a greater susceptibility to ill-health, and they did not act to reduce risks either in the work place or by not working at all. The failure of a State strategy to effect improvements in women's health (and in some limited cases men's) could thus be directed elsewhere.

Occupational Ill-health: the Failure of State Intervention

Even in terms of its own analysis of the problems of women's work, the State's response was both inadequate in extent and inappropriate in content. It failed to achieve either an improvement in the prevention of occupationally related ill-health, and it failed to achieve its social purposes of improving the quality of domestic life by returning women to the working-class family.

If one of the intentions of factory legislation was to prevent occupationally related ill-health and disease, then its approach was as Harold Tennant MP described it 'dilatory, mistaken and above all inadequate'.[60] This reference to industrial poisoning and the control of the 'dangerous trades' can be generalized to every aspect of occupational health risks. At least in the 'dangerous trades' there was some attempt at regulation and by 1914 rates of lead and phosphorous poisoning had substantially declined – although this was mainly due to a long-delayed prohibition of lead in pottery manufacture and of white or yellow phosphorous in match-making. On the other hand, conditions with respect to hours of work, ventilation, heating, heavy lifting, machine guarding and work-based welfare provision received relatively little attention. In those industries where the amelioration of poisoning was the primary aim, other conditions might have been improved as a by-product of measures directed at poisoning prevention, such as mechanical ventilation. Despite the exclusion from women in certain processes they continued to breathe white-lead dust or phosphorous fumes as they engaged in other work around the factory. In the Potteries, phthisis was destructive of both women's and men's health, but it was only in the later inquiry of 1910 that 'dusts' were even examined. The Committee concluded that conditions connected with dusts 'are far more serious and far more widespread than lead poisoning', but there is little evidence that this led to a departure in strategy. It was specific classes of worker, combined with particular problems within a limited number of industries, that received attention and this left many workers, women and men, untouched by regulation.

This suggests that there are two questions that require an answer in relation to the failure of the State's preventive strategy. Was regulation the 'right' approach to prevention? Was the problem not with regulation *per se*, but with its content and its limited application? If the answer to both these questions is 'yes', then the failure must lie elsewhere.

Different models of health promotion remain to this day contentious.[61] It has been argued that in this period there was a social and political climate which created pressure for the State to assume some responsibility for the amelioration of working conditions. Although this was still the 'early days' of State welfarism, a legislative approach was considered appropriate both because of this changed idea of the State's role, and the failure of voluntarism to effect improvement.[62] Although opposition remained in some quarters, notably among members of the feminist movement and among some employers, there was an acceptance of regulation as the 'right' preventative strategy in occupational disease. Outside of this, medical practitioners had little experience of alternative forms of preventive work. There was an increasing move toward the idea of education towards the end of this period, especially within the Factory Department itself, but this was a consequence of a return to voluntarism as offering more expansive and inclusive possibilities than the limited application of legislation.[63]

Of equal importance to legislation as the main form of State intervention was the role of investigation and enquiry. Although this often had a direct relationship on the direction of policy formation, it also served other significant purposes that were not in the services of prevention. It can be argued that investigation and enquiry obviated the need for legislation, being used as a political device to deflect agitation for State intervention elsewhere. By instituting enquiry, the State could still be seen to act. In the case of phosphorous necrosis in the match-making industry, the Home Secretary revealed his use of enquiry to delay legislation.[64] There is some indication of the motive for delaying legislation. It seems that legislation would have required a major departure in strategy: either to consider prohibition, or to give the Secretary of State absolute powers to deal with the 'dangerous trades' without arbitration. Despite indications that a restriction on employers' rights to arbitration was favoured by State officials, they were also fearful of the alarm this 'might excite'.[65] There is evidence here that the State did not act autonomously, and that the interests it sought most to protect were those of the capitalist class. If it could also demonstrate that it was acting to remedy the observed physical and social ills of women's work, then its own political purposes of being seen to serve wider political constituencies would also be achieved.

There were, however, evident problems with the content of legislation. There were limits to State action, particularly within the historical context outlined earlier, and it is probable that, although 'mistaken' in approach and content, improvements were sought through regulation. In occupational health, sanitary ideas on prevention remained high on the agenda. The dominant theme of regulation of the White Lead Industry in the early 1880s, and then subsequently with respect to the 'dangerous trades' in general, was the control of the working environment and controls around workers to try to secure it. Cleanliness of workspaces, air and bodies were expected to achieve considerable improvement. The State could be used to ensure conformity to some basic common standards of working conditions, through enshrining these standards in law. Unfortunately the law itself often proved difficult to use in meeting this ideal.

Widespread evasion as well as a liberal attitude toward the granting of exemption from regulation were commonplace. Evasion consisted of many different methods to circumvent restrictions, especially on hours and sanitary provision. Women trade union and labour activists continually argued that the often 'arbitrary and illogical exemptions' added considerably to the problems of detection.[66] Outside such direct attempts at evasion, however, were the difficulties caused by the language of regulation, which allowed for an interpretative reframing of the meaning of key provisions. This made prosecution difficult. These included the phrase 'knowingly employed' with respect to the regulation of the four-week period of post-confinement leave; the idea of 'reasonableness' which was embodied in sanitary legislation, and levels of fines under the 1896 Truck Act; or the 1901 legislation that required 'adequate' means to secure a 'reasonable' temperature. Many regulations also included a proviso as to 'as far as practicable' which provided for further evasion. These vague terms mitigated against the idea that the law provided a common set of standards for all employments included within the legislation's remit. As one contemporary commentator noted, 'people's ideas of what is "practicable", "harmless", even as to what is ventilation, differ'; and she argued that because 'we cannot trust it to anybody's own idea of what good ventilation is', what was required in this respect was an exact rule.[67]

Other factors contributed to difficulties in enforcement. Principal among these was the capacity of those whose responsibility it was to 'police' regulation to cope with the scale of the work. One of the rationales for the campaign to appoint women inspectors was that women workers had not benefited from male inspection. Even if a workplace *was* inspected, it was argued, women did not voice their grievances. As one woman unionist explained:

> I know from experience how scared they are of a man who comes as an official. If he questions them he can get nothing but the shortest answers and very seldom a voluntary statement.[68]

Despite the steady growth of women inspectors, there were still only seven of them by the end of the century. It was inevitable that inspection to ensure compliance with legal requirements would still be small relative to the scale of the problems.[69] Gertrude Tuckwell estimated that at the end of the century 107 inspectors served over 100 000 workplaces under regulation.[70] Women inspectors were frequently frustrated in their efforts, and exhausted as a result of undertaking this alongside their other responsibilities.

Outside of inspection within the Factory Department, other bodies who had statutory responsibilities for inspection, enforcement through prosecution, or identification and notification, also failed in their duties. Medical practitioners often failed to recognize and notify cases of industrial 'disease' and made cursory use of the requirements of medical inspection. Local authority sanitary bodies were also notably lax in the pursuit of the action required to meet the minimum standards set down for sanitary conditions, and in the inspection of workshops. May Abrahams noted in one report that action had been taken on only one case in the Lancashire and Cheshire Cotton Industry.[71]

Some of the problems with locally based enforcement were that it was not free of political favour, and the courts themselves were also influenced by, or, in the case of some magistrates, had local employment interests. This did not go unnoticed by contemporary commentators. In 1901, the Annual Report of the Women's Inspectorate[72] called for a change so that persons with an interest in the trade or occupation of the persons charged should not act as a JP in the hearing. In support they cited a case where a woman had worked on a 'mourning' clothes order from 8.30 am until 5.00 am the next day for a magistrate's clerk. The magistrate, who refused to sign the order, was an active partner in the business (and also the Mayor), while in the Chair was another workshop employer who had previously been cautioned for the irregular employment of a child.

One contemporary author summarized the difficulties all these issues posed to the realization of 'admirable intentions':

> The vague phraseology, the lack of a definite standard, the readiness to grant exemptions to certain trades, and under certain conditions, the large discretion left in the hands both of the Secretary of State and the Inspectors of Factories, these are amongst the signs of the contending elements among which the Acts represent a compromise.[73]

Confusion, compromise, concessions and prevarication characterized the State's efforts in respect to intervention in women's working conditions and the right of women to work. If the Factory Acts in general, and its 'protective' orientation with respect to women in particular, were to effect improvements in human life and health – 'care of a community' – then at best it was minimal. At worst it was a perpetuation of exploitative, unhealthy working conditions and the oppressive operation of male power that consigned women to few opportunities only for 'second-class', low-paid work, and the exhausting consequences of the 'double day'.

Women, Men and the State

What were the responses and possible consequences of State intervention through factory legislation on working men and women? The relationship of State intervention in women's work to the intentions or motives of those with political interests in the issue, and the consequences for women who were the 'subjects' of it are difficult to uncover. This is due in part to the difficulty of accessing information about ordinary men and women's work and lives. We can ascertain what activists, including trade unionists, thought and did, and the representations they made on behalf of other workers. However, there are dangers in interpreting both motives and outcomes of legislation in this way. Angela John[74] raised this issue in relation to men's attitudes toward the prohibition of women from underground coal-mining. In her critique of Jane Humphries' interpretation of men's involvement with the 1842 Act, she argues that particular sources can access only some men's views: and those voices heard for prohibition 'do not mean that miners "almost universally" opposed the work'. There may also be a discrepancy between expressed ideals and actual behaviour, and 'ambivalences and variations amongst the workforce'.

In addition to considering the attitudes of working men and women to legislation, there have been some attempts, both at the time and more recently, to assess the more general consequences of legislation. The analysis of both issues has been a matter of some dispute between feminist theorists of the topic, and this particular aspect is discussed in the conclusion. Here, an attempt is made to ascertain contemporary views of the impact of legislation.

There were contradictions in the State's approach to occupational health problems and the social control of women's lives through limits on workplace participation and the reinforcement of domestic ideology. If one purpose of the legislation was to limit the participation of women, and especially married women, in paid work, the evidence suggests this was largely unsuccessful. Data on marital status and women's employment shows little change in participation over this period. Exclusions from particular processes did not necessarily lead to a withdrawal from work itself. Accounts of women in the 'dangerous trades' indicated they often moved their place of employment or the kind of work they did if they were faced with actual or potential suspension. Similarly, prohibitions on night work or the length of the working day affected few women, and certainly not their participation at all. Economic circumstances and necessity, or customary practice consistent with local values and norms, were more important determinants than legislation.

Despite the increased strength of maternalist ideology in the early decades of the twentieth century, State intervention was minimal, and factory legislation itself failed to reflect the discursive importance attached to working mothers. The only regulation passed during this whole period was the 'unworkable' requirement about post-confinement leave of four weeks. Those measures which were gradually implemented with respect to infant welfare in the first two decades of the twentieth century, were aimed at all working-class mothers, and at infant-feeding practices, education, and domestic hygiene in particular, rather than factory work.[75] Supporters of both 'protective' legislation and the extension of State intervention continued to use maternal and infant health as a rationale. Sidney and Beatrice Webb, for example, called for the State to 'endow motherhood' alongside calls for factory legislation,[76] and Gertrude Tuckwell similarly argued:

> the state should see fit to intervene more fully between the claims of the little ones and the demands of labour, to interfere for the protection of family life, and restore the children to their homes.[77]

Considering the possible impact of legislation on employment, the empirical evidence we have suggests that there was little impact here either. There was no change in the sexual division of labour in terms of either women's subordinate status or in the general designation of work as suited to women or men. There were changes in particular industries and work processes, but substitutions of women for men, or men for women were usually due to changes in production methods or the introduction of machinery.[78] An investigation of women compositors[79] was unable to find a single instance of displacement due to legislation. The majority of employers were 'emphatic' that it did not affect the question of whether they employed women. However, an insistence by men on women earning less effectively confined them to other duties. It was also argued that what women most complained of was *irregular* hours rather than long hours.[80] A contemporary feminist critic of legislation argued that there was an illogicality in official thinking: that by decreasing women's hours by one hour a day, 'so she may choose to do her household duties', would lessen her hours overall.[81]

There were also indications that women's pay did not improve either, and restrictions on overtime might have limited potential earnings. Views differed on this: some informants told investigators they would have preferred a choice as to whether to work overtime,[82] while others pointed to the pay being so low it was not worth working overtime 'for a few pence more'.[83] Because working hours did not change much in this period, the effect on wages was not readily visible. In trying to identify the benefits that legislation might have brought women in employment, contemporary investigators argued it was difficult to identify these separately from other influences.

From the perspective of men, factory legislation can be viewed in a number of ways. It did not protect men from the health consequences of employment. The protective emphasis on 'classes' of employee in many instances left men working in the same industry as women but without any benefits of regulation. Where women were prohibited, as in processes in white-lead manufacture, men were expected to step in – and they died in increasing numbers as a result. Most controversy is around the interpretion of men's support for legislation. Although this is not as clear-cut, the most pervasive contemporary view was that men supported restrictions on women because they would benefit from it. It is the oft-quoted remark (attributed originally to Thomas Ashton, an Oldham Spinners representative)[84] that men obtained shorter hours for themselves from 'behind the petticoats of women'. The explanation offered was that men, aware that intervention in their labour would not be countenanced by the State, used the remaining route open to them outside collective organization: which was legislation for women. Such an argument would only hold, however, in industries where men were employed alongside women. As Gertrude Tuckwell concluded, a limitation on men's hours 'is due simply to the fact that their work was dependent on women'.[85] Other improvements in conditions could similarly have brought benefits to men, including the regulation, such as that in 1903, requiring all lead workers to be subject to medical inspection.

Another explanation for men's support for 'protective' legislation was that men feared competition. This was rarely the case, since men and women seldom did the same jobs, although employers might have used such fears to manage male labour. Clementina Black argued that competition was 'infinitismal', and further that 'the actions and designs of men were irrelevant' since the effects of legislation were not dependent on their aims or the means by which it was brought about.[86] In any case, even among trade union activists, women activists exerted greater influence over the direction of State intervention than men unionists. Although they favoured restrictions or prohibitions on women's work, they were not particularly militant in pursuit of such objectives. Unlike women unionists, they did not form alliances with middle-class men on important campaigns. Thus in the Anti-Sweating League, credited with playing a major role in the eventual passing of the 1909 Trades Boards Act, women unionists and feminist activists combined with middle-class men reformers and, Morris[87] claims, male unionists had relatively little involvement or influence.

It is important to recognize that expressed antagonism to women's work was an important component of the discourse that men entered in order to construct both political and gender identities. As Gray[88] argues, the real effects of legislation were not to exclude women, but to define the terms for their participation in waged factory labour, in which some balance had to be struck between waged work and the domestic role. Thus 'protective legislation continued to define normative gendered behaviour which included excluding women from the legitimate meanings of work, further entrenching the masculinity of work culture, work identities and the market'.[89]

The situation for women workers and State intervention in relation to working conditions was not unlike the contradictions which other areas of intervention posed for them. For example, Linda Gordon[90] has shown that the outrage expressed over intervention in the family frequently came from men because it was a threat to male authority. In the area of domestic violence, for example, or in making birth control available, State intervention also brought women some relief. Equally, 'protective legislation' represented restrictions on women's rights and opportunities, their access to economic resources and subjected them to increased surveillance. Because State intervention served to define women's indentities and lives as different to men, it can be viewed as patriarchal.[91] Catherine MacKinnon[92] argues that the State and State laws are 'male' to the extent that it is male viewpoints and experience that frame policy and are framed by it – and factory legislation was no exception.

In this discussion of the developing role of the State, and the way in which it was enshrined in the particular case of 'protective' legislation, a contradiction has been apparent. Those areas most prominent in *laissez-faire* ideas about non-interference, the family and economic relations, were to be the focus of State policy and emerging status apparatuses. It was not surprising, therefore, to find that the discourse around 'protection' should both affirm the intervention as ensuring the welfare of individuals and the nation State, while maintaining, as Rose has described it, 'the fiction of non-involvement'.[93] The framework for the increasing regulation of people's lives in various respects in this period can be seen encompassing a necessary moral dimension of economic regulation: and, as such, economic regulation was the regulation of women and the family at one and the same time. Legislative regulation as a means of dealing with occupational risk was certainly flawed in this historical context, and these flaws were related to the wider objectives of the State beyond prevention.

Notes

1   Jamieson, L. and Corr, H. (Eds) (1990) *State, Private Life and Political Change*, Introduction, pp.1–2.
2   Melling, J. (1992) 'Welfare capitalism and the origins of welfare states'.
3   Hall, S. and Schwartz, S. (1986) 'State and society, 1880–1930', in M. Langan and H. Schwartz (Eds).
4   Hall and Schwartz, *ibid.*, p.15.
5   Black, C. (1907) *Sweated Industry and the Minimum Wage*, p.*xxiv*.
6   Foucault, M. (1979) *Discipline and Punish.*
7   Mort, F. (1986) 'Purity, feminism and the state'.
8   Gray, R. (1987a) 'The language of factory reform', in Joyce, P. (Ed.).
9   In the Royal Commission on Labour, Clara Collet refers to the reputation of several groups of women workers, including Birmingham umbrella-and-screw girls as 'rough', PP XXXVII, 1893–4. Women inspectors' reports are littered with expressions of injury to morality.
10 Gray, R. (1987a) 'The language of factory reform'.
11 Shadwell, A. (1906) *Industrial Efficiency*, pp.1–4.
12 See, for example, Wohl, A. (1983) *Endangered Lives: Public Health in Victorian England* for an excellent summary of nineteenth-century interventions.
13 Hall, S. and Schwartz, B. (1986) 'State and society', p.18.
14 Mockett, H. (1988) 'A danger to the state': Women and factory legislation (1830–1850)'.
15 Humphries, J. (1981) 'Protective Legislation, the capitalist state and working-class men: the case of the 1842 Mines Act'; but see also John's reply (1981) to this article, questioning some aspects of the use of evidence and interpretation.
16 Cited in Hutchins, B. (1902) 'The historical development of the Factory Acts', in Webb, B. (Ed.)
17 *Ibid.*
18 Butler, J.E. (1874) 'Legislative restriction on the industry of women considered from the woman's point of view'.
19 Harrison, B. and Mockett, H. (1990) 'Women in the factory: the state and factory legislation in nineteenth-century Britain', in Jamieson, L. and Corr, H. (Eds).
20 *Hansard*, 1900, p.1512, my emphasis.
21 Levine, P. (1993) 'Consistent contradictions: prostitution and protective labour legislation in nineteenth-century England'.
22 Hutchins, B. and Harrison, A. (1903) *A History of Factory Legislation.*
23 Levine, P. (1993) p.19.
24 See May Abraham's Report to the Royal Commission of Labour on the Conditions of Work in White Lead Manufacture, PP XXXVII, 1892–3.
25 The remit given to the Assistant Lady Commissioners was 'the effects of women's industrial employment on their health, morality and home'. They were also instructed

'to inquire into the existence and causes of the exclusion of women from trades in which women's work is not unsuitable'. PP XXXVII, 1893–4, preamble.

26 See Morris, J. (1985) *Women workers and the Sweated Trades*; Schwartz, B. (1986b) 'The corporate economy 1890–1929', in Langan, M. and Schwartz, B. (Eds).

27 However, the Board of Trade was at the forefront of the development of statistical information from the 1830s. See Szreter, S. (1991) 'The GRO and the historians', and Goldman, L. (1991) 'Statistics and the science of society in early Victorian Britain'.

28 May Abraham, for example, served on the Dangerous Trades Committee after her eventual resignation from the inspectorate after marriage and pregnancy. Gertrude Tuckwell, Secretary of the WTUL, served on the 1910 Committee set up to investigate the dangers of lead and dusts in the Potteries. There are also examples of enquiry not directly related to work: Lucy Deane investigated the Boer War Concentration Camps and sat on the Committee of Inquiry into the Civil Service (1912) as well as various wartime committees.

29 See, for example, Hollis, P. (1979) *Women in Public*, and Harrison, B. 'Gender, the state and occupational health': (in press).

30 Weindling, P. (1985) 'Linking self-help and medical science: the social history of occupational health'.

31 Hall, S. and Schwartz, B. (1986) 'State and society' outline of the importance of these ideological strands within Fabian socialism in particular.

32 MacKinnon, C. (1989) *Toward a Feminist Theory of the State*. See especially the chapter on 'The liberal state'.

33 Hall, S. and Schwartz, B. (1986) 'State and society', pp.21–3.

34 Webb, B. (1902) *The Case for the Factory Acts*, p.18.

35 Annual Report of Her Majesty's Chief Inspector of Factories, Report of the Women's Inspectorate for 1897. Report by Miss Deane.

36 Melling, J. (1992) 'Welfare capitalism and the origins of welfare states', provides a brief overview and critique of their position. For a development of the Marxist view to encompass the discursive as well as the institutional basis of state organization and practice involving workers and employers, see Jessop, B. (1990) *State Theory: Putting the Capitalist State in its Place*.

37 Annual Report of Her Majesty's Chief Inspector of Factories for the Year 1893.

38 Annual Report of Her Majesty's Inspector of Factories for the Year 1894, PP XIV; 1895, p.17.

39 Rose, S. (1992) *Limited Livelihoods*, p.76.

40 PRO HO45/9845/B12393 D: Pages 22–6 contain some employers responses.

41 *Ibid.*, p.24, dated 11/2/95.

42 The delay was partly caused by Lord James granting master potters an opportunity to experiment.

43 Lown, J. (1990) *Women and Industrialisation* is a detailed study of Courtaulds; Rose, S. (1992) *Limited Livelihoods*, of these firms in general; and Satre, R. (1982) 'After the match-girls strike: Bryant and May in the 1890s'.

44 Annual Report of His Majesty's Women Inspectors of Factories for the Year 1907, PP X, 1908. This comment formed part of Miss Vines' report on p.236.

45 Report on Regulations in the Potteries by Inspectors Pendock and Werner, PP LXXI, 1914.

46 Report on the Various Lead Industries, PP XVII, 1893–4.

47 Report of the 1910 Inquiry on the Use of Lead, PP XXIX, 1910, p.101.

48 Annual Report of Her Majesty's Chief Inspector of Factories for the Year 1894, PP XIX, 1895.
49 PRO HO45/9922/B23725/7 file begins with a correspondence on this issue.
50 PRO HO45/9849/B12393 D: Memo on p.52.
51 A.G.C. Irvine to the Home Office in PRO HO45/9849/B1239 C p.15.
52 See his Annual Report for 1890, PP XIX, 1890–1.
53 Arlidge, T. (1892) *The Hygiene, Diseases and Mortality of Occupations*, p.4.
54 Reports on the inquests, and cuttings related to them from the Press are in HO45/9848/96988/B12393 A.
55 Annual Report of Her Majesty's Chief Inspector of Factories, Reports of the Women Inspectors for the Year 1896, PP XVII, 1897. Page 61 for comments to this effect from Miss Paterson, and those of Miss Squire on p.63.
56 PRO HO45/9849/B1239 C, p.8.
57 Annual Report of Her Majesty's Women Inspectors of Factories for the Year 1898, PP XII, 1899, p.129.
58 Annual Report for the Year 1897, PP XIV, 1898, p.103.
59 Crawford, R. (1977) 'You are dangerous to your health'.
60 *Hansard*, LXII, 1898, p.455.
61 Allsop, J. (1984) *Health Policy and the NHS*, Chapter 9.
62 See Thane, P. (1982) *Foundations of the Welfare State*. This also demonstrates that this voluntarism was still utilized in the pursuance of welfare policies, with the costs in some areas such as child welfare being met by the State.
63 Jones, H. (1985) 'An Inspector calls: health and safety at work in inter-war Britain', in Weindling, P. (Ed.). This shows that this trend found its way into more formal organizational outlets, such as The Industrial Museum.
64 PRO HO45/9849/B12393 D, dated 14/6/98, p.52.
65 *Ibid.*
66 Tuckwell, G. (1902) 'The more obvious defects of our factory code', in Webb, B. (Ed.) p.130–5.
67 Nash, R. (1897) *Public Health Laws*, pp.6–7.
68 Hicks, A. (1893) 'Secretary of Rope Workers Union', in *The Woman's Herald*, 30 March, p.83.
69 Jones, H. (1988) 'Women health workers: the case of the first women factory inspectors', argues that women inspectors not only served to depoliticize the issue of women's working conditions, but also agrees their impact could only be minimal, given the scale of the problems.
70 Tuckwell, G. (1902) 'The more obvious defects of our factory code', p.129.
71 Report to the Royal Commission of Labour, PP XXXVII, 1892–3.
72 PP XII, 1902.
73 Shadwell, A. (1906) *Industrial Efficiency*, p.155.
74 John, A.V. (1981) 'Letter' to *Feminist Review*, p.107.
75 Lewis, J. (1980a) *The Politics of Motherhood*; Dyhouse, C. (1979) 'Working-class mothers and infant mortality', and Davin, A. (1978) 'Imperialism and motherhood'. See also Thane, P. (1988) *Foundations of the Welfare State*.
76 Webb, S. and Webb, B. (1902) *Problems of Modern Industry*; Webb, B. (1902) 'The Case for the Factory Acts'.
77 Tuckwell, G. (1908) 'The regulation of women's work', in Tuckwell (Ed.), *Women in Industry*, p.25.

78 Harrison, A. (1904) *Women's Industries in Liverpool.*
79 Bradby, B. and Black, A. (1899) 'Women compositors and the Factory Acts'.
80 Harrison, A. (1904) *Women's Industries in Liverpool.*
81 Butler, J. (1874) 'The effects of legislation from a woman's point of view'.
82 MacDonald, J. Ramsay (1902) *Women in the Printing Trades.*
83 Harrison, A. (1904) *Women's Industries in Liverpool.*
84 See Webb, S. and Webb, B. (1894) *A History of Trade Unionism,* p.297. It appears unattributed in Strachey, R. *The Cause,* in Hewitt, M. (1958) *Wives and Mothers in Victorian Industry.*
85 Tuckwell, G. (1902) 'The more obvious defects of our Factory Code'.
86 Black, C. (1902) 'Some current objections to factory legislation for women'.
87 Morris, J. (1986b) *Women Workers and the Sweated Trades,* Chapter 8.
88 Gray, R. (1987a) 'The language of factory reform'.
89 See Valverde, M. (1988) 'Giving the female a domestic turn'; Levine, P. (1993) 'Consistent contradictions', and Rose, S. (1992) 'Limited livelihoods', especially p.130 for similar arguments.
90 Gordon, L. (1988) *Heroes of their Own Lives: The Politics and History of Family Violence.*
91 H. Hartmann (1979) provides this definition of patriarchy in her 'The unhappy marriage of Marxism and feminism'.
92 MacKinnon, C. (1988) *Toward a Feminist Theory of the State.*
93 Rose, S. (1992) *Limited Livelihoods,* p.51.

Chapter 6

Medical Men[1] and Women's Occupational Ill-health

An examination of questions of ill-health usually requires some attention to the role of the health professionals. The account of the problems of women's occupational ill-health earlier in this book indicated that medical knowledge and medical practitioners were involved. Outside of medicine, few other health practitioners were directly concerned with the issue. Sanitary inspectors were one exception and dentists were another in the case of the match-making industry. This involvement of medical professionals in questions of working conditions, industrial disease and the effects of industrial work on women's health was mainly a result of their direct involvement with State initiatives in terms of investigation or enquiry and in the roles assigned to medical practitioners in relation to legislative regulation. This aspect is, therefore, a central concern of this chapter.

However, as a form of knowledge and practice, medicine has long occupied a position of power and privilege, not all of which emanates 'from their exclusive jurisdiction over the label illness'.[2] Class and gender characteristics have not only been important in those historical and political processes through which doctors have been able to secure their place in the occupational structure.[3] They have also enabled doctors to exercise social power, medical perceptions to influence and become incorporated into broader social discourses and practitioners to acquire forms of social deference that are not directly a result of the state of medical knowledge *per se*.[4] If this argument has validity, we would expect to see that in this case doctors entered into the debates about women and employment, as they did about women and education,[5] because of the social rather than the medical issues at stake. The particular case of the health effects of factory or industrial work were only a part of this larger social discourse, which extended to middle-class women's aspirations to wider employment opportunities.

Medicine as a profession was still in its infancy at this time. Although the 1858 Medical Act had created a single medical register there were still many divisions in doctors' social backgrounds, forms of practice and how their medical services were administered. Inspite of developing knowledge and social status – and a growing demand for medical care from the expanding urban middle class – medical practitioners often still occupied both an economically insecure and a socially marginal status.[6] Some people in society still looked on doctoring as a trade and not every doctor had access to extra income through hospital appointments.[7] Those whose tradition of knowledge and practice had grown considerably in the nineteenth century, the medical officers of health, who had a secure place within local administration, found their status was being eroded by the growing prestige of clinical knowledge and practice mainly associated with individualized care and hospital-based practice.[8] These aspects of marginality are important to understand medical responses to women's health and medical involvement with occupational health questions.

Medical knowledge itself was also in its infancy. The cholera and typhoid epidemics of the nineteenth century had revealed many medical men's inability to understand the causes and thereby deliver any effective remedies. Many medical theories about health were based on impressions, prejudice and experiences, the latter sometimes enabling them to be rather more effective than the former.[9] Forms of treatment relied more on tradition than fresh knowledge or technological developments, as witnessed by the persistence of blood-letting well into the twentieth century.[10] Developments were not necessarily diffused to the level of individual practitioners – and even if they were aware of them, they did not always use them in their own practice. It has been argued that the improvements in health and the decline in mortality that became evident at the end of the nineteenth century owed little to medical intervention. Rather, improved social conditions, some of which were achieved through sanitary reform, rising incomes and improved diet, resulted in the rise in population.[11] Occupational-health knowledge and practice was not particularly well-developed either, but I explore the extent to which, as some commentators have claimed, the identification of 'industrial diseases' as a social and political priority also served medical professional interests.[12]

Early Debates

There were debates about the effects of factory labour on women from the earliest attempts to regulate their work and conditions in relation to their children and medical men were certainly involved in the debates. Although women were not included in legislation until the 1840s, the foundation was laid in the debates of the 1830s. There were objections to women working on the basis of their physical incapacity and on grounds of sexual morality. Medical arguments were used both for and against the labour of women in factories and, early on at least, medical grounds were largely rejected. The Factory Commission of 1833, for example, rejected any need to restrict women, since whatever 'the delicacy of the female organisation . . . [she] bears factory labour better than the male, and in regard to her own peculiar constitution and health, sustains no appreciable injury from it'.[13] Medical men also entered into discussion on the social grounds for the restriction of women in terms of both sexual morality and the breakdown of family relationships.[14] Some thought that the poor morality of factory women adversely affected their fertility; others pointed to the consequent neglect of domestic economy.[15] There was certainly no medical consensus, but this is understandable given the context in which medical men developed and expressed their views.

Important fora for such discussions and pamphlets were the local philosophical, statistical and literary societies and gentlemens' clubs. The position of individual practitioners within local social networks and the nature of their middle-class client base were important influences on whether or not medical men entered such debates.[16] In many cases, their own practice, especially if they served on charity or friendly-society panels or did poor-law dispensing, closely involved them with the working-class poor and the effects of working conditions. Some of the earliest prominent men in the field of occupational medicine had this kind of experience, among them Thackrah, Kay and Robert Baker who left medicine to become a factory inspector in 1834.[17]

As divisions of opinion continued on the possible dangers of women's work in industrial manufacture, it was accepted that women were, like children, in need of 'protection'. From the 1840s onwards they were included within the legislation on these terms. Medical opinion continued to focus on whether to extend or to limit the application of the 'principle' but provided no questioning of the principle itself.

Before the 1880s, medical involvement was within the debates about 'protective legislation' and the use of certifying surgeons to inspect children in employment and certify them fit. There was one other main area in which medical practitioners became involved: through their role within local administration of public health and at the national level through the office of the Medical Officer to the Privy Council and the Local Government Board.[18] The major sanitary investigations of the first half of the nineteenth century had revealed the extent to which occupations seemed to be a factor in mortality. Some medical officers of health in particular, such as Chadwick and then Greenhow and Simon, undertook systematic investigations into the dangers of particular occupations as well as occupational mortality in general.[19] When he moved to his position as Medical Officer at the Privy Council in 1860, Simon extended investigation into occupational health, using his annual reports to build up his case for legislation. He was, as Wohl describes it, 'to rejoice prematurely' at the regulation gained in the 1864 and 1867 Acts and the 1878 consolidation measures.[20] Simon and his colleagues gave no special attention to the case of women except for the specific instance of infant mortality, (see Chapter 3) although Simon was pleased that at least they were 'protected from certain dangerous processes'.[21] These were only small moves in the regulation of danger and the failure of implementation and enforcement resulted in little change in the risk to women of dangerous employments.

Lee[22] has argued that industrial medicine was 'stillborn in the age of sanitary medicine', a reference not so much to the fact that it was 'sanitarians' who took an interest in the subject, but rather because the development of knowledge simply did not occur. Leading figures clung to issues of the past, defending the traditional role of the certifying surgeons and emphasizing the control of infectious diseases. The validity of Lee's argument is supported by the extent to which there was a focus on sanitary matters in relation to factory reform and in a tendency to look for factors outside the factory itself as being responsible for the poor health of operatives. Commenting on Lee's characterization of this early development of industrial medicine, Gray has pointed to a divergence in the languages of medicine and factory reform.[23] While there may indeed be two such languages, the eventual 'success' of medicine in securing a role for itself in relation to reform in this later period was because it could articulate the case for a strategy to be pursued by drawing on non-medical discourse. This discourse was shared with promoters of State intervention in general and in the specific case of women's work. So while Gray is right to emphasize that in the early period 'forms of regulation did not provide any secure institutional base for the practice of such a discipline'[24] later the relationship to regulation was important as a base, however small. The development of workmen's compensation in relation to scheduled diseases provided a language linking the factory to industrial medicine, albeit around the adult male worker.[25]

In the 1880s when medical opinion discussed proposals to restrict the work of women in pit-brow work, the social dimensions of the question were as important as any possible dangers or benefits of the work. Local practitioners spoke of the 'healthy nature of the work', which was linked to it being outdoors. As John outlines[26] a considerable number of risks were attached to the work, but these were neglected in favour of more generalized and 'idealized' expectations. Most of the dangers came from management's neglect and whether or not accidents occurred was more likely to be related to levels of experience than gender. Work in the mines was subject to the moral argument for restriction; doctors joined others in complaining about its 'defeminizing' aspects. In mining, arguments about strength and the ability to do the work were confused with the political issues of women's right to work.

In the Service of the State

Robert Baker's constant appeals to the Home Department to use medical expertise to undertake special investigation into matters such as the health effects of dusts had gone unheeded earlier in the century.[27] The increased agitation and the State's response to the 'dangerous trades' gave particular impetus to the involvement of medical expertise in relation to State-initiated investigation. By the early 1890s some doctors had developed their expertise in the field of industrial diseases, notably Thomas Arlidge, a practitioner in the Staffordshire Potteries who by 1892 had already published a standard text on the subject[28] and Thomas Oliver, physician at Newcastle Infirmary. These and other practitioners were already known to the Factory Department. It was common practice for officials to consult local practitioners and factory inspectors often used medical opinion and local evidence that practitioners had collected to confirm their own observations and opinions in their reports to the Factory Department. For women inspectors this was probably even more important since, as peripatetic inspectors, they were less able to build up their own local knowledge. Gray[29] maintained a different status accrued to metropolitan as opposed to local practitioners. Those who were used by the State in high-profile positions associated with enquiry were 'metropolitan' because they were attached to large city infirmaries, but they had also acquired some of their expertise from local situations. In other respects, however, factory inspectors and later investigations of infant mortality relied more heavily on local practitioners, believing that they had more information to give. The legitimation of professional medical men through an association with the local network or the national State could work at different levels and might also depend on other social and ideological alliances that acted as forms of patronage.[30]

With the expansion of State enquiry in the 1890s, practitioners with metropolitan status but local knowledge were called on to act as committee members. Both Arlidge and Oliver represented medical expertise on the 1893 Committees of Inquiry into the Potteries and the various lead industries respectively.[31] On the Potteries Committee of Inquiry, other medical representatives had also been selected because they were active practitioners in the Potteries themselves. This continued to be an important basis for the use of medical expertise in enquiry on behalf of the State. Oliver, for example, in his association with the Newcastle Infirmary, had encountered many cases of lead-poisoning, since Newcastle was one of the centres of lead manufacture. Data from Oliver continued to find its way into the Factory and Home Departments and in 1891 he invited himself to act on behalf of the Home Department at the International Conference on Hygiene in Madrid, since he was 'well qualified to speak for the country on such questions'.[32] Oliver went on to be the 'accepted' medical expert on lead-poisoning[33] and also served as the principal medical expert in relation to the match industry and phosphorous necrosis,[34] although the State also drew here on dental expertise. Doctors themselves laid claim to such roles, emphasizing the value of prevention within a context of extremes of human suffering. A.P. Laurie called for a consultative committee of experts in the Factory Department:

> noble as the work of curing disease undoubtedly is, that of preventing disease is nobler, and there are thousands in our manufacturing cities the victims of industrial conditions, living lives of hopeless ill health who are looking for deliverance ... obtained for them by the calm, clear intellect of the man [*sic*] of science with a burning compassion for the suffering of their fellows, a combination of qualities which is to be found most frequently in the medical profession.[35]

Such claims may also have been important in establishing the legitimacy of occupational health as a form of medical practice, but they probably operated within the broader humanitarian discourse of reform rather than earn doctors any expansion in their practice. The State had already decided that medical and scientific expertise would play a role in policy and administration. A further indication that forms of 'scientific' knowledge would be increasingly employed in relation to occupational health issues was the use of chemists for lead enquiries, in particular. By the turn of the century, engineers were also used in matters related to accidents, machine-guarding and ventilation.

One of the major ways in which the medical practitioner had become involved with State administration of factory regulation was through medical inspection. From the 1890s many people believed that medical inspection had proved to be one of the most effective aspects of the 'special' rules instituted in relation to those trades scheduled as 'dangerous' under the 1891 legislation. The special rules set up in 1883 in relation to the white lead industry required 'periodic medical inspection'. The 1893 Committee recommended that as a result of the benefits that had been gained from this, a further rule should be added. This required the medical examination and certification of women as to their age and fitness before employment and their re-certification if they had been absent through illness. This should occur also where women were employed in the enamelling of iron plates.[36]

These perceived benefits of earlier medical inspection were not evident to everyone. In her report to the Labour Commission, May Abraham noted that there were cases where the doctor visited once a week but did not examine anyone. In another case, 'periodic' meant once a year, when only men were examined.[37] Medical inspection thus suffered the same fate as many other areas of regulation: it was often less than diligently implemented or enforced. There were also repeated examples where inspection had occurred, but practitioners either did not observe the symptoms or considered them to be so minor as not to warrant suspension. In the inquest on the death of the enameller, Lydia Cox, the practitioner, Mr Ravenshill, testified that he 'regards it as very difficult to detect illness in advance'. In the case of the last two inquests he 'had passed one of the women, in ignorance of a very severe previous illness . . . and the other had only slight symptoms'.[38] In a report on the death of Annie Hicks, a 19-year-old white lead worker, the doctor had testified to her 'good health'. On one occasion she had looked very pale and had been 'stopped' but two months later she returned 'pale but well'. In this case, doctors reported that a foreman in the firm induced women to take a short time out to avoid medical inspection.[39]

Union representatives were also critical of medical inspection for many of the same reasons, complaining to the 1910 Committee on the Potteries, for example, that insufficient time was devoted to medical examinations. Others felt the independent position of the certifying surgeon to be compromised by private practice.[40] These observed weaknesses in the system did not undermine either official or expert support for such measures, since it seemed the measures themselves were not intrinsically flawed.

Medical opinion contributed to a consensus that workers themselves were mainly to blame for their ill-health. As a result, the surveillance of health status increased. The 1895 Act required medical practitioners to notify cases of industrial poisoning from 1896. Certifying surgeons found their roles extended to the investigation and notification of disease in relation to scheduled industries and accidents. The rules were modified to increase the frequency of medical inspection to monthly, but it was principally women who were subject to medical inspection. This was undoubtedly a direct outcome of the acceptance of medical opinion that women were more at risk from their employments and, in the case of lead, were more susceptible to poisoning.

The acceptance of a role for medical practice in relation to State and factory legislation is revealed by the attention it received in the medical press. There are few discussions of occupational health issues in either *The Lancet* or the *British Medical Journal* outside this context. Although there were matters of clinical interest with respect to reproductive health or predisposition, these were not debated in this context. The State used the medical press to try to inform practitioners of the requirements to notify. The medical press provided commentary on the success or otherwise of legislative regulation to press its own claims for an increased role in this regard. In 1882 *The Lancet* called for an enquiry into lead on the grounds that physicians were continuing to notice cases in hospital out-patient departments, hinting there was 'laxity' somewhere that was responsible.[41] The analysis of the problem, it suggested, was often right; the difficulties lay with the solutions. Inspectors were overburdened and there was a body of expertise which could be drawn on further – the certifying surgeons.

These demands by and on behalf of certifying surgeons that their expertise and experience could be put to greater use[42] might also have been a result of divisions in status and competing claims within the profession for a stake in the nation's health. The exhortations about the value of medical expertise was also evident in the debates about physical deterioration in the first decade of the twentieth century. These included the Interdepartmental Committee of Inquiry in 1904, fuelling the development of personal health services, limited as those were.[43] But medical professionals did not confine their criticism of factory legislation to the problems of enforcement. Increasingly, medical opinion began to push for prohibition on lead and there was a vociferous attack on pottery manufacturers over their use of arbitration to attempt to defeat the introduction of lead with lower solubility.

The concerns about women's physical deterioration and infant mortality demonstrated how the ill-health consequences of work were not only those of industrial diseases or the effects of working conditions. More doctors were probably engaged with this issue than with the working conditions themselves. As the principal initiatives for health and welfare were within local administration, local medical officers of health, especially in industrial towns, would have found them difficult to avoid. Many were engaged with local enquiries and initiatives on infant welfare. As with the opportunities offered by the State enquiry into the 'dangerous trades' for medical men to assume a national profile, this was also the case in relation to infant mortality. The position of the Medical Officer to the Privy Council of the Local Government Board continued to provide an impetus to national enquiry and in 1907 a medical officer was appointed to the Board of Education. In the early decades of the twentieth century, two men who had begun as local medical officers of health occupied these positions: Arthur Newsholme and George Newman. Both men were at the centre of developing the statistical analysis of the causes and especially the variability of infant deaths.

Doctors did not significantly depart from Robert Baker's earlier belief that 'very considerable mischief arises with women going out to work, not merely on the mother but also on the child'.[44] The difficulty was that its causality in infant mortality could not be directly linked to any physiological or clinical outcomes and most doctors agreed that social and environmental aspects were implicated. In the now-classic examination of the medical arguments by Margaret Hewitt, she concludes that 'beyond doubt, the employment of mothers was a threat to health and well-being of their babies. . . . Yet the problem still remains as to whether these disadvantages were counterbalanced by other factors.'[45] It is also possible that we may over-emphasize the importance attributed to employment. For example, Davin points out that only one paper at the 1906 conference on infant mortality was on women's employment.[46] While Newman, in particular, and Newsholme both referred to the 'evil' of industrial employment of mothers, the latter did not consider it was clearly a cause of mortality. Recent evaluations[47] have suggested he did not 'go with the crowd' on this, even though he did agree that maternal negligence and infant feeding were important factors. Within a local context, doctors were involved in giving prescriptive advice to mothers, especially those considered most 'at risk', but they often did so without a knowledge base for it. For example, there were different views on aspects of feeding, and questions of ante-natal care and medical aspects of birth had little interest for doctors.[48] Obstetric expertise was even less in evidence than occupational medicine.

The Medical Construction of Knowledge of Women's Occupational Ill-health

Medical knowledge about occupational ill-health was still undeveloped and often minimal except among those who had developed some specialist expertise as a result of the geographical location of their practice. Even those who did have experience exhibited a great deal of indifference and lack of understanding of either specific diseases or of the mechanisms of causality. This continued to be a matter for debate among physicians; difficulties in diagnosis proved problematic for both the theory of effective prevention and for doctors' practise with respect to occupational health problems. To the extent that medical knowledge remained impressionistic and speculative, an opportunity was provided for regulation to proceed on already-accepted principles and for medical expertise to be used to support the social basis of the legislation.[49]

In the case of lead-poisoning there were problems for practitioners in deciding whether the wide range of symptoms, that might have other causes, were indeed examples of poisoning. The Chief Medical Inspector noted in his report in 1899 that lead-poisoning did not present 'the same unmistakable signs that an acute infectious disease like smallpox does. No absolute definition of lead poisoning is possible and each practitioner . . . must form his own standard'.[50] Even the commonly accepted sign of a blue line on the gums was not present in all cases. Given the prominence of medical perceptions of hysteria (also with a plethora of symptoms) as a common nervous complaint among women at this time,[51] it was not surprising that, as the *British Medical Journal* claimed,[52] symptoms of lead-poisoning in young women would often initially be considered as hysteria. This difficulty in diagnosis would have impacted on the accuracy of poisoning notification, but medical uncertainty could also be used as a basis for keeping women in work rather than excluding them – which they and their employers often wanted – and it was used as a defence in those cases where death brought medical 'failure' to public notice. Lead was not unique in this: the same arguments were mounted with respect to phosphorous where, although its symptomology was more specific, there was considerable evidence of poor dental health that might have produced similar symptoms.[53] Some medical experts argued that the reason they had not notified cases was because they were unsure about them. In one prosecution case, the defence offered the excuse that the worker had complained of toothache not of phosphorous necrosis.[54]

A further area of difficulty that impinged on the appropriateness of preventive measures in these two cases of lead and phosphorous was the route of transmission. In both cases, opinion eventually settled on inhalation but the possibility of ingestion and then absorption through the body was retained. In the event both these means were reflected in regulations about ventilation and protective clothing in lead work and protective clothing, cleanliness and rules about food consumption in the match industry. The continuing adherence to the idea that ingestion of lead and phosphorous occurred was again possibly because of the strong tendency to level accusations against workers' own habits and practices. They could hardly be responsible for air quality, but they continued to chew tobacco (in the case of men), eat food in workrooms, and were dirty and unkempt. It is perhaps ironic that Oliver later observed lead-poisoning in the wives of house painters caused by washing their overalls.[55]

The speculative nature of medical theorizing can also be seen in the debates about both phosphorous and lead-poisoning, as medical experts were required to explain the differential rates and why not all the workers were poisoned. This is revealed by some of the witnesses to the 1893 Committee. One doctor, who did not think women were susceptible, nevertheless argued:

> But if I were a manager I would not employ women with large eyes, and what you call melting eyes, that is to say full of tears – liquid eyes are susceptible to the dust of white lead, and it causes brain disease and frequently blindness.[56]

Another witness suggested that the few cases he observed 'seemed to take it in turn to be ill'.[57] One member of the Committee, Mr Laurie, was to comment later that most local doctors had very little information to give and that 'evidently their attention had never been especially turned to the question'.[58] So although there were differing opinions about susceptibility, evidence, from physicians such as Oliver from his infirmary which received support from notification data (although flawed), combined with his position as a key medical expert and enabled the theory of female susceptibility to lead-poisoning to be pursued. Although Oliver admitted there were other factors that were important, he did not waver from his belief in female susceptibility. With the substitution of women in white lead processes and the consequent increase in male poisoning, Oliver argued that this was mainly because of the casualness of male labour, a group who were 'more careless, less cleanly and more intemperate'.[59]

The American occupational physician, Alice Hamilton, in her investigation of lead-based industries[60] argued that the excess of American rates over British ones was due to the latter's success with hygiene regulations, including better ventilation. She further challenged British ideas of female susceptibility: a close examination of her data led to the conclusion that where there were higher rates in women these were a result of economic and other disadvantages. When women and men were of the same class, they suffered equally. Oliver accepted that poverty and the other disadvantages which Hamilton alluded to, such as lack of food, were factors in lead-poisoning, but what was unique about a woman's constitution was her biology. It was the impact on the menstrual cycle and reproductive organs that was primarily responsible for their predisposition.[61]

Susceptibility arguments were a prominent strand of medical arguments in relation to occupational ill-health. In the case of phosphorous this was thought by some dental experts to lie in the state of dental health, and by others, Oliver included, in the state of constitutional health. There was, however, also an interest in the inverse of this equation: whether factory employment, or work in the 'dangerous trades' specifically, led to a deterioration in the constitutional health of operatives.

The existence of medical disagreements as to whether susceptibility or poor constitutional heath were brought to factory employment or were a consequence of such employment was irrelevant to the pursuit of legislative protection for women. If they were not susceptible in the first place it was necessary to prevent them from becoming so, and if they were susceptible then they would need to be prevented from working or protected from possible injury if they did.

It is evident that the Committee on Physical Deterioration did consider that women and factory employment might be a factor in assessing the extent to which there was a case for deterioration.[62] These debates were less central, however, than a consideration of an enormous increase in urban living, a decline in fertility (mainly among the middle-class) and thereby, as many Eugenicists and Social Darwinists believed, a larger pool of the 'unfit'.[63] The essence of the medical debate about physical deterioration was whether it indicated a need for further reform, or whether these reforms had themselves contributed to a 'weakening' of the national stock of health by permitting the unfit to survive.[64] The latter would have been a major blow to social and public health reformers, but it was only a minority of medical practitioners who gave any legitimacy to the pessimistic view of the national health. However, although Wohl argues the Committee's report gave further impetus to reform, particularly to the quality of town life, this was accompanied by a shift in thinking away from public health measures and towards personal health.[65] In the factory context medical inspection was an early indicator of this. In prioritizing the raising of the standards of physical health of the working class, social policy turned less to the environment and more to those measures which might improve the health of the next generation. Ironically, the provision of personal health services and welfare measures was mainly for infants and children, and as a consequence women's health, even as a factor in children's health, was marginalized.[66]

Doctors' support for wider perceptions about such issues as the 'negligence' or carelessness of workers, the characteristics of the female labour force and the impact of factory work on their ability to perform their domestic duties, served important ideological purposes. Doctors were continually to support arguments that the preventative measures that were in place were rendered ineffective because of the actions of workers themselves. 'I fear the dangerous practice of sucking sweets, etc., while at work has not yet disappeared', one doctor commented to a factory inspector. A letter from another reported on a failure of young women who 'would rather leave than make such a guy of herself' by wearing a respirator as indicative of the systematic neglect of precautionary measures, while another young woman did not consult on having symptoms of colic 'for the exquisite reason she did not like doctors'.[67] Dr Alexander Hay argued: 'I don't see why we should not have complete immunity from illness if the workers themselves would only avail themselves of the means which are provided for their own protection'.[68] Nor did doctors depart from a view that women should not be employed at all. As Robert Baker had told an audience earlier in the century, 'our homes, our hearth, our comforts are perfectly dependent on the qualifications of the female character'.[69] Middle-class men continued to see paid work, particularly in factories, as an unsuitable occupation for women. In this way doctors served to preserve patriarchal interests in the family and in the workplace.

Doctors and Industry

While the State provided a major focus for medical practice in relation to occupational health, a by-product of factory legislation was that it opened up some opportunities for doctors to practise in industry. Even if this were not the case, through their State role doctors had to deal with employers in their localities. Both cases led to difficulties for medical practitioners and was to earn them a great deal of criticism. The problem with their occupational health practice was not so much the lack of knowledge or 'unaccountable ignorance' the inspectors had levelled at some of their number,[70] rather they were perceived not to be neutral. If they were seen to protect employers' interests, they could also be seen as working against the State.

The scandal over undisclosed cases of phosphorous necrosis was one example where medical men were seen to work in an employer's interests. As the *Daily Chronicle* argued in the case of Bryant and May:

> the conduct of the doctor who under such circumstances 'is not positive' and therefore returns a certificate which ignores the main fact, so inconvenient to his employers, ought to be considered. There is a Medical Council that can do these things if it chooses.[71]

Dr Cunningham had written to the Home Secretary that he disagreed with Dr Garman of Bryant and May who allowed for continued working after tooth extraction 'contrary to the best official opinion'.[72] Dr Garman had also been criticized earlier in the 1890s when Clara Collet indicated she not did place much reliance on his evidence.[73] In the same industry at a later death, the certifying surgeon referred to the failure of the works doctor as indicative that 'his examinations cannot be of much use'.[74] Workers who consulted practitioners other than the works doctor lost their entitlement to sickness benefit.[75] Ironically, those firms who employed their own doctors often did so out of a genuine desire to provide health and welfare for their workforce – and Bryant and May had a reputation for this kind of paternalistic approach. Their doctors may have found it difficult to be other than loyal since this provided a secure income; interestingly, Dr Garman's son also worked for Bryant and May in the same capacity.

Dependency on local employers for income no doubt also accounts for an exchange in the *British Medical Journal* in the early 1900s when it was very critical of pottery employers. This led the Staffordshire Branch of the BMA 'with due regard to the whole interests of the district' to disassociate itself from the opinions expressed and conclusions reached.[76] But while individual and local networks of practitioners may have found it difficult to be critical of employers, it is clear that many employers had little time for medical interference in their industries. Nor did the medical profession have any sympathy for employers who, in their view, failed to look after the health of their workforce.

The hostility of employers to medical inspection was part of their general objections to State interference with their production and potential labour market. They also had to bear the cost of medical inspection, a factor that Alexander Redgrave had anticipated in the early 1880s might make it difficult to get such measures introduced.[77] The medical inspector presented a report from one of the certifying surgeons in the Potteries that he had 'experienced difficulty in convincing employers of the value of monthly medical inspection. They have been inclined to regard it as a unnecessary expense.'[78] Employers also mounted attacks on 'expertise' itself, claiming some privileges for practical as opposed to scientific knowledge and in some cases for that expertise to be 'local'. In a deputation to object to proposed rules following the 1893 inquiry, pottery manufacturers accused the Committee 'of public servants and advocates of regulation' of being not 'full, free and public'. This was in part a reference to perceived secrecy, but they had also taken evidence from medical men who had had no recent experience as certifying surgeons and they omitted to obtain it in the 'case of one of the oldest and most experienced certifying surgeons in the district'.[79]

Later, similar arguments about local expertise were used in the debates about the impact of lead-free glazes on the quality and competitiveness of china and pottery ware. Hence employers resorted to arbitration on proposed rules about the use of lead in glazes. This in turn put the medical profession itself on the attack. The *British Medical Journal* had noted in 1900 that the 'pottery manufacturers are not given to reform. Experience shows that they are a conservative body and move but slowly.'[80] In 1901 Lord James suspended the arbitration hearing for 18 months which *The Lancet* viewed 'with dismay'[81] and the *British Medical Journal* denounced, as 'the pottery manufacturers are jubilant for they think they have beaten the Home Office'.[82] How could a trade be considered by Lord James to be conducted with 'credit to the country' when it 'had 400 cases four years ago, 100 last year and since January this year 87 cases with 4 deaths?'. This leading article had already caused local practitioners some discomfort. At the meeting of the Staffordshire Branch of the BMA, a resolution was passed recognizing the continuing evil of lead-poisoning but equally accusing the article of being 'misleading, inaccurate, unfair, and contrary to the evidence given at the recent arbitration hearings'.[83]

However, despite some distinctions between the assumed neutrality of doctors employed on behalf of the State and the interests of those employed in industry, neither parties acted without some concern for their own livelihoods outside their role within State and industry. At the same time it is important not to overstate the 'power' of medical professionals to influence or shift opinion. In fact, most medically led campaigns to tighten up employers' responsibilities failed to have much impact either here or on State intervention generally.

Medical Surveillance: Success or Failure?

On balance, despite the arguments made for it, medical inspection and health surveillance of women workers was a failure. There are a number of reasons why. The first was doctors' ignorance.[84] Those aspects discussed above suggest that doctors did not often possess the knowledge that would have allowed them to make judgments about either the possibility that women were at risk, or already had symptoms of a disease. Another difficulty was the economic and class marginality of doctors which impinged on practitioners' judgments as to potential suspensions of workers. It has been argued that doctors at this time found themselves colluding with women in legitimating their sickness and thereby undermining patriarchal control within the family. In this case doctors' collusion with employers may have compromised their professional autonomy.[85]

At the outset a certification of fitness would have been difficult, considering the low standards of health in general, and the establishment of any kind of norm was probably quite arbitrary. It seems likely that what happened was, unless there was some obvious visible symptomology, certification went through, and that suspension was a 'fall-back' position. It is also evident that doctors did not regard 'slight' symptoms as reasons for suspension. Over and above these obstacles, both certification and suspension were difficult because of strategies which women themselves employed to defeat medical surveillance and attempts to restrict their work. If they were able, they would conceal any symptoms they had. In many instances they would leave the factory at the first signs of illness, wait until the symptoms were past and then either return or seek employment in another factory. In industries like match-making or enamelling of iron plates, case studies revealed women who employed both of these tactics in order to remain in work.[86] Factory inspector Henderson informed the Home Department that employers in lead manufacture had tried to defeat this practice by passing on information about rejected workers, to find that they presented themselves for work with false names and addresses.[87] Whether women could move and find alternative employment, depended on local labour markets, and whether there were concentrations of manufacturers in the same industry, as with pottery manufacture, or whether there were alternative forms of employment for women as in the east end of London. If that was not possible, then women had other alternatives, in particular homework or domestic service, or forms of casual employment. To this extent women often left the factory for employments that were as equally damaging to their health. In practice it seems very few exclusions or suspensions occurred, although accurate information on this is difficult to find. In the Annual Report of the Medical Inspector for 1900, Dr Arlidge had inspected 17 651 workers and had suspended 29, 19 of whom worked in lead processes, and earlier, although individual practitioners claimed that women had been advised to leave, in one case this amounted to only 31 over a one-year period.[88] It is difficult to see how, other than by operating as a 'threat' which served to remove some women from 'dangerous processes', that the claims made for the value of medical inspection can be justified.

Furthermore, medical inspection may have brought minimal benefits to women's health. If women were ill and either excluded themselves or were suspended, they were rarely offered medical treatment. The only access many working-class women had at this time to free health care was as an in- or outpatient at some of the voluntary hospitals. In some firms, it seems they received sickness benefit.[89] Later (after 1906) some were eligible for compensation under workers' compensation legislation, although this was primarily to benefit men. In addition, however, such health surveillance only occurred in scheduled industries, and thus it left the majority of women's work places and the health risks attendant on them outside of medical scrutiny or remedy.

It must be argued that the humanitarian values that were claimed to underlie the motives of the State's sponsorship for medical inspection and medical men's involvement in its practice ignored its oppressive dimensions. For all of the constant complaints that men made about the extent to which factory work was contrary to women's sensitivities, these did not seem to be considered in relation to medical inspection. There was still a problem about the 'decency' of male doctors in the examination of women clients, and in fact it often did not occur. Only women factory inspectors, it seems, were conscious of this problem. They campaigned for some time to have private medical rooms provided and succeeded in 1913. Issues of proprietary aside, the social relations of medical inspection in working situations exemplified the power of men and middle-class interests in the social control of women.

Medical inspection suffered from the same inadequacies as other forms of legislative regulation in that it was an individualistic solution to the collective problem of industrial working conditions. It focused on the possibility that there were sick individuals rather than sick work places. It was a strategy pursued because it was thought necessary to 'weed out' the constitutionally unfit for work, and thus enabled questions of prohibition, long hours of work or any other aspects of industrial production to remain relatively unscathed.

The employment of medical expertise in the service of State investigation should not be seen entirely in a negative light. While involvement with State inquiry gave opportunities for 'industrial diseases' to take the centre stage and for knowledge about them to develop, it also constrained it. The growth of the medical specialism may have been hindered because ultimately State service confined the use of medical expertize to a narrow and essentially social agenda.[90] Such a development was probably more readily aided by workmen's compensation which provided a basis for the recognition that industrial diseases could be treated as accidents, an injury to workers arising directly from their employment.

The tenor of the medical response was of compromise. They were often in favour of the exclusion of women or at least married women but accepted that instead the work should be surrounded with safeguards. Equally they supported the prohibition of substances that would have eliminated problems, but considered it was 'unlikely to happen' so that alternatives were to continue which essentially maintained the status quo.[91] State officials, it seems were only prepared to accept medical expertise to the extent that it remained within its own frame of reference.

Notes

1 I have deliberately used the term medical men here to reflect the gender of the occupation. While some women successfully became medical practitioners by the end of the nineteenth century, men were the occupational health specialists.

2 See Freidson (1970) *Profession of Medicine* p.251.

3 Witz (1992) *Professions and Patriarchy*.

4 See Turner (1987) *Medical Power and Social Knowledge*.

5 See Burstyn (1980) *Victorian Education and the Idea of Womanhood* and Purvis (1991) *A History of Women's Education in England*.

6 Several writers have noted these aspects of nineteenth-century medical professionalism: Inkster (1977) 'Marginal men: aspects of the role of the medical community in Sheffield, 1790–1850' Peterson (1978) *The Medical Profession in Mid-Victorian London*; Woodward (1984) 'Medicine and the city: the nineteenth-century experience'; and Waddington (1984) 'The development of medicine as a modern profession'.

7 For an account of doctors' relationship to poor-law administration, see Smith (1979) *The People's Health* Chapter 5.

8 Ibid., p.417. Lewis (1986a) *What Price Community Medicine? Philosophy, Practice and Politics of Public Health since 1919* notes this as a starting point for her later analysis.

9 In the case of occupational ill-health, ample evidence of a lack of knowledge is provided by medical witnesses to Committees of Inquiry in the early 1890s.

10 Smith (1979) *The People's Health*.

11 The classic thesis on this is McKeown (1971) 'An historical appraisal of the medical task'. For continuing debates around contributions to mortality decline see Szreter (1988) 'The importance of social intervention in Britain's mortality decline *c*. 1850–1914: a reinterpretation of the role of public health'.

12 Lee (1973) *The Emergence of Occupational Medicine in Victorian England*.

13 PP XXI, 1833, p.6.

14 Mockett (1988) '"A danger to the State": women and factory legislation 1830–50'.

15 See medical witnesses to Sadler's Select Committee in 1832, PP XV, 1831–2, also discussed in Mockett (1988) and Gray (1991) 'Medical men, industrial labour and the State 1830–50'.

16 See Gray (1991) and an earlier unpublished paper (1987b), with the same title, for an excellent overview of medical involvement in the early debates.

17 Rosen (1952–3) 'Charles Turner Thackrah in the agitation for early factory reform'; Lee (1964) 'Robert Baker: the first doctor in the factory department'; Rose (1971) 'The doctor and the industrial revolution'; and Gray (1991).

18 Wohl (1983) *Endangered Lives: Public Health in Victorian England.*

19 Chadwick (1842) 'Report on the sanitary condition of the British labouring population', reprinted in Flinn (1965); Greenhow (1858) 'Papers Relating to the Sanitary State of the People of England'; and Simon's reports to the Privy Council, all cited in Wohl (1982).

20 Wohl (1983) p.263.

21 Ibid.

22 Lee (1964) 'Robert Baker: the first doctor in the factory department' p.164.

23 Gray (1987b) 'Medical men, industrial labour and the State in nineteenth-century Britain' p.32.

24 Gray (1991) p.33.

25 See Gray (1987a) pp.33–4; and Bartrip (1985) 'The rise and decline of workmen's compensation'.

26 John (1984b) *By the Sweat of their Brow.*

27 Lee (1964) 'Robert Baker'.

28 Arlidge (1892) *The Hygiene, Diseases and Mortality of Occupations.*

29 This is most clearly argued in his 1988 paper presented to the Annual BSA Conference.

30 Gray (1987a) p.2.

31 PP XVII, 1893–4.

32 PRO/HO45/B26315. He also offered to pay his own expenses.

33 See his text *Lead Poisoning: From the Legal, Medical and Social Points of View* (1914).

34 Included in this were a number of visits Oliver made to match-making factories in Europe. The State agreed to sponsor these although they were not always taken on its behalf.

35 Laurie (1895) 'The medical profession and the unhealthy trades', *British Medical Journal* 5 October, p.835.

36 *Report of the Committee on the Various Lead Industries*, PP XVII, 1893–4.

37 Abraham (1893–4) 'Report on the Conditions of Work in the White Lead Industry', in *Reports of the Assistant Lady Commissioners' Royal Commission on Labour*, PP XXVII.

38 Reported in PRO/HO45/9848/B12393C.

39 Report by May Abraham to the Chief Inspector, in PRO/HO45/9848/B12393A.

40 PP XXIX (1910) *Evidence of Samuel Clowes of the Organisation of the National Amalgamated Society of Male and Female Pottery Operatives* pp.185–6.

41 *The Lancet*, 8 April 1882, Vol. 1, p.575.

42 The Association of Certifying Factory Surgeons continually reiterated calls for industrial hygiene as a branch of State medicine. See Deardon (1923) 'What medical science can do for industry'.

43 See Woodward (1984) 'Medicine and the city'.

44 In *Evidence to the Commission on Factory and Workshops 1875*, cited in Hewitt (1958) *Wives and Mothers in Victorian Industry* p.176.

45 Hewitt (1958) p.189.

46 Davin (1978) 'Imperialism and motherhood' p.31.

47 See Woods, Watterson and Woodward (1989) 'The causes of rapid infant mortality decline' p.115.

48 Oakley (1984) *The Captured Womb.*

49 Harrison (1991) 'Women's health or social control? The role of the medical profession

in relation to factory legislation in late-nineteenth-century Britain'; Gray (1991) 'Medical men, industrial labour and the State in Britain 1830–1850'.

50 *Annual Report of the Medical Inspector for 1899*, PP XI, 1900.

51 See Smith-Rosenberg (1972) 'The hysterical woman: sex roles and role conflict in nineteenth-century America'; Showalter (1987) *The Female Malady*.

52 'Lead poisoning in the Potteries', *British Medical Journal* (1896) p.237.

53 Harrison (1995a) 'The politics of occupational health in late-nineteenth-century Britain: the case of the match-making industry'.

54 PRO/HO45/9849/12393D, a defence of Dr Garman's son in relation to an employee at Bryant and May.

55 Oliver (1914) *Lead Poisoning; Legal, Medical and Social Points of View*.

56 PP XVII (1893–4) Minute 6736, Witness Mr John Ives Vaughan.

57 Ibid., Witness Dr Williams.

58 Laurie (1895) 'The medical profession and the unhealthy trades' p.833.

59 Oliver (1902) 'Lead and its compounds' in his *The Dangerous Trades* p.296.

60 Hamilton (1912) 'Lead poisoning in potteries, tile works and porcelain, enamel and sanitary ware factories'.

61 Thorpe/Oliver's *Report on the Potteries* in 1899 gave considerable emphasis to the link with reproductive biology, PP XII.

62 *Report of the Committee and the Minutes of Evidence*, PP XXXII, 1904.

63 Porter (1991) '"Enemies of the race": biologism, environmentalism and public health in Edwardian England'.

64 Wohl (1983) *Endangered Lives* pp.332–9.

65 Ibid., p.339.

66 For a general overview, see Harrison (1995) 'Women's Health' and also accounts of the development of the Infant Health and Welfare Movement such as Lewis (1980a) *The Politics of Motherhood*, Davin, (1978) 'Imperialism and motherhood' and Dwork (1987) *War is Good for Babies and Other Young Children*.

67 Letter from Mr Irvine, MRCS, 13 November 1894, PRO/HO45/B12393C p.15. As a reference to habits such as sucking sweets.

68 Cited by Mr Henderson in PRO/HO45/9848/B12393A.

69 Cited in Lee (1964) 'Robert Baker' pp.92–3.

70 Lucy Deane made this accusation in the 1898 Report with Rose Squire on the Match Industry, PP XIV.

71 *Daily Chronicle*, 2 May 1898 in PRO/HO45/9848/B12393D.

72 In a letter to Home Secretary Ridley, in PRO/HO45, ibid.

73 In her *Report on Conditions of Work in London for the Royal Commission on Labour*, PP XXVII (1893–4).

74 PRO/HO45/9848/B12393D, p.35.

75 Again there is evidence of this in relation to match-making in the files PRO/HO45/ 9848/B12393D and in Inspectors' Reports about cases of lead-poisoning.

76 *British Medical Journal* 15 March 1902, p.685.

77 In his *Reports on Regulation of the White Lead Industry*, PP XVIII (1882) and PP XVIII (1883).

78 Dr Hill of Tunstall in the *Annual Report of the Medical Inspector for 1900*, PP XI, 1901.

79 PRO/HO45/9851/B12393E, p.53.

80 *British Medical Journal*, 8 September 1900, p.681.

81 Cited in Meiklejohn (1963) 'The successful prevention of lead poisoning in the glazing of earthenware in the North Staffordshire Potteries' p.178.

82 *British Medical Journal*, 30 November 1901, pp.1616–17.
83 *British Medical Journal*, 15 March 1902, p.685. The meeting was held in December 1901.
84 *Annual Report for 1897*, PP XIV, 1898.
85 This argument has been mounted in relation to a number of disease categories affection women sufferers in the later nineteenth century. See Harrison (1995) for an overview.
86 Herbert Burrows of the Matchmakers Union cites some examples in London match-making, PRO/HO45/9848/B12393D.
87 PRO/HO45/9848/B12393D report on Newcastle also noted that Elisabeth Rafferty had 'lied' about her age.
88 *Annual Report of the Medical Inspector for 1900*, PP X1. The earlier example was that of the statistics supplied by a Dr Smith for 1895–6, cited in a report by Inspector Jackson to the Home Department PRO/HO45/9849/B12393C.
89 This was the case in Bryant and May matchworks and in some enamelling and lead industries.
90 Harrison (1991) 'Women's health or social control?'
91 This was the conclusion of the 1899 *Thorpe/Oliver Report on the Potteries*, PP XII.

Chapter 7

'Missionaries of the State'[1]: Women Factory Inspectors and Women at Work

As agitation mounted in the 1880s and 1890s for improvements in industrial conditions and the debates around the need for the 'protection' of women continued unabated, there was a strong argument that the failure of factory legislation thus far could be attributed to a failure in its enforcement. Ensuring compliance and prosecuting offenders were the chief responsibilities of the Factory Department through its inspectorate, so the inadequacy of enforcement was placed firmly at their door. There were too few inspectors. Some people, particularly trade unionists, questioned whether the best people were being selected. They argued that inspectors should be chosen who had 'practical' experience of working conditions. Those who were recruited in the nineteenth century were mainly working-class men from white-collar or industrial jobs. However, the failure of inspection of women workers was seen as a result of the gender of factory inspectors and, from the 1870s, there were increasing calls for the appointment of women inspectors. In the early channelling of these demands through the TUC and women's organizations it was thought that these women too should have 'practical' experience.

Mounting the Campaign

The calls for the appointment of women inspectors by women's organizations at this time provides something of a paradox. In the 1870s and 1880s all sections of the women's movement, including women unionists, were opposed to 'protective' legislation and the necessity for State interference in women's work. They considered that the solution to poor conditions essentially lay in organizing women. At the same time they clearly felt that existing legislation and inspection had failed them. In articulating that failure they frequently drew on the same discourse that argued for 'protection', that women workers had special 'needs'. This did not go unnoticed by men trade unionists at the TUC. In the debate on a resolution before the 1878 Congress, Henry Broadhurst observed:

> that the Congress in their fight to obtain the passage of the Factory and Workshop Acts encountered great opposition from women's organisations, and it seemed most extraordinary that, having opposed the Factory Acts, the lady delegates should now ask to be placed in a position to see that the Acts were (not) administered.[2]

The parentheses are used here to indicate that although pointing to the seeming inconsistency in position, Broadhurst was indicating that the appointment of women inspectors could result in widespread evasion. In this and subsequent congresses, resolutions called for the appointment of women, for the appointments to have responsibility for workplaces where women and children were employed and for them to be 'practical' women with experience of trades already covered by legislation.[3]

The campaign gathered force toward the end of the 1880s and into the early 1890s. Individual women unionists, such as Clementina Black (who frequently wrote to the Home Office in a personal capacity) and a wide variety of women's organizations kept up the pressure on the Home Department with repeated letters, petitions and deputations.[4] The London Women's Trade Council in its representation to the Home Office in 1890 argued that women workers were unwilling to communicate with men inspectors,[5] a factor noted in 1893 by Amie Hicks, Secretary of the Ropeworkers Union.[6] Women's trades or rooms where women worked, it was claimed, were often excluded from routine inspection. Like many other witnesses to the Royal Commission of Labour (1892–3) Amie Hicks maintained that the abuses and failures of the existing system could only be put right by 'women inspectors'.[7] By the early 1890s there were also calls within the House of Commons. Mr Leng MP found that the question he addressed to the Home Secretary as to 'whether he has any powers at present to appoint female inspectors of factories and workshops'[8] was rejected on the grounds of 'administrative economy and practicability'.[9]

The arguments used against the appointment of women to the inspectorate and the counter-claims made by their supporters reveal the pervasiveness of an ideological construction of gender difference in 'natural abilities', its relationship to the separate spheres of home and the paid labour market and the kinds of work women did when they were in paid employment. The work of factory inspection was defined as not being 'suitable work for a woman'. In response to the early demands for women inspectors, Alexander Redgrave, Chief Inspector of Factories, commented in his 1878 Report that he would:

> doubt very much whether the office of a factory inspector is one suitable for a woman . . . Factories would really be incompatible with the gentle and home loving character of a woman . . . I cannot conceive that such functions would commend themselves to a woman or that she could successfully discharge them.[10]

There were specific aspects of the work of factory inspection for women that were considered problematic. First, it was argued that women inspectors would inevitably be asked to inspect workplaces where men and boys were employed: this was considered to be inappropriate. The basis for this inappropriateness did not seem to lie in any a moral objection (that is of women mixing with men) but in the fact that men were unwilling to accept a situation where women would be in a position of authority over them. Second, objections centred on arguments about women inspecting industries involving machine-based production. Textile districts, for example, were full of 'crowded machinery' which would create two problems: how could women inspect machines and machine-based work, since they did not understand them, and how could they guarantee their own safety because of their dress?

The requirements of inspection were also unsuitable for women in other ways, especially visits to factories at night. A Home Office memo to Mr Leng who was evidently to the forefront of parliamentary pressure, put it thus:

> Presuming that a Factory Inspector were to be appointed to workshops in which women are employed, one of the duties would be to inspect them at night – even after 10.00 pm. Could they, as the inspectors are now doing, pass an hour or more after that time of night in the purlieus of Shoreditch and Whitechapel?[11]

These views about the unsuitability of women for the job of inspection reinforced objections made on administrative grounds: there would be unnecessary duplication because women would have the same duties as men. Thus, even if women could have been considered competent, it would be inefficient to use them. These arguments combined to protect factory inspection as a male preserve.

In examining the case mounted by the protagonists for women factory inspectors, an oppositional politics operated within the same conventional discourse that emphasized women's 'natural' talents and abilities. The difference was that men had argued that these talents were best employed within the domestic domain; women and their supporters, on the other hand, claimed these 'womanly' attributes would be particularly suited to serving women workers and in overcoming the existing defects in male factory inspection. Objections to their dress, for example, were countered by the assertion that this meant women would be better judges of the space required for them to work safely. Recognizing that there were social divisions between the two genders, the issue of 'sensitivity' was raised to suggest that only women could enter bedrooms at night in order to detect overtime working and, for similar reasons, women would be in a better position to receive complaints and investigate sanitary matters.[12]

When the argument for women inspectors was conceded and their work subject to constant scrutiny both within and outside official circles, these ideas of gendered expertise – the special claims for the value of women in the service of women and the potential and real conflict with men and male jurisdiction over inspection – continued to be evident. Women were not to operate within the factory inspectorate on the same basis as men until 1921.[13] These ideas were also directly experienced by women who became factory inspectors at the outset and in their day-to-day working lives. Rose Squire recalled, 'Only by effort of memory is it possible now to recall the disapproval and even dismay with which the news was received among relatives and friends that a young woman in the family had become an inspector.' It was, she suggests, viewed as 'not quite nice', 'an unladylike occupation'.[14]

Activists and reformers whose campaign for women factory inspectors was conducted largely in terms of existing patriarchal relations allowed those relations to remain intact. Thus in the inspectorate, as elsewhere, ideas that masculine or feminine attributes were suited to particular kinds of work continued to contribute to and reproduce the sexual division of labour. However, given the pervasive nature of these ideological constructions and socially constituted identities, it would be more politically pragmatic to challenge the results of these ideas rather than the ideas themselves. Witz[15] has shown how gender-based struggles within professional groups in the healthcare division of labour at this time had similar features. A consequence of such strategies, as with 'protective' legislation itself, were that they confirmed sexual difference as a legitimate basis of social difference and thereby per-petuate the structures of women's oppression. At the same time it might be argued, that a pragmatic and acceptable form of politics is to turn accepted categoriza-tions to women's advantage. The extent to which the women's factory inspectorate were able to provide some oppositional struggle not just to late nineteenth century gender relations, but also the exploitation of working-class women and their labour is a concern of this chapter.

Eventual Success

In 1893 Asquith, the Home Secretary, continued to receive deputations about the desirability of appointing women inspectors. He was sympathetic as he put it, 'to the movement to extend the area of female employment' and 'I hope I may be able . . . to do something'.[16] He believed there was already evidence of the value of women through those who had served on school boards and boards of guardians. There were by now important precedents of women doing this kind of work which undoubtedly smoothed the way.

As early as 1873, the Head of the Local Government Board (LGB) appointed Mrs Senior to provide 'a woman's point of view on the education of girls at pauper schools'. The Head of the LGB took steps to ensure this position was permanent since 'many of the officials could not endure the appointment and it was the greatest trial for them'.[17] In 1883, a Miss Mason was appointed as an Inspector of Boarded-out Children and in 1890 a woman was appointed as Inspector for Domestic Subjects by the Board of Education. Some local authorities, notably in London, had also appointed women to posts as sanitary inspectors.[18] More import-ant than any of these precedents was the Royal Commission on Labour 1891–2. The Commission recognized that the work and working conditions of women and girls required investigation as issues in their own right – and it considered this investigation should be conducted by women. Four Assistant Lady Commissioners were appointed and their reports constituted a separate section of the final report. The Commission was crucial in providing documented evidence about conditions and in placing issues of women's occupational ill-health more firmly on the polit-ical agenda.The Commission gave other employment opportunities to women as clerks and précis writers, and these forms of employment routed some women to employment as factory inspectors.[19] However, in anticipation that the Commission report would favour the appointment of women to the inspectorate, the Home Secretary decided to act rather than wait for its final recommendations.

Asquith's support for the appointment of women as factory inspectors accepted the same arguments that had been used by the Royal Commission for its own separate investigations of women by women, using the same ideas of gendered expertise:

> that there could not be free and frank communication between female operatives on the one side and the male inspector on the other. In addition to that there was the peculiar knowledge, the intuitive and instinctive knowledge which, without complaint and without inquiry a woman necessarily had as to the wants of her own sex.[20]

In addition to Asquith's more sympathetic views, other personnel changes, notably the retirement of Sir Alexander Redgrave as Chief Inspector of Factories, also paved the way, although opposition within the civil service was still considerable. Asquith later recalled: 'It was considered by state officials at the time to be a terrible proposition, they shook their heads and they did not sleep at night.'[21]

Following their association with the Royal Commission, May Abraham and Mary Paterson were duly appointed as the first two women inspectors by Asquith in 1893. Given the opposition to the appointment of women within the Home and Factory Departments and the emphasis on administrative difficulties within the expressed reservations, it is not surprising that the admission of women to the factory inspectorate and the way in which they would work within it would be on a different basis than men. It was only these first two inspectors, however, who did not have to sit the civil-service examinations, although these 'regular' admissions' procedures were less important than experience and networks in who was considered for entry after these two initial appointees. Asquith established a separate branch of the inspectorate. This was a peripatetic one whose women worked directly to the Chief Inspector. Women inspectors were given a brief, alongside other Factory Inspectors, to 'promote and enforce the uniform observance of the Factory and Workshop Acts'. But they also had a specific brief to investigate, inspect and regulate factories and workshops where women and children were employed. In Sprague-Oram, the new Chief Inspector, they had a supporter who, according to McFeeley,[22] not only defended them but gave them both responsibility and considerable freedom to design their work. In his first report of their work he commended them thus:

> Being of the opinion that the field of employment for women within the limits of their own special capacities and aptitudes, should be as wide and as large as you can possibly make it, and that there is no field in which they could be more fruitfully employed than in looking after the health and industrial conditions under which their fellow women labour in factories and workshops, you appointed two ladies as inspectors whose labours have already been found to be most useful.[23]

In the first decade of their work the peripatetic mode of organization and operation was to be continually defended. In addition to calls for more appointments to be made, campaigners also argued the case for some women to be stationed in particular districts where there were high concentrations of women workers.[24] This particularly applied to the Potteries. It also became a prominent theme within the agitation around the 'dangerous trades' where women were seen to be particularly at risk. As with the debates prior to their appointment this option was always rejected, usually on the grounds of problems related to male jurisdiction and efficiency. Women inspectors, in retrospect, defended it on the basis that it minimized direct conflict with male colleagues. From their perspective it would have given them some protection, although hostility, suspicion and even sabotage of their work still occurred. Ironically, the peripatetic role itself resulted in 'bold, unexpected and sporadic inroads into any district . . . and was fraught with the possibilities of friction', according to one women inspector.[25] While undoubtedly the rationale for this different mode of organization and operation was a response to male fears and did not completely vitiate them, it may also have given women inspectors opportunities for considerable autonomy, as well as freedom from day-to-day male control over their work, especially given their Chief's attitude toward them. However, there were constant threats not just to the peripatetic principle but to those spheres of influence they acquired. From the outset there were some areas that were defined as outside their expertise. The investigation of accidents and issues of machine-guarding was one of them.[26]

Becoming a Woman Factory Inspector

Becoming a woman factory inspector was unusual for several reasons. Despite the fact that by this time there was a well-established feminist campaign for extended employment opportunities for women – and middle-class women in particular – inspecting factories was still considered to be an inappropriate occupation. However, such feminist activism did make available a discourse that gave legitimacy to middle-class women's aspirations.[27] Women who entered public service work arenas had developed their personal aspirations within middle-class families who placed great value on providing education for their daughters.[28] Early recruits to the factory inspectorate had been educated often to university level. They were active members of various societies in the public domain, including health and suffrage. There was also an economic necessity for them to do paid work. May Abraham, for example, had come to England when her family in Dublin fell on hard times following the death of her father. Lucy Deane, Rose Squire and Adelaide Anderson, who became part of the 'pioneering five', came from similar backgrounds.[29] These women also had important social connections, however, and either through education or their paid work had developed relevant experience and knowledge of working conditions and factory legislation.

Contrary to the long campaign of trade unionists and labour women campaigners for women with 'practical knowledge' of women's working conditions to be appointed, in their terms envisaging perhaps working-class trade-union activists, the appointments were decidedly middle-class. McFeeley, in her account of the inspectorate, notes that this issue was raised by labour activists over the proposed appointment of the Girton-educated Adelaide Anderson as the third inspector, although the protests went unheeded.[30] The reference to the term 'Lady Inspector', she suggests, firmly placed inspection as a middle-class occupation. However, the term probably reflected the terminology of the time, as Rose Squire pointed out.[31] They were initially female inspectors, then lady inspectors and finally women inspectors: Rose saw this as a reflection of the changing position of women. Hilda Martindale, on becoming a senior lady inspector in 1908, noted these were still the days of 'a lady' although she had emerged from being 'a female'.[32]

There are other points about class that are relevant here, however. It might not have been a particularly viable alternative to have found working-class women with industrial work experience who could have occupied these positions – at least, not once it was required they sit the examinations. Lady Dilke, President of the WTUL, maintained that office-work experience and report-writing skills were essential and that working women may be 'utterly lacking in tact'.[33] This should not be taken to indicate that her views were correct. Some women who were active in labour organizations were extremely articulate and knowledgeable about working conditions and might have performed the duties with competence. The civil service examination might have been an obstacle, but it was probably the intention of the Home Office that middle-class women should be recruited. The middle-class women who were appointed, especially in the early years, did have direct experience of working conditions, either through their work, their philanthropic activities or their political ones and this was often in the context of direct investigation of working conditions. Both Lucy Deane and Rose Squire had worked together as sanitary inspectors with special responsibility for women's workshops in the London Borough of Kensington and Chelsea.

The network of people in trade-union and labour organizations and in liberal political circles were used in the initial appointments and provided some support for women's initiation into the politics of the Factory Department. The home of Sir Charles and Lady Dilke was the setting for many meetings in connection with initial introductions,[34] but similar meetings continued throughout the 1890s especially as women inspectors felt their positions to be under threat. Although they were not permitted to take 'political' positions on their work or on issues around legislation, they continued to use these networks in ways that at least indirectly operated politically. They were, for example, permitted to lecture, give classes and explain about their work and the Factory Acts. Beatrice Webb organized the publication of their articles and other 'supporters' provided platforms for them to lecture. Although they also spoke at women's organizations opposed to the legislation, they found not being able to fight their case directly in this context difficult.[35] The other important way in which these networks were important to them was in the prosecution of certain legislative changes through the political process. Rose Squire, in particular, pointed to the time she spent attempting to get laundries included in the 1895 legislation (just before her appointment she had helped the inspectorate to prepare their case on laundries) although it also reminded her of the injustice of women's lack of power:

> it seemed to me irksome that men, for the most part ignorant of the meaning of the words they uttered, took part in the discussion, while I, who knew so much, had to pass a few hasty sentences . . . to . . . members hurrying out of their seats to be put wise.[36]

Despite some occasional internal differences between the women factory inspectors, strong links of mutual respect and affection developed between them, partly out of a sense of being pioneers and partly because of their centralized administration. Numbers for the first five years remained small but these early members were to have a long association both with the inspectorate and each other. Violet Markham in her biography of May Tennant (Abraham) notes that she described Lucy Deane as 'a trusted colleague and dear friend for life'.[37] Hilda Martindale, who joined later in 1901, described Adelaide Anderson as 'outstanding . . . she at once gave me responsibility'.[38] But in spite of some small increases in number, there were still only 18 women inspectors following the increase permitted by Gladstone in 1908 (see Appendix 1).

Working Days and Working Nights

Women inspectors were to confound their critics and acquire almost unprecedented status as 'celebrated' public officials. Some understanding of the practice of female inspection is however important in an assessment of their contribution to the understanding of and improvements in working conditions and women's health.

Even in the early years of small staff numbers, the scale of the work seems considerable. Thousands of miles were travelled every year, covering the whole of the United Kingdom. In 1896, May Abraham travelled 9921 miles, Mary Paterson 11 764 and Lucy Deane and Adelaide Anderson (who joined that year) 4156 and 3556 miles respectively.[39] In 1899 Mary Paterson covered 15 847 miles.[40] This can be explained partly by the watching brief she kept on Scotland, but between 8000 and 10 000 miles per inspector in any one year was not uncommon. Visits were also numerous. In 1895 these included 2358 factories, 4599 workshops and 4500 other visits.[41] In later years the average rose to around 6000 to 7000 factories, 3000 to 4000 workshops and additional visits covering homes, local authorities, hospitals and courts. Written complaints, in the region of 300 to 400 in the early years rose to 729 in 1901[42] and 2025 by 1910.[43]

The increase in complaints was due both to an increased awareness by working women themselves of their existence, combined with a lessening of fear in doing so and the use made of the complaint mechanism by women's labour organizations, especially the WTUL, on behalf of women workers. The kinds of work investigated were enormously varied: one year alone might cover rag-sorting, fur-pulling, yarn-dyeing, brush-making, laundry work, the manufacture of blue and black lead, fish-curing, the rubber industry, licking labels, artificial flower-making, the use of naphtha, flock-mattress stuffing, outwork and the employment of children.[44] The work, Hilda Martindale commented later, 'was almost breathless in its variety'.[45] But these reported details about the work of women inspectors, although seemingly impressive, obscures its limitations in both amount and impact.

The first limitation for their practice came from the prescription of their role within State regulation. This meant that in their capacity of ensuring compliance with factory legislation, those workplaces and workers who came under their scrutiny were regulated. The kinds of problems the reports describe and the statistics on matters such as complaints and prosecutions were to a large extent the results of their 'policing' role. Since regulation mainly covered the hours of work, decent sanitary provision and the special rules surrounding the 'dangerous trades', these remained at the forefront of their work. Although they were given a remit for special enquiry, which provided opportunities on their own behalf to conduct investigations into unregulated areas of women's work, they were often required to conduct such investigations into problems which were circumscribed by official considerations.

The inspectors' own frustrations with the limitations on their powers imposed by factory legislation led them to advocate further extensions of legislation as one line of remedy. They would constantly reiterate such demands. Given the slow progress of legislation and an ambivalence which they shared with other supporters of State intervention about its effectiveness, they thought they would use their position whenever possible to engage in preventive and educative work. The aim was to use their visits to persuade employers of the benefits that would result from changing unhealthy practices or introducing measures that would benefit workers and employer alike. This led to one MP in 1903 objecting to the fact that they went beyond their province of seeing the laws were obeyed by doing 'missionary work'.[46] Between 1898 and 1914 they brought 4962 cases to the courts, securing convictions in 4715. But the Chief Lady Inspector, Adelaide Anderson,[47] commenting on these figures, noted that from 1911, 'the tendency was to place more reliance on conferences and persuasion'. The prosecutions during this period only represented 1974 occupiers, a very small number considering the scale of employment and contravention that were observed.

The women's inspectorate was very short staffed, particularly given the scale of the problems with which they were expected to deal. For this and other reasons, Helen Jones[48] has argued that the very existence of women inspectors also served to depoliticize the issue of women's working conditions, and the success of the women's inspectorate as health and welfare workers must be in doubt. Such a view is valid to the extent that State intervention itself was paradoxically a means of defusing political demands and mediating between different interests, and officials of the state are circumscribed by their role as State functionaries which requires a stance of seeming political neutrality. Lucy Deane recalls in her diary a conversation with May Abraham, prior to her acceptance into the inspectorate, when she was advised to 'keep clear of public speaking or sympathy with any political or Trade Unions etc. because the government cannot employ a "party" woman.'[49] However, it would also be wrong to imply that the strategies pursued by the women's inspectorate were never able to realize some beneficial outcome or achieve radical shifts in thinking. Unfortunately I think it was not the operation of the inspectorate during this period that allowed this; but the opportunities provided by the exceptional circumstances of welfare provision in relation to women's war work to which many of them later attended to. Even here, however, the achievements were often short-lived.[50]

Perspectives on Women's Occupational Health

The annual reports of the women's inspectorate provide us with some of the most comprehensive source material on the conditions of women at work and the possible impact of these conditions on their health and wellbeing. They also offer insights into the lives led by many working-class women. To the extent that women inspectors felt able to enter into the private worlds of women, as they often did by visiting them at home and by living in their communities, there was the opportunity for relationships that enabled women to talk about their experiences. In their contemporary context the reports were given considerable coverage in feminist periodicals and the local and national press. The complimentary view that these commentaries give of the inspectorate's work reflected genuine admiration both for their work, and its usefulness in the political struggles being waged around industrial and welfare reform. One such example described:

> The exhaustive character of these reports and the human interest with which they throb, show how admirably the Lady Officials have done their work, and with what thoroughness they have investigated complaints received[51]

and referring to their earlier reports Violet Markham remarked:

> It is impossible to read these early reports of the Women's Inspectorate and to realise the disgraceful conditions they often found, and not to ask oneself what, prior to their appointment, the men inspectors had been doing?[52]

Such comments emphasize a public perception of the value of women with duties and responsibilities for women.

At the same time, it is important to be cautious about the interpretation of these kinds of data. Although women inspectors were not as remote from the reality of women's working conditions as some other middle-class commentators on women's work, the class differences between themselves and working women were still considerable and would have impacted on the relationship between women workers and women inspectors. There was a deference on the part of women workers that marked not just class but their official status. Many women communicated with inspectors because they hoped something might be done about their own circumstances. They were not prepared to take the inspector's side, for example, by acting as witnesses: this would also put their own position in jeopardy, not just in their employment but also within their own communities. So the social and economic arguments that were the basis for why women inspectors were required at the outset also impinged directly on their ability to pursue aspects of their work. The existence of women inspectors did not mean an end to workers' experienced and real vulnerability. As Hilda Martindale records in the context of the enormous difficulties of collecting evidence and taking prosecutions: 'however skilful a worker may be, she finds it very hard indeed to get another situation if she has been dismissed through telling the truth to the inspector, she is regarded as a spy'.[53]

It is arguable whether the presence of women inspectors did empower women or not. Their own view implies that this was the case: it did make women more aware of their rights under legislation. Complaining or using the inspectorate, which showed a steady increase year by year, was indicative of women being more assertive in seeking redress. Hilda Martindale cites one example of a group of 80 women who marched on her office when she was stationed in Ireland, demanding to know 'what she could do for them'.[54] Adelaide Anderson concluded that women workers became bolder and that greater self-expression and self-help among them was due to the confidence built-up between workers, women factory inspectors and the work of leading women organizers.[55] Groups such as laundry women had been more open in their protests as their involvement in the WTUL rally of 1891 indicated. Anderson reported that 'the fourteen hour day met with outbursts of indignation from women who would "like to see how men would stand fourteen hours of this work in the heat and steam"'.[56] Against this are the continued indications that even though women felt more ready to complain, they were often fearful that their complaint would be discovered. 'Please mem, when you come never make any calls or let anyone know where you gained this letter' was typical of letters Hilda Martindale received that asked her to 'say nothing'.[57] In 1902 Mary Paterson expressed the view that 'acquiescing at first in conditions she feels powerless to improve, gradually ceases to feel them as an offense to her'.[58] Because not all women had the benefit of an inspector's response to their problems, or that often she could not effect change in any case, the scale of empowerment was probably small.

To what extent did women factory inspectors merely confirm 'official' views or were they able to develop and present an alternative perspective on occupational ill-health? Elements of both these alternatives were probably discernible in the perspectives they took on a variety of issues. The fact that they exhibited more conservative thinking about the causes of illness or remedy or about the women at work was a result of their own middle-class origins and the extent to which aspects of Victorian and Edwardian social values were widely held. It may also have been necessary for them not 'to rock the boat' as part of a delicate political balance that was necessary to ensure their own position while they pursued some limited but more radical reforms. They were certainly conscious of having to act 'politically' and of the difficulties of doing so. Although as civil servants they were supposed to be politically neutral, they did not entirely give up their links with feminist and labour organizations, although they used them and presented themselves in these contexts in an 'official' capacity. But, as with other aspects of their role, they developed a certain political acumen in their pursuit of their own ideas of occupational health. Lucy Deane describes a discussion over dinner with May Tennant about Deane's investigation into lead-poisoning in the Potteries. May Tennant advised her to collect comparative statistics to 'blunt the risk of making lead-poisoning a women's problem'.[59]

There were two important respects in which women inspectors challenged the approach to occupational health reflected in State intervention and, to some extent, the approach of medical experts. Although they considered the 'dangerous trades' posed risks to women's health, they were more concerned about those aspects of working conditions which led to its gradual undermining. They implied that to some extent the 'dangerous trades' were a diversion from this. In her retrospective account, Adelaide Anderson argued that hours of work was one such issue which suffered and that there were factories, such as a 'white work factory' with a high incidence of phthisis, 'where the steady undermining of health that went on was really greater than in many a factory under special rules'.[60] The second challenge lay in their wider interpretation of 'working conditions'. Traditionally it was low pay, poor sanitation, long hours, dangerous dusts and fumes and machinery, lack of ventilation and extremes of temperature that were generally accepted as being related to ill-health, although not all these received recognition in legislative control. In these aspects of occupational ill-health they acquired a reputation as 'experts' in their own right, as their contribution to one of the leading medical texts on the subject demonstrated.[61]

Equally, however, they also drew attention to new work dangers, such as asbestos-spinning, 'which in those days was met by incredulity' recalls Hilda Martindale.[62] However, inspectors' perceptions about the organization and social relations of work, in which gender was a major factor, were more radical. A recognition of women's relative powerlessness in the labour market and the disadvantages they brought with them from inequality outside the industrial system, in turn compounding other aspects of occupational health risks, were issues which inspectors put and kept on the agenda. However, while their own analyses pointed to these factors in wellbeing, it is not possible to assess whether any changes came about as a consequence. While their testimony as expert witnesses to many committees of enquiry may have been important in keeping women's interests to the forefront, it was unlikely to have changed the discourse substantially. The extent to which more radical demands to restrict women's work on the grounds of health were not met, was probably as much to do with the State's own interests as it was the arguments of women against them.

Gender Divisions in the Service of the State

There were aspects of the bureaucratic organization of the inspectorate and the day-to-day experience of work in which the ability of women to be inspectors without the direct control of men was constantly under scrutiny. Energies which could have been given over to inspection were inevitably diverted to dealing with their own working circumstances. From the first appointments some restriction of women's responsibilities in terms of gender and expertise was evident over the issue of accidents and related questions of the fencing and guarding of machinery. There was an assumption that accidents were primarily a problem within forms of male employment, but it was also assumed that women would not know about machines.[63] Ideas of gendered expertise continued to be evident elsewhere. Rose Squire remembers that a woman inspector was 'to a certain extent handicapped in arguing a factory was not in a cleanly state, being thought to have the bias of her sex in favour of much cleaning',[64] and Lucy Deane recorded male inspectors who viewed her as a 'fusser' in respect of machine guarding.[65] Those special enquires also indicated that their expertise was considered distinct. In 1908 they were given specific duties with respect to sanitary inspection, child labour and the employment of women after childbirth. Over and above these specific examples, the general case for gendered expertise never wavered: that women inspectors would be concerned with those industries and those factories and workshops where women and girls were employed. Such ideas of gendered expertise would in some instances benefit working women and in others limit their access to the women's inspectorate.

Another area where patriarchal values directly affected employment opportunities for women and the retention of experienced women within the factory inspectorate, was over the marriage bar. At the time the inspectorate had been formed there had been no marriage bar, but it was not long before the pressures around married women working and the regulation of this within the civil service itself was to impinge upon them. May Abraham married Harold Tennant in 1896, and by 1897 she was pregnant. Deane documents in her diary that she continued working despite the social pressures put upon her by her husband's family: 'she evidently wants to keep on her superintendship, and most of her family object while the authorities are doubtful as the possibilities of her doing it.'[66] Earlier the diary suggests that Anderson and Deane discussed ways of organizing the work in an effort to keep her in the service. In the event, May Tennant resigned following the death of her small stepson.

In 1894 the Treasury proposed that regulations which gave a gratuity to women who were required to leave the service on marriage, principally among the clerical ranks of the Post Office, should be extended to other parts of the service.[67] There is some evidence that the Factory Department resisted such a proposal. Internal memoranda[68] reveal that the Chief Inspector informed the Treasury (in 1896) that it would be undesirable to have a rule which required 'female inspectors to resign on marriage'. In the ensuing correspondence he argued for the 'exceptional' nature of the qualifications needed for inspecting women's work places that 'it may happen the Secretary of State should appoint a married lady'. It was, he argued, that 'the nature of the duties are so very different from government employed women in the post office or as typists in other departments', and that the case for married women in inspecting was evident in respect of the appointment of such as Assistant Commissioners for Education in 1894 and 1895. The Treasury continued to press for a marriage bar, and in the event a compromise was reached that retirement on marriage should apply to all future appointments 'unless the

Secretary of State considered it desirable to retain them.'[69] The records suggest that factory inspection did become an occupation for single women (see Appendix 1).

It was not long before the women's inspectorate acquired a distinct professional and administrative identity. However, such power and status as they did acquire was always tenuous. Within a relatively short period their branch was to be reviewed by a Committee whose concern was the organization, staffing and working brief of the inspectorate. These matters were returned to several times throughout the 1893–1921 period.[70] These reviews were always viewed by women inspectors as a threat, although by the time the separate inspectorate was abolished in 1921 there were divisions between long-serving seniors and more recently appointed juniors who favoured reorganization and merger with the male inspectorate.

In this period the committee returned again and again to the question of dual inspection and the friction between men and women. The first review of 1896 seems to have been prompted by men's concerns about the independent authority of women, rather than any real instances of conflict or duplication. It was possible for these issues to be raised because the women had lost their two early supporters after the 1895 election, Asquith from the Home Office, and Sprague-Oram as Chief Inspector of Factories. There was opposition from men to the appointment of May Abraham as Superintending Inspector, and McFeeley[71] and Lucy Deane's diary suggest that there was considerable 'back room' politics, utilizing their friends in parliament, to secure their newly won position and defeat moves from the men's inspectorate. However, they were not entirely successful. As a consequence of the 1896 review they were instructed to consult and communicate directly with men district inspectors.[72] The role of Superintending Inspector was lost on the retirement of May Abraham (now Tennant), in 1897 when it was replaced by a Principal Lady Inspector. In addition the women's inspectorate lost the power to prosecute, and to order structural alterations in work places to remedy deficiencies in ventilation or sanitation.

May Tennant's anger at these changes was demonstrated publicly in *The Fortnightly* when she attacked these moves as undermining the ability of women inspectors by making improvements dependent on the cooperation of men.[73] The *English Woman's Review*, which was often ambivalent on the role of inspectors because of their own opposition to legislation, saluted this outburst making 'their annoyances thus public . . . may yet hope . . . the Women's Inspectorate will become more essential to the department . . . (and) overcome the prejudice of their opponents'.[74] Adelaide Anderson, who had assumed the position of Principal Lady Inspector, had the power to prosecute restored, but in 1898 the Committee was of the view that the women inspectors had not offered any relief to the district inspectors and there were still problems of demarcation.[75]

By the end of the 1890s there were initial signs that there might be some 'official' support for the idea of localization, either in the form of 'block' inspection or working in special districts. In 1900, although still stationed in headquarters, Lucy Deane began working in west London, and it was recommended one inspector be stationed in Ireland. In 1904 Hilda Martindale spent eight months here and then four months in the Potteries. The pursuit of localization was still cautious, but by 1907 there was a push for reorganization on localized lines, using the argument that the peripatetic system was too expensive.[76] The Principal Lady Inspector continued her opposition to changes in their mode of operation, pointing out that there were additional hardships for women consequent on requiring them to be mobile on a permanent basis, in that it isolated them from colleagues, family and friends.[77] Women inspectors were also worried about friction and asked that they be given definite duties and positions within districts. In the event some localization resulted although the separate branch was maintained.

There is little doubt that the committee sought to meet men's concerns rather than women's. The assumption was that if there was friction then remedy had to be sought in the way the women operated, not the men. It is also evident that women's opposition to any change reflected their own fears about loss of autonomy and more overt conflict with male colleagues. For Adelaide Anderson in particular, the dispersal of her inspectors was a threat to her own authority and control and undermined her management style.[78] The change she argued, would not only seriously injure their work, but destroy the Branch as a Branch. The impact on her own self-esteem was hinted at in a memo to the Chief Inspector in 1908:

> The care and trouble caused by this imposition on me of excessive work with decreased control of its rate and amount, and decreased opportunity of conferring with my staff have been accompanied by insomnia and as soon as it is possible to arrange matters I must ask for a few months rest.[79]

Later, she appears to have become more sanguine about reorganization, concluding in her annual report of 1909 that local residency had been a success in making inspectors more accessible and complaints more readily dealt with.[80] Equally, her locally based inspectors, despite their initial misgivings also expressed enthusiasm, not least because they acquired a new authority for the training and supervision of junior members, and more opportunities for team work.[81]

On a day to day basis women inspectors experienced conflict with men, including forms of sabotage where men colleagues would send them to places already inspected, which served to annoy employers in particular. Lucy Deane's journal gives examples of these kinds of hostilities. She was also critical of men's lack of enthusiasm for the job treating it simply as a means of earning a livelihood. Despite frustrations with their men colleagues, many of the women invested their work with a reforming zeal and enthusiasm that in part was a product of their unique position. Rose Squire and Hilda Martindale both made reference to reorganization in their accounts of the women's inspectorate, and seemed to indicate that it often depended on who those male colleagues were. Rose Squire commented:

> I think that, broadly speaking, it occasioned in the mind of the majority of men a sense of irritation that a set of women inspectors not subject to their direction and control (and women at that!) should be circulating in their districts; to the women it caused at times a galling sense of limitation of function and of isolation from the main current of departmental practice and policy vested in the men's organisation.[82]

Hilda Martindale describing her residency in the Potteries confided that 'I have to admit that my relationship with him (the District Inspector) at times was somewhat difficult; but we both tried to work harmoniously together.'[83]

Localization provided evidence that women could work away from family and friends, and in fact this argument had always been somewhat spurious as their peripatetic status had required them to be away from their home base for considerable periods. The threat to the power vested in 'headquarters' and the Principal Lady Inspector, and day to day autonomous working was probably much more important in women's opposition to this constant scrutiny of their work and their defense of the status quo. Divisional operation no doubt laid the groundwork for considering even more radical forms of reorganization, but the First World War was to intervene.[84]

There has been a tendency to celebrate the work of the women's factory inspectorate, understandable perhaps given the uniqueness of women's involvement in this official capacity, and thus to characterize women's ministrations on behalf of women in a positive light. There were also the plaudits heaped upon them in the contemporary context by supporters of regulatory approaches to the problems of working conditions. Certainly in their own writing, journal's and retrospective accounts there is indicated a conviction, perhaps typical of a proselytizing 'missionary' that they could take some credit for a changed perspective on occupational ill-health. Referring to Adelaide Anderson's account, Hilda Martindale commented:

> Anderson is undoubtedly right. The early years of the twentieth century
> saw what was unquestionably the most remarkable development that had
> ever yet been attempted in any age, in any country in applying scientific
> knowledge and care to the protection of workers from industrial disease
> and injury.[85]

At the time that the inspectorate was to disappear as a separate entity, Adelaide Anderson was to wonder 'why our predecessors so long grudged to the woman worker the help which only a woman can give.'[86] They were a unique experiment in factory administration; and factory administration was at this time to take a new and more concerted direction in health and safety.

The contribution of women factory inspectors has been neglected within the context of accounts of late nineteenth-century feminism and labour activism, as if it were not possible to countenance such middle-class women state officials in this light. A corrective is required to both this and the over-celebratory tendencies. The achievements of the women's factory inspectorate were in increasing knowledge and awareness of the plight of many working-class women in industrial and workshop employment; and of the many ways in which work, and wider social and economic factors produced ill-health. Their effectiveness however was undermined by its circumscription within a flawed State strategy, and by the reproduction of gender relations within factory inspection and in a constitution of women's relation to the spheres of home and work.

Within the possibilities and priorities for middle-class women in terms of feminist struggle, it is evident that their analysis and practice shared much with contemporary feminism. Occupational health was often to be subsumed in other struggles around work, and in those around health and health care. It may well be, as Jones argued,[87] the major achievement of the women's inspectorate was in breaking the ground for middle-class professional women in the civil service. It would be a mistake, however, to under-estimate the value of their 'blue-books' to developing a new political role for the State in welfare reform, and informing the consciousness of 'first wave' feminism about working conditions and working women's lives.

Notes

1 There were repeated references to the women factory inspectors in these terms in newspapers and periodicals. Hilda Martindale cites a *Daily News* reference to 'a missionary of the state' that protects the 'human element' in industry in her *From One Generation to Another* (1944a) p.86. Adelaide Anderson, in her retrospective account of the inspectorate *Women in the Factory* (1922) cites a reference to a Canon Scott Holland in which he refers to inspectors as 'missionaries of order and health' *Commonwealth*, March 1896.

2 *Eleventh Annual Report of the Trades Union Congress 1878*, p.82.

3 See further *Annual Reports of the Trades Union Congress* from 1879 to the end of the 1880s.

4 See PRO HO45/B8031/5 for many examples of these.

5 PRO/HO45/B1137AF.

6 *The Woman's Herald*, 30 March 1893.

7 *Report* and *Minutes of Evidence*, PP XXVII, 1893–4.

8 PRO HO45/9819/B8031/5.

9 Ibid. This version is taken from a report in *The Times*, 27 January 1991.

10 *Annual Report for 1878*, PP XL, 1879, pp.189–90.

11 Memo dated 11 November 1891 in PRO/HO45/9818/B8031/5.

12 Examples of all these lines of anti- and pro-argument can be found in the files PRO/HO45/9818/B8031/5 and PRO/HO45/B1137AF, as well as in the debates of the Trade Union Congress and Women's periodicals such as *English Woman's Journal*.

13 For an overview of the whole period of the Women's Inspectorate, see McFeeley (1988) *Lady Inspectors*; Omori (1986) 'British factory inspectorate as women's profession 1893–1921'; and Harrison (1995c) 'Gender, the State and occupational ill-health'.

14 Squire (1927) *Thirty Years in the Public Service* p.17.

15 Witz (1992) *Professions and Patriarchy* especially draws attention to the gender-based strategies of occupational closure employed by both women and men, and countervailing strategies to contest exclusion.

16 In an address to the National Liberal Federation 1893, cited in Martindale (1938) *Women Servants of the State*.

17 Martindale (1938) ibid., p.30.

18 Ibid. Discussion of these early appointments of women can also be found in Hollis (1979) *Women in Public*; Holcombe (1973) *Victorian Ladies at Work* Chapter VII.

19 May Abraham and Mary Paterson, the first two to be appointed (1893) were an Assistant

Lady Commissioner and clerk and précis writer respectively. Adelaide Anderson (1894) and Anna Tracey (1897) were both clerks and précis writers.

20 *The Times*, 25 January 1893.
21 From his personal memoirs and also an address to the House of Commons, 5 August 1921, cited in Martindale (1938) *Women Servants of the State*.
22 McFeeley (1988) *Lady Inspectors* Chapter 3.
23 *Annual Report for 1893*, PP XX1, 1894.
24 PRO HO45/9933/B26610 for the correspondence and other materials pertaining to the campaign for women inspector(s) in the Potteries.
25 Squire (1927) *Thirty Years in the Public Service* p.34.
26 Harrison (1993a) 'Are accidents gender-neutral?' argues that because machine expertise was gendered, this impacted on both the idea of the industrial accident as belonging to men's work and to women inspectors being denied responsibility for the inspection of machines and accident investigation.
27 See Levine (1988) *Victorian Feminism 1850–1900*.
28 There are a number of specific examples within the inspectorate and in the case of Clara Collet. For the importance of social origins of particular kinds in 'first wave feminism' see Banks (1986) *Becoming a Feminist*. For a general discussion see Dyhouse (1989) *Feminism and the Family in England*.
29 See Fawcett collection of biographical notes; Markham (1949) 'May Tennant: a portrait'; Martindale (1948) *Some Victorian Portraits and Others*; Squire (1927) *Thirty Years in the Public Service*; McFeeley (1988) *Lady Inspectors*.
30 McFeeley (1988) *Lady Inspectors* pp.24–5. The appointment of Lucy Deane at the same time also confirmed the preference for educated women.
31 Squire (1927) *Thirty Years in the Public Service* p.36.
32 Martindale (1944a) *From One Generation to Another*.
33 Dilke (1895) *The Industrial Position of Women*.
34 This is highlighted in Lucy Deane's diary account of her efforts to get herself considered for the inspectorate. See entries from late 1893 through to March 1894.
35 McFeeley (1988) *Lady Inspectors* pp.48–9.
36 Squire (1927) *Thirty Years in the Public Service* p.26.
37 Markham (1949) *May Tenant: A Portrait* p.25.
38 Martindale (1944a) *From One Generation to Another* p.74.
39 *Annual Report for 1896*, PP XVII, 1897. These figures and those relating to the numbers and types of inspections, prosecutions and enquiries were provided at the beginning of each yearly report.
40 *Annual Report for 1899*, PP II, 1900. Most of this travel would have been by train.
41 *Annual Report for 1895*, PP XIX, 1896.
42 *Annual Report for 1901*, PP XII, 1902.
43 *Annual Report for 1910*, PP XXII, 1911.
44 *Annual Report for 1895*, PP XIX, 1896.
45 Martindale (1944a) *From One Generation to Another* p.82.
46 Mr Collings to the House of Commons on 29 June 1903. Cited by Adelaide Anderson (1922) *Women in the Factory* as the only complaint about their work.
47 Anderson (1922) *Women in the Factory* Chapter VI.
48 Jones (1988) 'Women health workers'.
49 Deane (1893) *Business Diary* entry, 27 October.
50 Thane (1982) *Foundations of the Welfare State* notes in general terms how there were innovations in welfare that provided precedents for later developments, but were also

a long time coming, such as family allowance. Rose Squire (1927) in her retrospective account of her years in the inspectorate and public service also notes the administrative difficulties there were in securing satisfactory industrial conditions: Chapter XI.

51 *Lancashire Post*, 17 August 1908, in the Gertrude Tuckwell Collection.
52 Markham (1949) *May Tennant* p.27.
53 Martindale (1944a) *From One Generation to Another* p.77.
54 Martindale (1944a) ibid., p.96.
55 Anderson (1922) *Women in the Factory* Chapter 1.
56 *Annual Report for 1896*, PP XVII, 1897, p.97.
57 Martindale (1944a) *From One Generation to Another* pp.90–100 gives a number of examples of letters to this effect.
58 *Annual Report for 1902*, PP XII, 1903.
59 *Lucy Deane's Diary*, entry 26 April 1897.
60 Anderson (1922) *Women in the Factory* p.48.
61 Oliver (Ed.) (1902) *The Dangerous Trades*. This includes chapters by Rose Squire, Mary Paterson, Lucy Deane and May Tennant.
62 Martindale (1944a) *From One Generation to Another* p.150.
63 Harrison (1993a) 'Are accidents gender neutral?' examines these issues in more detail.
64 Squire (1927) *Thirty Years in the Public Service* p.45.
65 *Annual Report for 1904* PP X, 1905.
66 Deane (1896) diary entry 5 October.
67 Holcombe (1973) *Victorian Ladies at Work*.
68 PRO, HO45/9933/B26610 contains all the notes and correspondence on this issue.
69 Ibid.
70 See McFeeley (1988) *Lady Inspectors*, and Omori (1986) 'British factory inspectorate as woman's profession'.
71 McFeeley (1988) *Lady Inspectors* pp.46–7 and Lucy Deane's Diary entries for the first three months of 1896.
72 PRO/HO45/9910/B21173 contains details of exchanges on this issue.
73 Tennant (1898) 'The women's factory department' pp.150–1 and McFeeley (1988) also documents these exchanges pp.60–2.
74 *EWR* (1898) 15 July, p.214.
75 LAB 15/5.
76 LAB 15/5, and these administrative and jurisdiction issues are also discussed in Omori (1986).
77 PRO/HO45/10327/B13295.
78 McFeeley (1988) *Lady Inspectors* pp.114–5.
79 PRO/HO45/10553/B164207.
80 *Annual Report for 1909*, PP XXI, 1910.
81 Martindale (1944a) *From One Generation to Another* p.149.
82 Squire (1927) *Thirty Years in the Public Service* p.133.
83 Martindale (1944a) *From One Generation to Another* p.85.
84 For details of the remaining years of the inspectorate, including organizational issues see, Omori (1986), McFeeley (1988) and Harrison (1995c).
85 Martindale (1944a) *From One Generation to Another* p.151.
86 Anderson (1922) *Women in the Factory*, preface.
87 Jones (1988) 'Women health workers' p.182.

Chapter 8

Women, Feminism and the Politics of 'Protective' Legislation

Outside of suffrage, 'protective' legislation was one of most important foci for feminist politics during the period of 'first wave' feminism in the late Victorian and early twentieth-century period. Suffrage also provided a context for the position that sections of the women's movement took toward State intervention in general and 'protective' labour legislation in particular. 'Protective' legislation also gave rise to divisions between women in their analysis of both the problem of and possible remedy for women's working conditions. These divisions reflected different views of what was the right political strategy for activists to pursue in the light of their disenfranchisement from the mainstream political process and national policy-making.

The concern with 'protective' legislation centred on two major aspects: the extent to which, consistent with ideas of both a *laissez-faire* approach to economic life and that civil liberties were endangered by State laws, there should be any State interference at all with women's employment; and the extent to which a legislative approach to the regulation of industrial life – one which essentially defined women as 'like children', a class in need of some form of 'special protection' – was effective as a solution to women's exploitation and their poor working conditions and thence was a politically acceptable strategy to pursue. Both gender and class issues entered into feminist politics around these dimensions of the State, women at work and their working conditions.

At the outset the debates about 'protective' legislation and other feminist activism around work and working conditions were not centred on occupational ill-health itself. So to what extent did occupational health issues feature as part of these wider concerns and how did feminist activism contribute to a constitution of the problem of women's occupational ill-health? These are important concerns if feminist scholarship is to appreciate what Walby[1] called the 'large multi-faceted, long-lived and highly effective phenomena that was "first-wave" feminism'. This chapter also assesses how working women themselves 'felt' about their working conditions and the struggles going on around them.

The approach to analysing the positions women took on 'protective' legislation taken here is different to the one taken by previous feminist scholars whose principal interest in this issue has often been to inform different projects. This has been evident in work concerned with the women's movement or feminism at this time, divisions within feminist politics[2] or as part of studies of women's trade unionism or the historical gender-segregation of work.[3] 'Protective' legislation has thus been given a particular meaning and significance. All these issues are also pertinent to my analysis, but I have a central interest in the extent to which these other struggles can be seen as occupational health struggles, not just ones about questions of civil rights, equal work opportunities, women's autonomous organiza- tion and economic independence or the collective unionization of working-class women. We must also ask whether 'protective legislation' was the only domain for a feminist analysis and political practice in respect of these kinds of health issues. The case for the toll work took on the health and wellbeing of women workers has been made in the first section of this book, and the extent to which 'industrial diseases', reproductive and maternal/infant health and a perceived crisis in the health of the nation, entered both an official and public discourse about the employ- ment of women was considerable. It might be expected, therefore, that feminists would have responded to these concerns also.

Lining up on 'Protective' Legislation

Before the 1880s there was united opposition to the idea of State intervention in women's labour. There were broadly two kinds of groups, although any divisions are to some extent artificial. There were those feminists who emphasized the equal- ity of women and men and those who emphasized their differences. The former will be called equal rights feminists, the latter social feminists.[4] Olive Banks[5] identifies a third group: women whose activism initially developed from within the evangel- ical movement and contained some elements of both other strands – an emphasis on human rights on the one hand and women's unique capacities and talents on the other. This group did not accept women as subordinate to men but were among the most conservative in their support of women's domestic role. On 'protective' legis- lation this group was less evident.

Despite a considerable amount of unity of analysis and purpose up to the 1890s, some of which remained the two broad groupings on which I focus my analysis were to become more distinct. The source of this was the issue of 'protect- ive' legislation itself. However, despite distinct ideological positions and a differ- ence in political organization and strategy around work, negative consequences and positive effects were common to both. Women's structurally subordinate position in the labour market and to a lesser extent the Victorian 'ideal' that women should not work at all were confirmed. A theoretical if not always practically realized unity in gender as a class and the possibility of autonomous, self-determined forms of organization was emphasised.

The organizational base for the equal rights feminists was formed in the 1860s and 1870s. Organizations such as the Society for Promoting the Employment of Women (SPEW) and the Vigilance Association for the Defence of Personal Rights (VA) combined philanthropic work with concerns to widen women's employment opportunities and oppose any legal restrictions on them. An important vehicle for publicizing their campaigns was the *English Woman's Journal* which later became the *Englishwoman's Review* (ER).[6] This had been launched in the 1850s by Bessie Parker and Barbara Leigh Smith Bodichon. The journal and SPEW (with its founder Jessie Boucherett) shared an office in Langham Place and equal rights feminists came to be known as 'the Langham Place' set. An employment bureau for women also operated on the premises. Jessie Boucherett was the first editor of EWR, followed by Helen Blackburn. These women became the most conspicuous advocates of the group's expressed opposition to factory legislation.[7]

Originally the aim of the journal was to cover women's issues, but in 1866 it took on a more specific focus with its subtitle 'A Journal of Women's Work'. The leading article presented the work to be done as 'to deal with the evils which press so heavily on our female working population' and 'the need for discovering wider opportunities for women of the lower middle class'.[8] In large measure, however, the 'evils' and 'distress' dealt with were those relating to the lack of work rather than the nature of working conditions and it was a decidedly middle-class publication during its first few decades. Even with its concerns to find 'respectable', suitable occupations for women and the need for education and training so that these were attainable, there seems to have been little awareness of the possible health consequences of such work. Feminists had to fight for the right to enter many white-collar or 'professional' occupations against a backdrop which insisted their 'health status' debarred them from work in the first place.[9] However, despite a primary focus on middle-class employment, from the late 1870s, when the Women's Protection and Provident League (WPPL) acted as an umbrella women's trade-union organization, there was more coverage of issues concerning working-class women. From this time, too, as further legislation was proposed around work that applied to women as well as children and young persons, 'protective' legislation was a principal focus.

The social feminists were connected with trade unions in general or women's trade-union organizations and socialist political organizations, whose primary concern was to organize women workers and to form women's unions. They were more sympathetic to the development of the Welfare State, although at this time they did not support 'protective' legislation because it was discriminatory. This aspect of State intervention was viewed as problematic even when their opposition to intervention *per se* declined. In the 1880s, prominent figures in the WPPL, such as Emma Paterson and Clementina Black, opposed State intervention in women's work. This was most evident in the context of trade-union politics where they found themselves having to defend women's right to work against male unionists attempts to restrict them. In the Trades Union Congress (TUC) male unionists frequently called on the State to exclude women from employment, or from employment in particular trades. In 1887 Clementina Black, in opposing a motion calling for 'the prevention of the employment of females in the chain- and nail-making trades' argued:

> that women did suffer the physical evils was no doubt true. But there was not one injury which Mr Juggins had instanced that could not be capped by a worse story of the women employed in trades no one dreamed of

forbidding, such as needlework and matchbox making. Why not? There was no need to ask. Men did not work at these trades and suffered nothing from the competition of women.[10]

Equal rights feminists supported unionization as a means of seeking redress for women's working conditions – and in any case they supported any form of organization of women for women. As with the social feminists they suspected that State intervention was instigated by men because of their fear of competition. Jessie Boucherett commented on the *House of Lords Select Committee on Sweating Report* that:

> the Committee acknowledges men's complaints are not genuine, and then proceeds to endorse them, and recommends that these poor women should be forbidden . . . Legislation for the assumed object of preventing women from over-working themselves, and for the very real object of competing with men is unfair.[11]

However, the example of chain- and nail-making was unusual. In general men's attitude toward 'protective' legislation was more ambivalent. They probably supported it when there was a fear of competition but in many cases, because of the sexual segregation of jobs that often coincided with views of the 'natural' attributes of women, there was neither competition for jobs nor a depression of male wages. However, many male trade unionists advocated restrictions on women because they thought that ideally women should not work. Some social feminists came to the view that men favoured 'protective' legislation because it was a means of achieving improvements in their own conditions.[12]

For the equal rights feminists, factory legislation was only one example of laws that made women defenceless and dependent. They opposed all forms of patriarchal control that exacerbated women's economic and political powerlessness. This more general stance on State intervention enabled them to join forces with social feminists on the specific case of women's work. In the late 1880s they did so around the campaign to prohibit women from 'pit-brow' work.[13] Feminists supported those arguing against restriction and they mobilized support of other local women to the cause. The Mayoress of Wigan informed a women's conference in Liverpool that:

> the work of these women is very healthy. I have never, even in the country, seen women looking so robust and vigorous. They have been styled 'The Colliery Amazons and Venuses', the former on account of their strength, the latter for their splendid development and beautiful teeth.[14]

Although social feminists at this time had repeatedly brought forward resolutions to the TUC for the appointment of women inspectors, this was another issue on which the two groups were united. However, the appointment of women as factory inspectors presented a paradox for equal rights feminists, because without factory legislation there was essentially no role for them. Social feminists had initially supported the idea that working women with practical experience of industrial conditions should be appointed to such positions and in the event it would be middle-class and professional women. Equal rights feminists, despite their continued support for the inspectorate, saw the issue differently. There was still the possibility of redefining the role as one which limited inspection to all work places where conditions had been agreed voluntarily through collective action and because such appointments could be seen as a public health measure. There would also be support for women inspectors, in their later internal 'battles' in the Factory Department over role and organization, consistent with their position on all discrimination.[15]

Division and Dissent

By the end of the 1880s there began to be a shift in position within social feminism on the question of State intervention. This gave rise to a sometimes verbally acrimonious split with equal rights feminists. The latter did not alter their position, remaining steadfast in their opposition to a male legislature imposing its will on a disenfranchised class – women. Several factors gave an impetus to the change in thinking within social feminism. It was not simply the change in leadership of the WPPL after the death of Emma Paterson in 1886. Paterson herself had moved some way from implacable opposition to legislation and her successor, Lady Emilia Dilke, certainly saw a role for the State. The attempts to unionize women were generally thought to have been disappointing. There were some successes: more women were visible at the TUC and there was the high-profile successful industrial action by the match girls in 1888, but these went against the general trend.[16] The reasons for the difficulties in organizing women were in turn a product of the conditions of their work that collective organization hoped to solve. Exploitation, long hours and lack of power, as well as the wider responsibilities women had within their families, left neither time nor energy even if there was the will. As far as women workers in the East End of London were concerned, one woman suggested that few could 'spare time or thought beyond'.[17] As a result, hope in unionism as the main means of redress was, for the time being, abandoned.

Union activism continued, principally in the form of umbrella organizations. The WPPL gave way to the Women's Trade Union and Provident League (WTUPL) in 1889 and dropped the Provident in 1891 to become the Women's Trade Union League (WTUL). There was a break from the WTUPL of some members including Clementina Black, Amie Hicks and Clara James, to form the Women's Trade Union Association (WTUA) in 1889. A further and related factor in the change in attitude toward 'protective' legislation was that social feminists were becoming increasingly acquainted with actual working conditions. In Clementina Black's words they were 'shocked and horrified' by what they saw.[18] Some familiarity had been acquired in the process of organizing, but a number of feminist and socialist organizations had also begun to undertake investigations of their own – different forms of enquiry into work and living conditions – and these continued to be a major source of information about women's lives in the early decades of the twentieth century. This was especially so with the Women's Industrial Council (WIC), the Women's Cooperative Guild (WCG) and the Fabian Women's Group (FWG).[19]

Some women had chosen to see for themselves in an individual capacity. Beatrice Webb worked for some time as a seamstress.[20] Either within this context or elsewhere, individual women built up considerable expertise in social investigation and statistical analysis, including Barbara Hutchins, Amy Harrison and Clara Collet who had helped Charles Booth with his poverty study and then joined the Board of Trade as a Labour Correspondent after her service on the Royal Commission on Labour. This tradition continued to be an important weapon in feminist struggles to publicize and improve conditions for working women. In addition to the benefits of expertise acquired here, social feminism illustrates how feminist activism moved around the various organizational outlets. There were also considerable overlaps in membership. Some members of the WPPL set up the WTUA, which then merged with the WIC. Members of the WTUPL and then the WTUL and the later National Federation of Working Women formed in 1906, also had links with the WIC and the FWG as well as party political organizations such as the Independent Labour Party (ILP).

In accounting for the shift in social feminist thinking, the growth of union consciousness, influenced by 'new unionism', was also important. Although organizing women was not seen to offer a sufficient practical remedy for women's grievances, belief in its principle did not waver. Many socialists favoured State intervention not only as a necessary constraint on the excesses of capitalist industrial production but as a precondition for organization itself. The example often used was that of women textile workers whose hours had been regulated from early in the century. Beatrice Webb claimed it was only when 'they were saved from the unhealthy conditions and excessive hours . . . that they began to combine in Trade Unions, to join Friendly Societies and to form Cooperative stores'.[21]

From the 1890s social feminists increasingly saw legislation as a means of obtaining some amelioration for working women. They accepted that women's relatively powerless position meant that some special 'protection' might be warranted. Phillipa Levine[22] argues that there were two distinct groups here: those who gave whole-hearted support to State intervention, viewing it as essentially benevolent; and those who supported 'protective' legislation but not its gendered basis. There were few enthusiasts who did not also have reservations about its oppressive potential and sought to have conditions improved for all. Beatrice Webb, about whom there is some controversy in any case as to her feminist credentials,[23] was perhaps the exception: she saw State intervention in the form of 'protective' legislation as necessary for a more progressive economic life.

Many feminists remained sceptical of the motives of men who supported it. Madeleine Greenwood told one audience: 'I believe at the bottom of all the agitation in favour of interference with women's labour, is the feeling that it would be better for women not to work at all outside her home.'[24] On many occasions it was argued that legislation should not be gender specific, since conditions needed to be improved for every worker. As Enid Stacey put it:

a great injustice will be done if state interference deals with them intimately and leaves men pretty much alone. Socialists urge that the state has power to regulate individuals *qua* individuals but not *qua* women.[25]

Barbara Hutchins argued that the idea of 'protecting certain classes of workers because they are not free agents is more and more felt to be irrelevant' and that critics of the Factory Acts had overemphasized the focus on sex-specific measures. The Acts of 1891 and 1895, she claimed, 'show signs of a recognition . . . that the grounds of interference with industry are considerations of public health and safety'.[26] There were also supporters of legislation who considered it was not just sex-specific but class-specific. Jane Brownlow demonstrated this by pointing out that:

No legislator has yet attempted to make laws preventing women from taking night work when nursing, or acting or dancing, no one has yet proposed to restrict the number of hours given to her work overtime by the female teacher in an elementary or secondary school.[27]

There was thus suspicion about the 'benefits' men claimed for legislation and for many supporters and opponents a questioning of motives that were deeply entwined with suffrage. Class as well as gender featured as important dimensions of social feminists' political programmes, especially for those who were Fabians.

Equal rights feminists remained consistently opposed to interference. In 1891, Jessie Boucherett, Helen Blackburn and Ada Heather-Biggs formed the Women's Employment Defence League (WEDL) specifically to fight 'protective' legislation. Their hostility to male unionists and the male legislature now extended to social feminists whom they accused of colluding with them. In April 1894, in an attack on a speech by Beatrice Webb, the ER suggested the British workwoman was 'most in danger from those who are most anxious to serve her'.[28] In 1899, when there was some correspondence between equal rights feminists, Helen Blackburn and Millicent Fawcett, and two investigators into the effects of the Factory Acts on women compositors,[29] Fawcett had replied:

I think that every proposal affecting the labour of women which is vigorously pushed by men's trades is itself suspect and ought to be narrowly watched by all who wish to see the industrial position of women improved.[30]

Social feminists in their turn accused equal rights feminists of collusion – in this case with employers who exploited women – and also of exposing women to unnecessary dangers in the workplace. There was a suspicion that they did not understand the problems of women in industry, so the 'freedom' for which they fought was for middle-class women, not for their working-class 'sisters'. In one such attack on opponents of legislation Beatrice Webb suggested that 'evidently many ladies of education and position superstitiously clinging to the same belief' because they had 'no practical experience'. 'In the life of the wage-earning class', she argued, 'absence of regulation does not mean personal freedom.'[31] Another social feminist pointed out that:

However gladly some of us may overwork ourselves when engaged in writing novels or painting pictures, it is quite certain that no woman keeps a sewing machine going, or pastes matchboxes or pulls rabbit fur for 14–16 hours a day because she likes doing it.[32]

There is indication outside of such publicly expressed opposition that the political differences also extended to personal antagonisms. In her diary, Lucy Deane whose political leanings were with social feminism, wrote an entry in November 1896 which refers to 'a view' that 'suffrage will be captured by the "Heather-Biggs" and rampant sex-equality people if we don't'. Later that same year after a meeting with the activist Isabella Ford, Deane refers to her view 'that the Fawcett and Heather-Biggs School of Industrial Theories is dying out'.[33] Lady Emilia Dilke, of the WTUL, also refers to those 'who have been called "the shrieking sisterhood" and "wild women"' as having 'retarded the advance of public opinion toward reform'.[34]

Fabian women in particular mounted a defence of the Factory Acts in the broader context of the overall improvement of the efficiency of industry. They directed their campaign at employers who were fearful of the consequences of restraints on their competitiveness and thence profitability. Opponents were informed that workers – and women in particular – were caught in a permanent position of inequality, unable to bargain without those cherished personal liberties. 'What freedom,' asked Constance Smith, 'can there be where the life of one of the parties is at stake? But the first step upward she is incapable of making unless the State helps her make it.'[35] If the health of operatives was improved, Webb argued, so would efficiency and profit. Sweating in particular was singled out for its social and economic costs. Improvements were not going to happen voluntarily. So, Barbara Hutchins argued, it 'was better to make the conditions of industry fit for women than to drive them out' and for the State to set these standards:

The working woman, the victim of that very unrestricted competition which her better off sister was demanding; before all things needed improved wages and conditions of work for which State protection and combination with men was essential.[36]

Having put some measure of faith in State intervention as a means of increasing women's physical strength and wellbeing, there continued to be frustrations in what it delivered. More legislation, fewer exemptions and effective enforcement were the continuing refrain. Gertrude Tuckwell of the WTUL bemoaned 'a national habit of mind' where 'we move slowly remedying proved evils, instead of anticipating their occurrence, and slowly building up the necessary safeguards against existing abuses instead of limiting their growth'.[37] Barbara Hutchins similarly argued that legislation was 'timid, cautious, tentative and slow' and had 'lagged far behind the ideals of its promoters and the needs of the classes most concerned'.[38]

These divisions within nineteenth-century feminism over 'protective' legislation have been characterized as differences in class. This may have been because class had a particular rhetorical value within social feminist politics. It was important in claiming their sphere of interest and in demarcating them from equal rights feminists. Despite their own predominately middle-class origins, social feminists argued that they were promoting working-class women's interests. Joan Scott[39] has argued that such an appropriation of class has served to undermine the importance of gender in labour politics. Phillipa Levine[40] has emphasized that class differences may have been less significant than those between women who worked and those who did not. In women's own writing of this period there is an indication that this was a more salient aspect of women's self-identity.[41] Thus the category working women is more pertinent to the concerns of feminist politics than that of working-class women. But work probably did not feature as a central identifying characteristic of working-class women's lives, nor could questions of employment opportunity and choice be considered outside the boundaries of economic subsistence. More recent feminist analyses have, therefore considered that it was gender as a class that informed both equal rights and social feminists despite their differences.[42]

While the main achievement of the Langham Place heritage may have been its demonstration that women could enter into debates about public affairs and providing an example of new modes of behaviour for younger middle-class women, they also needed employment opportunities. They consistently supported employment goals as the right for every woman and they were correct in recognizing that a State strategy which ultimately aimed to restrict the employment of women was one that would perpetuate discrimination both within the labour market and elsewhere. The logic of their position sometimes left them open to ridicule, particularly on the specific issue of poor working conditions, but that needs to be considered in the broader context of what were viable strategies for relatively new feminist politics. There were undoubtedly ways in which class as well as gender both united and pulled feminists in different directions, but it may be more useful to see these divisions between women as ideological.

Olive Banks[43] argues that ultimately social feminists were not only divided from other feminists by their socialism, but that their politics also compromised their feminism. There is support for this view in the developing analysis of activists such as Beatrice Webb and Barbara Hutchins and those whose political allegiances were moving from Liberal to Labour, although the FWG maintained a clear theoretical rejection of women's dependence on men in the family and economy.[44] It was particularly evident in the general acceptance of the 'minimum wage' legislation as the remedy for the 'sweated' trades, since this would obviate the necessity for women to work at all.[45] Clearly there were also shortcomings in this approach: it failed to address women's structural weakness in the labour market, the sexual segregation of jobs and issues of economic dependency, while it confirmed the traditional patriarchal view of the family.[46]

Feminism, Work and the 'Protection' of Health

The debates about the results of industrial work for women had from the outset drawn on the possible impact it might have on women's health, although this was always secondary to the social concern that they should not be working at all because their primary responsibility was for the welfare of their families. However, explicit arguments about health consequences could always be used to achieve the social purposes of restriction, and 'protective' legislation was certainly viewed by equal rights feminists in these terms. In addition, despite their support for it, social feminists sought the reform of industrial conditions as something that ought to pursued for all workers. In this sense the strategy pursued by social feminists failed to challenge the social basis of the legislation and confirmed women's disadvantage in the labour market, and which also had limited success in improving conditions for men or women.

Feminist activism was inevitably drawn into the concerns about the 'dangerous trades'. Social feminists were in the forefront of agitation around the white-lead industry, but they opposed restriction and especially any suggestion that married women should be prohibited. Social feminists were quite particular about what kinds of measure should be included in 'protective' legislation and both groups of feminists agreed on the kinds of prevention that would be effective but not discriminatory. Amie Hicks argued: 'now why instead of allowing a woman to be temporarily displaced . . . do not people agitate for alterations in the conditions of the unhealthy trades?'[47] Ada Heather-Biggs called upon those attending the Women's Liberal Association 'to suggest that it should be the methods of manufacture which should be altered in the trades'.[48] Madeleine Greenwood, who supported legislation, argued that 'they should insist on employers rendering their work as innocuous as is possible to make it [the Potteries] and the same applies to the match trade'.[49] An important example of social feminist opposition to the tenor of official regulation was Gertrude Tuckwell's dissent as a member of the Committee that examined the health dangers in the Potteries: their report in 1910 recommended restrictions on workers and not a prohibition on lead.[50]

The opposition of equal rights feminists to any legislative interference posed some difficulties in their response to the hazards and health effects of work. On a number of occasions, the ER argued that 'every employment has its illness', a reference in this case to phosphorous necrosis.[51] On the possibility that work might damage women's health they thought that, as in other areas of social life, it was for women themselves to choose if they could do the work; 'a woman could decide herself if her strength is equal to the job'.[52] They did not try to deny that the result might be illness and debility, although they asserted this was often overstated, that poverty was a more important factor in illness and that being deprived of employment would further exacerbate that poverty. In the context of a discussion of the Royal Commission of Labour reports, Jessie Boucherett commented on the chain-making trade:

> [they] . . . made no complaint of loss of health, which confirmed my impression that when women get plenty of good food, they can do a surprising amount of work without suffering and that half of the illness supposed to be caused by hard work is really caused by a combination of hard work and poor food.[53]

Two SPEW members undertook an investigation of the white-lead trade in New-castle in 1895. They argued that 'some look pale and sickly, but many of them had good complexions and looked quite healthy' and a medical witness was used to surmise that 'the evil effects from working with lead could in most cases be avoided by care and cleanliness'. Their article disputed claims that prohibition would not bring about hardship. In fact, the authors saw 'no alternative but the workhouse'.[54]

Social feminists did not disagree with the view that other factors besides work in women's lives damaged their health. They were equally concerned about the impact of poverty in 'pushing women into the labour market' and trapping them into poor conditions and 'sweated' workshops in particular. They also accepted a view shared by medical experts and factory inspectors that the extra deprivations suffered by women undermined their general health in ways that predisposed them to the results of hazards, long hours and other working conditions. In recognition of the importance of poverty, social feminists pursued issues of wages and gender-segregated jobs that left women as the worst paid and most exploited sector of the adult workforce. Equal rights feminists argued: 'it is a mockery to talk of raising the standard of comfort in the home by lowering the status of women who make the home',[55] and thus both groups contended that 'protective' legislation should not be about prohibiting women from much-needed work.

Equal rights feminists who consistently thought that male fears of competition were evident in legislation around the 'dangerous trades' as well as in the hours of work exploited inconsistencies in State regulation. Jessie Boucherett, noted that in the Potteries majolica painting, done by women, was 'the most dangerous part of the trade', and the explanation for not recommending restriction she argued; 'seems to be that men are not at present prepared to take the places of the paintresses . . . but are anxious to get rid of Glost Placers'.[56] In 1899, SPEW sent a memorial to Sir Matthew Ridley Bart at the Home Department, calling on him to consider adopting similar precautions to those in Europe, instead of following recommendations that women be dismissed.[57] The overall tenor of equal rights feminist campaigns around legislation, were, as Feurer[58] has argued, to eschew health problems in favour of more abstract principles.

Outside of the pursuit or opposition to 'protective' legislation there were only a limited number of ways in which feminist activism dealt with occupational health issues. There were few opportunities for women to lead by example, although the Victoria Printing Press, set up by Emily Faithfull was a model of good working conditions. 'She insisted upon open windows and regular periods of relaxation to safeguard her work women from the industrial diseases which were then prevalent among printers.'[59] Feminist activities around occupational ill-health were mainly a by-product of the legislative issue. The attention many organizations, in particular WIC or the WTUL, gave to channelling and anonymizing complaints about conditions or infringements of the Factory Acts to the Home Office or to Factory Inspectors arose out of their belief that more efficient inspection was required if the benefits of legislation were to be better realized. Similarly, the activities of an organization such as WIC, which embarked on an extensive educational programme of lectures, conferences, circulating material, writing and publishing often focused these specifically on the Factory Acts.[60]

WIC was also a result of union activists' relative disillusionment with the attempts to organize women into trade unions as a means of redress for their grievances. Leading members of the Women's Trade Union Association (WTUA) looked to a different form of political organization. The central *raison d'être* of the Council was the systematic investigation of the conditions of working women. In the conference to inaugurate the Council, this information was 'to promote such action as may be conducive to their improvement'. This was viewed by the leadership in terms of acting as a pressure group on government officials to bring about change.[61] Such lobbying has been seen by some analysts as an important strand of trade-union activism.[62]

The close alliance of organizations such as WIC with social feminist' concerns about the Factory Acts could have had an impact on raising consciousness about occupational health issues generally. There were a range of activities that might have improved working women's health status. For example, WIC wanted to develop educational provision for working-class girls both technically and socially. This was in line with gendered and class assumptions about work and women's needs. Technical training for working-class girls amounted to domestic service or factory work, for middle-class girls training in commercial subjects. Although technical classes were seen as a remedy for the large pool of unskilled labour they would be 'in the great industries peculiar to women': domestic industries, laundry work and the needle trades.[63]

The second major strand of their educational programme was to develop social skills so that women could 'be better equipped for wifehood and motherhood'.[64] Here WIC joined mainstream thinking about the need for working-class girls to train in domestic economy in order to do their duty to a future generation: a practical contribution to the pressing problem of infant mortality, despite a recognition that women often needed to work. WIC formed clubs which served these educational purposes, but could also be used to provide forms of 'healthy' leisure. Physical education was provided as were opportunities for girls to have seaside holidays. The clubs attracted working-class girls and certainly made a contribution to their health and wellbeing. One meeting in 1905 where Dr Ethel Vaughan spoke on 'Health at home and in the workshop' was attended by 127 people from 27 different clubs.[65] These would have given many young women some respite from their very poor living conditions. However, the clubs flourished mainly in London although the idea of girls' clubs were put into practice elsewhere, including some set up by working firms themselves. Bryant and May, Courtaulds, and Cadbury were examples of this kind of paternalistic provision.[66]

While it might be considered that an equal rights analysis gave rise to the most serious obstacles to a strategy for dealing with occupational ill-health in women, there were clearly many problems with the social feminists' approach to the issue of working conditions. Many contemporary accounts have emphasized their failure to develop an analysis and strategy to challenge sexual divisions at work and in the home. Mappen argues that WIC 'brought the needs of a group of working-class women to the public eye, only to clothe the solutions to these problems in Victorian rhetoric'.[67] This failure was centrally related to their support for the concept of the family wage, which was seen as the key to eliminating the problem of 'sweating'. Increasingly, social feminists joined with men to demand support for unemployed men and the establishment of a minimum wage, in order that women would not have to enter the labour market at all. In doing so they were not only reinforcing the economic dependence of wives on husbands, but neglecting those women for whom a family wage would be irrelevant. It was to be the basis for the direction that social policy and the development of the Welfare State would take so it was not surprising that in the post-First World War period, family allowances took centre stage of the feminist agenda.[68]

Feminist analysis seemed equally unable to consider such issues as the impact of work on maternal and infant health outside of established discourse both about the 'natural' and 'proper' sphere of women's work for the care of children and the idea that working conditions for women in some measure contributed to their degeneration. There were also concerns among feminists about the restrictions on women's work opportunities, especially any prohibition on married women which would exacerbate ill-health, as additional sources of income might provide a better lifestyle. Gertrude Tuckwell argued:

> it is essential the State should intervene and that it is in the interests of its future citizens the mother should be restored to care for them. Yet to deprive her of her power of earning without compensation would be an injustice . . . thus some system of insurance must go hand in hand with the measures tending in this direction.[69]

Consistent with Beatrice Webb's view of factory legislation as necessary to economic prosperity was the health of the labour force, which included the health of future generations, 'the capital stock of the nation'. Such concerns were not particular to feminist and other women activists or professionals. Sectors of the State, the medical profession and reformers shared them and probably tempered the more extreme demands for prohibition. These arguments for intervention were visible in the social feminist campaigns around 'sweated' labour and homework. There was a conflict between concerns for women's working conditions and the health of future generations in activists' pronouncements on the issue. Whether, as Margaret MacDonald did, they favoured licensing because it might ensure 'the woman of the house used a little soap and water and made her beds each morning'[70], or supported Clementina Black's call for the 'minimum wage' to reduce the need for women to work, considerations for the health of mothers and their responsibilities for children abounded.

It is surprising that outside the Women's Cooperative Guild's campaign on maternity[71] and also to some extent the FWG's investigations into household management,[72] there was little political articulation of other policy directions required to realize improvements in women's and mothers' health or domestic economy. Some feminists, such as Anna Martin, mounted a defence of mothers and their domestic skills.[73] Josephine Butler was one of the few to note in the early years of the debates about legislative restriction that reducing the hours of work in industry merely enabled women to work equally hard as unpaid domestic servants. It was, she said:

> obvious that whatever be the causes of infant mortality in factory districts, they cannot be removed by compelling women to arrive at the mills at 7.00 am instead of 6.00 [and] if the principle of legislative interference is on grounds of physical welfare, their children's health and comfort of homes, its application cannot be limited to factories.[74]

Women, Trade Unionism and Working Conditions

While the perceived failure of organization in the form of women's trade unionism was an impetus for demands for State intervention and support for 'protective' legislation in the 1890s and early 1900s, much had been achieved both before and during this period by women's trade unionism or unionists. Women unionists and unionist-based organizations were at the core of feminist activism around women's work, working conditions and 'protective' legislation. Prominent women unionists were also active in a broader spectrum of feminist and labour politics and this allowed them to pursue some of trade unionism's traditional political aims in other contexts. Encouraging women to join a union remained an important goal and although actual union membership was very low throughout the 1880s and 1890s and many unions had a short life,[75] organization was still pursued and had some successes at different times and in different parts of the country throughout the period. In the early-twentieth century, new unions sprang up among the expanding 'white blouse' and professional areas of women's work.

In the decades up to the 1880s there had been little in the way of women's auto-nomous organization into trade unions, although many women had been recruited into men's unions where there had been a long tradition of women's work, not-ably in the cotton and textile industries. This also enabled women not only to benefit from collective agreements here, but also to engage early on with suffrage issues.[76] It was within the context of trade unionism, however, that the opposition of men to women's employment and women's opposition to men's attempts to restrict their employment opportunities, were most clearly articulated. By 1881, with 10 women in the TUC, women were able to experience and directly confront male opposition. As Solden[77] shows, women experienced considerable hostility in these early years. But they also had some successes. In particular they were able to persuade Congress to support the campaign for women to be appointed to the inspectorate, although this indicated the extent to which their views of women's need for 'protection' were developing. In the 1880s, the strike of women in the match industry provided a focus for new unions. This pattern of exploiting indus-trial unrest was one that activists continued to exploit into the twentieth century.[78]

The umbrella union organizations provided women in different trades with some form of organization and collective representation, often when there was no women's union for the trade or the union would not admit women, as many still did not. However, women in any TUC affiliated union could also become a member of these organizations. Providing some association for women without the benefit of alternative union membership was one advantage, but more importantly these fostered policy development and enabled the energies of the women's union leadership to be concentrated. The provision of a base with resources of experience and, less so, money – a perpetual problem for women's unionism and its autonomy from men – allowed for some regional development. Opportunities provided in this context for women's involvement facilitated the formation of individual unions. Julia Varley, for example, left the NFWW to become the first woman organizer in Birmingham for the Worker's union in 1912 and the NFWW itself merged with the General and Municipal Workers Union in 1913.[79]

In the decade immediately preceding the First World War, women's trade unionism was directly sponsored by legislation itself, although not in the way that social feminists had always claimed, by improving conditions to the extent that women would have the strength and economic power to organize. The passing of the Trade Boards Act 1909 and the broader social and economic conditions in which women workers found themselves, in particular the falling value of wages and rising unemployment in some trades, led to an increasingly politicized context which women organizers were able to utilize. A series of strikes in women's trades around food-processing and manufacture, in 1910 and 1911, led to the formation of a number of new women's unions, often after trade-union activists had stepped in and negotiated for them. While some strikes were successful in achieving strikers' aims, others were less so.[80] One disadvantage of this mode of organizing was that in practice it was a product of women outside the trade and workplace concerned. This probably directly impacted on the degree to which local women sustained unionism at this level. Thom has suggested that in the 1907–1914 period, when these strikes took place, women's industrial unrest owed something to the politics of suffrage: the use of militancy, propaganda and the production of materials and ephemera – although some leading women unionists, notably Mary McArthur, played down the sex-specific nature of this unrest.

The Trade Boards Acts stimulated unionism directly because it was mainly in women's trades that the Boards were initially set up. Gertrude Tuckwell argued they were a basis for union growth and that unionism also had a role in their establishment. The agitation prior to the Bill had involved leading women trade unionists, although their activity was more often through their association with the Anti-Sweating League, for example Clementina Black, or through their attempts to represent the interests of homeworkers, as with Mary McArthur. There were differences here too between women over the possible remedies for sweating: was it to be the minimum wage or a system of licensing?[81] Overall, however, women's unionism retained a strong belief in the State as an agent of change. Trade unions would have a mediating role in this. Thom argues that as a result:

> The Trade Board route to improvement in the condition of women in industry was emphatically not one which challenged the social and political order, it was one that asked for women's participation in it.[82]

This is hardly surprising. In every arena of social and political life, the exclusion of women was fundamental to any analysis and strategy. However, in so far as trade unionism can be regarded as effective in ameliorating working conditions and in its impact on women's health, then a different evaluation is needed. While women's unionism was important in campaigns around the 'dangerous trades' and achieved some success, notably in relation to employers' attempts to defeat the introduction of leadless glazes in the potteries,[83] it was rarely the basis for either organization or militancy. It was precisely because of unionism's central concerns with pay that many other problems of working conditions were neglected.

Pay was perceived to be responsible for the problems of 'sweated' work and there is little in the agitation around the minimum wage to suggest that pay and poor conditions were seen as issues of occupational health, outside of those about 'national efficiency'. While pay is obviously important to securing the material conditions necessary to health – and thus pay campaigns can be seen indirectly as health campaigns – they can also be digressionary. In middle-class employment, the growing unionism of this time centred on such issues as equal pay, pensions, promotional opportunities and the marriage bar.[84] Only in the accusations of 'malingering' made after the high level of claims by women after the introduction of the National Insurance Act of 1911 did women unionists enter more general health issues. Mary McArthur pointed out that 'people who are underfed, badly housed and overworked are seldom in a state of physical efficiency . . . and that where industry pays starvation wages . . . it levies a tax on the community'.[85]

The difficulty with examining trade unionism as an effective form of collective organization among women workers and its success or potential success in achieving changes in the conditions that damaged women's health is that it has been dominated by accounts of its leading activists and their role in constituting both problem and solution. The majority have focused on the organizational and political aspects of trade unionism itself, to chronicle its successes and its failures. It is also very difficult in this specific area of feminist politics to access working women's experiences of either the effects on their health or their views on the relative success of different forms of action to deal with the problems. As Eleanor Gordon's detailed study of women jute workers in Scotland demonstrates, the degree and types of resistance by women workers has been subordinated by accounts which have ignored the connections of work and home.[86] Between 1889 and 1906, official statistics show women involved in 82 strikes in Dundee's jute industry, the majority of which were initiated by women and only involved them.[87] So women did employ forms of resistance outside formal organizations. Their own acceptance of gendered subordination does not mean they did not 'see themselves as workers with common interests' nor that as women and as workers they would not find their own response.[88]

Working Women, Legislation and Health

Both sides in the debate about the effects of work on health and attitudes toward intervention were usually able to find women or the voices of women themselves to support their line of argument, which they did on many occasions. Sometimes these would be somewhat spurious, as in Jessie Boucherett's claim that chain-makers, shop assistants and others who had been investigated by the Royal Commission on Labour, made no complaint: it was difficult, she said 'to get female assistants to complain and shows they are not anxious for legislation'.[89] The lack of visible complaint did not mean there was none. Shop assistants frequently complained to the women's inspectorate and wrote to the press in support of a restriction on shop hours. When they mounted a successful campaign to exclude laundries from hours-of-work legislation, equal rights feminists had argued laundresses did not seek interference, while in addition to the success of the WTUL rally, a woman inspector reported that her arrival in one large laundry was greeted with loud applause. There were women workers who felt that women inspectors could use their power to redress conditions, as the letters of complaint and demonstrations to them so graphically illustrated.[90] Women exhibited an awareness of the particular damaging aspects and some knowledge of what was illegal. The interlinking of feminist organizations with the publicity and educative activities around the Factory Acts and their mediating function between women workers and the State gave women a channel through which to seek redress.

Just as accessing voices through feminist organisations and their political activities causes problems for ascertaining the extent to which they 'spoke' for women's own views, it is difficult also for the researcher to assess what working-class women's own views were from other sources. In many instances these views were constituted by a context in which they were given or presented, and this was nearly always for the pursuit of political objectives. In the context of inquiry and investigation there were regulatory objectives and these also constrained the way in which women would account for such matters as their health, their working conditions and their views of 'protective' legislation. It is evident that in many instances where women were witnesses in official inquiry an intimidatory situation existed; the presence of mainly men inquirers and often also their employers. The views expressed were also dependent on what was asked for, and to this extent, the 'official' agenda, or 'private' agenda's of inquiry members determined the topic to be discussed. For example, in the Committee's concerned with lead industries or the potteries women were asked about health, symptoms, pregnancy histories, sickness absence and so on, while the Select Committee on Home Work (1907) was more concerned with pay, attitudes to homework, and so questions about health rarely arose. Despite these limitations some testimony of workers has provided views of their health, and lay explanations for ill-health as the case of lead poisoning demonstrated. It will not always be the case that where women and 'officials' shared views of how to 'protect oneself against lead poisoning' that this indicated women were 'toeing the line', but rather that such discourses were culturally pervasive and that women equally used them to make sense of their circumstances.

Women's expressed views of 'protective legislation' are more problematic. In the case of official enquiries it seems that women workers themselves were rarely asked their opinion on this issue, although men were. In the 1910 Inquiry into the Potteries, Joseph Lovatt, the General Secretary of the Society of Amalgamated

Pottery Workers, when asked about the employment of women in lead processes, argued that the union thought it should be made illegal. He was repeatedly questioned on what women members of the union thought about this and whether they had been consulted. From the women who attended the discussion he said 'we did not hear any objections'. But when he was pressed by Gertrude Tuckwell on whether women would support such a drastic measure, he replied that women in the society would accord with such a view but 'with regard to some of the women who have been employed in this business, if we were to ask them I may as well say frankly that probably many of them would object'.[91] Other male union officials said that women would not wish to be 'dislodged', although as the majority view of their union was to safeguard the health of women, restrictions were desirable.[92] Gertrude Tuckwell pointed out to Samuel Clowes, an organizer for this union that, with only 1000 women members and approximately 660 in lead processes, even if they did speak for all of them it would be for less than one-third of the women in lead processes.[93] In Gertrude Tuckwell's persistent questioning of male unionists there is the clear suspicion that she did not think they 'speak for women'.

One investigation conducted within the auspices of the WIC and the British Association that did pursue women's attitudes to 'protective' legislation was J. Ramsay MacDonald's *Women in the Printing Trades*.[94] The report found women to be in favour of restrictions, in this case hours of work, although there were differences between those who were new to the industry and those who had experienced work prior to legislation. Some newer employees regretted the restriction on overtime, but overall the fears of equal rights feminists that legislation would lead to a loss of jobs had not, he argued, been realized. But despite the activism of some working women in using legislation to better conditions, there would undoubtedly also have been some ambivalence toward it. Clementina Black claimed that from a simple fear of survival many women were suspicious of legislative protection. Anna Martin, who had considerable knowledge of working women in London, noted in relation to proposals to restrict married women:

> they know from their own experience the wholesale ruin that would result, under the present industrial system, from the passing of such a law . . . the women are appalled at the idea of their liberty of action in this matter being forcibly taken away from them.[95]

Rose Squire, a woman factory inspector, observed that into the early twentieth century, women had become impatient of restriction unless it was shared with men.[96]

Ultimately the various views that women might have had were influenced by the traditions of women's work, labour–market opportunities, the extent of unionism, the realities of their own and their families' circumstances and the meaning of work for themselves. We should not over-emphasize the invisibility of women's voices and their patterns of resistance. Ada Nield Chew's use of the press to publicize women's grievances and the use of fictionalized genres are well-known,[97] but other women also used local papers in this way and subjectivity and identity as working women were revealed in other forms of writing.[98]

Feminist activism in relation to occupational ill-health was a result of organization and political analyses that focused on employment opportunities for all women and the conditions of work that mainly focused on factories, workshops and the home as locations for working-class women's work. The changes observed reflected a constant working-out of the success and failure of alternative modes of organization and the development of new ideas of ameliorative strategies in relation to working conditions in particular. The principal change was therefore from the belief that organization in the form of women's trade unions or of women into male unions could achieve improvements by voluntary means, to a recognition that the degree of exploitation and powerlessness which women workers had required securing some improvements through State intervention and legal safeguards. The health dimension of work was only one dimension of feminism's engagement with 'protective' legislation. To some extent the divisions within feminism on the issue of State intervention might have precluded a unity on many other issues, including a recognition of patriarchal interests in preserving a structure of employment that continued to disadvantage women in the labour market; and a recognition of how this disadvantage had health implications for women workers. Unfortunately, this allowed the State, male unionists and occupational-health doctors to continue to pursue a strategy that was ineffectual either in tackling occupational health problems or the social purposes of controlling women's participation in the paid labour market.

It is important to understand feminist priorities within the historical circumstances in which feminist politics had to operate. Outside of struggles around the entry into medicine, and later the developing interest in birth control, health was not a major concern for feminists, and this is not surprising given the highly 'private' nature of health matters, and the lack of any institutional base which might have been a focus for such activism. Work, family life and suffrage on the other hand more clearly articulated women's powerless position and their specific grievance within the public domain.

It was inevitable that the pursuit of feminist objectives in relation to these issues, as well as those related to improving working conditions, would be led from those in the middle-class: for working-class women themselves, as Lydia Vaughan 'a working woman' described in relation to the East End of London, there was the reality of:

The constant moiling and toiling, the dread of debt and sickness, the constant strains to make ends meet by making 20 shillings go as far as 25 shillings. How can such a woman spare time or thought beyond?[99]

But these feminists provided important examples not just for other middle-class women but for working-class women too, some of whom became activists,[100] while others benefited from unionization, an increased knowledge of industrial and civic matters, the opportunities for sociability and the available outlets for the expression of their grievances. The fact that this might in the end have been for relatively small numbers and that the scale of problems faced by women who did not work were also enormous should not detract from these achievements.

Similarly, the criticism of both analysis and strategy that left traditional sexual divisions intact was also an attempt to seek some refinements to the narrow proscriptive roles of domestic ideology. To what extent would it have been possible for a practical politics to have espoused options for women outside the family context, given the value that both middle-class and working-class women gave to family life?[101] To do so did not mean that dependency or economic insecurity could not be raised as real concerns. The FWG clearly rejected a view of a 'parasitic relation of women to men' and 'women's enslavement in the economy and family'.[102]

It may have been unfortunate that many such analyses in relation to both work and family life remained theoretical, but the challenges to patriarchy and the possibility of gender-based politics were certainly realized within 'first wave' feminism. If women thereby gained any sense of having increased control over their lives, then this would also have contributed to their wellbeing. For working-class women, 'protective' legislation and the work of the factory inspectorate, helped by feminist organizations, also achieved some limited reforms of their working conditions.

Notes

1 Walby (1990a) 'From private to public patriarchy: the periodisation of British history' p.97.

2 See Banks (1981) *Faces of Feminism*; Feurer (1988) 'The meaning of "sisterhood": the British women's movement and protective labour legislation 1870–1900'; and Levine (1988) *Victorian Feminism 1850–1900*.

3 See Walby (1986) *Patriarchy at Work*.

4 This is the same division used by Feurer (1988) in her analysis. The former are also sometimes called liberal feminists and the latter welfare feminists; see Dale and Foster (1986) *Feminists and State Welfare*.

5 Banks (1981) *Faces of Feminism*.

6 For an overview of these and other feminist and women's periodicals, see Doughan (1987) 'Periodicals by, for, and about women in Britain' and Levine (1990) '"The humanising influences of five o'clock tea": Victorian feminist periodicals.' On the *English Woman's Journal* and *Review*, see the introduction to Murray, A.M. and Clarke, J.H. (1985) *The English Woman's Review of Social and Industrial Questions*.

7 In addition to their many articles in the ER, see Boucherett and Blackburn (1896) *The Condition of Women and the Factory Acts* which particularly responds to the 1895 legislation.

8 Murray, A.M. and Clarke, J.H. (1985) The introduction.

9 Harrison (1981) 'Women's health and the women's movement 1840–1940' provides an overview of how health was itself important to feminism at this time and gives details of medical hostility to women's challenges to their disadvantaged position.

10 *Women's Union Journal* 15 October 1887, 141, XII, p.76.

11 Report in ER following the publication of the Fifth Report of the House of Lords Committee, 16 June 1890, p.247.

12 See Strachey (1923) *The Cause*.

13 John (1984b) *By The Sweat of Their Brow.*
14 Paper read at Conference Convened by the Liverpool Ladies Union of Workers Among Women and Girls (1892), p.148.
15 ER 15 July 1898, p.214.
16 These aspects of early trade-union organization and industrial disputes are documented in a number of histories including Drake (1920) *Women in Trade Unions*; Lewenhak (1977) *Women and Trade Unions*; and Solden (1978) *Women in British Trade Unions.*
17 Lydia Vaughan, 'A protest against seeing indifference', *Shafts* 3 December 1892, p.74.
18 Black (1889) 'The organisation of working women', *Fortnightly Review*, XLVI, p.689.
19 Mappen (1985) *Helping Women at Work* and Mappen (1986) 'Strategists for change: social feminist approaches to the problems of women's work'.
20 Caine (1985) 'Beatrice Webb and 'the woman question'.
21 Webb (1902) 'Women and the Factory Acts', pp.90–1.
22 Levine (1988) *Victorian Feminism 1850–1900.*
23 Rubenstein (1986) *Before the Suffragettes* and Harrison (1992) 'A different world for women' have both suggested Webb was anti-feminist. Levine (1988) argues that in later years she regretted her spoken hostility.
24 In a speech delivered to the Society of Women Employed in Bookbinding and reported in *Shafts*, March 1896, p.23.
25 Cited in Levine (1988) *Victorian Feminism* p.120.
26 Hutchins (1902) 'The historical development of the Factory Acts', in Webb (Ed.) *The Case for the Factory Acts* pp.122–3.
27 Brownlow (1896) 'Women and factory legislation'.
28 'The British workwoman in danger', ER 16 April 1894, p.79.
29 Bradby and Black (1899) 'Women compositors and the Factory Acts'.
30 In EWR, 15 April 1899, p.54.
31 These are taken from her article on 'Women and the Factory Acts' (1902), pp.84–5.
32 Smith (1908) 'The minimum wage', in Tuckwell (Ed.) p.28.
33 *The Business Diaries of Lucy Deane Streatfield*, entries for 26 November and 4 December 1896.
34 Dilke (1894) in her introduction to Bulley and Whiteley *Women's Work.*
35 Smith (1908) 'The minimum wage', in Tuckwell (Ed.) *The Industrial Position of Women.*
36 (My emphasis) Hutchins (1915) *Women in Modern Industry* p.196.
37 Tuckwell (1902) 'The more obvious defects of our factory code', in Webb (Ed.) p.128.
38 Hutchins (1902) 'The historical development of the Factory Acts', in Webb (Ed.).
39 Scott (1987) 'On language, gender and working-class history'.
40 Levine (1988) *Victorian Feminism 1850–1900.*
41 Swindells (1985) *Victorian Writing and Working Women* argues that in the case of working women autobiographers, the category working-class is not the conscious identity within the genre.
42 See Feurer (1988) 'The meaning of "sisterhood" '; Levine (1988) *Victorian Feminism 1850–1900*; and Rose (1992) *Limited Livelihoods.*
43 Banks (1981) *Faces of Feminism.*
44 Mappen (1986) 'Strategists for change'; and Dyhouse (1989) *Feminism and the Family in England 1880–1939.*
45 Morris (1986b) *Women Workers and the Sweated Trades.*
46 Lewis and Davies (1991) 'Protective legislation in Britain 1870–1990'.

47 In *Shafts*, March 1896, p.81.

48 *Shafts*, March 1897, p.100.

49 *Shafts*, May–June 1897, p.107.

50 Memorandum from Gertrude Tuckwell, PP XXIX, 1910.

51 ER, 1894, p.193.

52 ER, June 1890, p.243.

53 ER, 1894, p.149.

54 Ogle-Moore and Hare (1896) 'Report to SPEW on work of women in white lead trade', in Boucherett and Blackburn *The Condition of Working Women and the Factory Acts.*

55 ER, April 1891, p.75.

56 'Lead poison in pottery work', ER 15 April 1899, pp.98–102.

57 ER, 15 July 1899 p.204.

58 Feurer (1988) 'The meaning of "sisterhood" '.

59 Levine *Victorian Feminism* p.89.

60 Mappen (1985) *Helping Women at Work: The Women's Industrial Council.*

61 Lewenhak (1977) *Women and Trade Unions.*

62 Ibid., pp.17–18.

63 Ibid., p.23.

64 *Annual Report* 1903–4, p.24.

65 Ibid., p.27.

66 See Milicent Fawcett's defence of Bryant and May in ER, 15 October 1898, p.287, where she points to the company's policy of girls' clubs. See also Lown (1990) *Women and Industrialisation* (for Courtaulds) and Rose (1992) *Limited Livelihoods* for Cadbury and other examples of paternalistic provision.

67 Mappen (1985) *Helping Women at Work* p.25.

68 Land (1985) 'The introduction of family allowances: an act of historic justice?', in Ungerson (Ed.) *Women and Social Policy.*

69 Tuckwell (1908) *Women in Industry* p.20.

70 Cited in Mappen (1986) 'Strategists for change' p.247.

71 Davies (1915) *Maternity: Letters from Working Women.*

72 See Reeves (1913) *Round About a Pound a Week.*

73 Martin (1913) *The Mother and Social Reform.*

74 Butler (1874) *Legislative Restrictions on the Industry of Women from the Women's Point of View.*

75 Lewenhak (1977) *Women and Trade Unions* p.71 suggests that membership of all-female societies numbered around 2500 in 1886. In 1892, 142 000 women were in trade unions but about half were in the cotton industry.

76 Liddington and Norris (1978) *One Hand Tied Behind Us*; Liddington (1979) 'Women cotton workers and the suffrage campaign', in Burman (Ed.).

77 Solden (1978) *Women in British Trade Unions.*

78 Solden ibid. documents the activity around the 'match-girls' strike and the militancy of 1910–11. The union of match-makers is indicative of the sometimes short life of women's unions. It folded in 1903.

79 Thom (1986) 'The bundle of sticks: women trade unionists and collective organisation before 1918', in John (Ed.) *Unequal Opportunities.*

80 Dundee jute workers among them. See Gordon (1987) 'Women, work and collective action'.

81 See Mappen (1986) 'Strategists for change'.

82 Thom (1986) p.274.
83 Constance Smith and Mona Wilson led this campaign. See Solden (1978).
84 Solden (1978); Holcombe (1973) *Victorian Ladies at Work*.
85 Cited in Solden (1978) pp.68–9.
86 Gordon (1987) 'Women, work and collective action', p.27.
87 Ibid., p.40.
88 This is the tenor of Gordon's conclusions, pp.44–5. It emphasizes the importance of the point made earlier of looking for new categories that more appropriately reflect women's experience.
89 ER, 1894, XXV, p.10.
90 Martindale (1944a) *From One Generation to Another* p.91.
91 *Minutes of Evidence*, PP XXIX (1910) p.173, see Minute 5636.
92 Ibid., *Evidence of Jabez Booth*, p.184.
93 Ibid., p.185.
94 MacDonald (1902) *Women in the Printing Trades*.
95 Martin (1911) *The Married Working Woman*, pp.41–2.
96 Squire (1927) *Thirty Years in the Public Service* p.65.
97 Chew (1982) *The Life and Writings of Ada Nield Chew*.
98 Swindells (1985) *Victorian Writing and Working Women*.
99 *Shafts*, 3 December 1892, p.74.
100 See Liddington and Norris (1978) *One Hand Tied Behind Us*; Chew (1982) *The Life and Writing of Ada Nield Chew*, especially Anna Davin's assessment of the latter in the introduction to these collected writings.
101 Nicholson (1986) *Gender and History: The Limits of Social Theory in the Age of the Family*.
102 Dyhouse (1988) *Feminism and the Family in England 1880–1939*.

Chapter 9

A Concluding Discussion: Toward a Feminist Analysis of the State, Women's Paid Work and Occupational Ill-health

This conclusion aims to bring together a number of strands this study has raised in exploring working women's health in the paid labour market. Many problems of poor working conditions generally and hazards associated with particular kinds of work gave rise to occupational ill-health. Working women of all classes and in all kinds of work were confronted with such problems and suffered the consequences throughout the period. In addition to the experience of work and work-related ill-health, women's work was also represented as a problem within a set of mutually constitutive discursive frameworks that drew on wider social values. There were a variety of responses, both conceptual and practical, from different groups or sections of society. From the perspective of the various interest groups, the potential threats of working conditions to women's health were framed in particular ways. Such definitions provided a basis for action.

But other important themes emerged in these discussions. There was some interdependence between specific occupational health issues and those concerns that can be seen as the health of the wider society so that the idea of 'health' extended beyond the physical status of the population to the moral and social health of society. 'Disease' metaphors were often used to describe 'pathological' features of the industrial system, such as 'sweated' labour. These in turn were seen as endangering the social system. Necessarily the link between economy and society in the production of physical and social ill-health was further framed within 'ideals' of appropriate behaviour and gender roles, both in relation to paid work and the domestic domain or family household. The health of the economy and society was thus inextricably linked to the perceived health of the family. While these relationships extended across the class divide, so that middle-class women did not escape accusations of being poor mothers[1] or their primary responsibility for the domestic sphere,[2] it was working-class family life that was most subject to scrutiny in the context of the industrial system. Here we have an indication of the extent to which the values of the bourgeoisie attained and sought to maintain its political hegemony. The effect of this conflation of economic and family life was that the problems of women at work became at the same time a problem of women who worked.

An important vehicle for representations of women's work as a danger to the social fabric was the changing role of the State with respect to its intervention in all areas of social life: in working out a political *modus operandi* that would enable some measure of 'protection' not just of vulnerable groups within the population but of the community as a whole – the beginning of a conception in which the nation required a Nation State. The development of this new field of political endeavour inevitably provided for new forms of administration. Among these was a unique long-term experiment in the use of women as factory inspectors, whose public and personal rationales as state 'servants'[3] were defined in terms of women's own particular 'needs' and interests. The State also provided a focus for new and different strategies on the part of political interests. New political actors and actresses were evident in reaction, resistance and cooperation.[4] Feminism itself exhibited this kind of diversity within its changing membership and political priorities, although as disenfranchisement particularly signalled the oppressive quality of late Victorian and Edwardian social relations in terms of class and gender, unsurprisingly it was a primary focus for feminist activism. There were also new sites for the development or acquisition of social power. The importance of knowledge about the causes and possible solutions to observed problems provided for opportunities in which the expert – those with claims to 'scientific' knowledge – acquired a new status to speak not just about their own subject, but on social dimensions independent of that knowledge, including the position of women in society.

Questions about occupational ill-health in women workers thus requires an examination of theoretical and empirical questions about gender relations and women's oppression in late nineteenth-century and early twentieth-century Britain. These issues have been to the forefront of feminist scholarship for many years.

Preventing Occupational Ill-health: A Failed Approach?

The nineteenth century witnessed a growth in the awareness of the damaging consequences of some kinds of work for those operatives engaged in them. In the early years of the century such a focus was limited in two main ways. First, while there was a visible discourse that encompassed the idea of occupational health damage, the agitation for reform was mainly couched in terms of the hours of labour. Second, such harmful consequences were not viewed as affecting all workers, but specifically children. It was around the question of intervention and the reform of the factory as unsuitable for children that representations were made suggesting that factory work might also be harmful to women.

In the early period this potential harm was often construed as impinging on the health of the domestic domain, rather than on women's ability to withstand the rigours of factory labour.[5] However, there was no consensus on the effects industrial work could have on health and there were disputes on both these 'clinical' questions and on the social dimensions that medical, sanitary and factory inspectors pronounced upon.[6] In this early period, too, political struggles by male workers, especially over the length of the working day, were for shorter hours for everyone.[7] The potential strain of industrial work on the health of the workforce was countered by arguments of the strain that alterations in working conditions would bring: thus the grounds for non-interference were also well-rehearsed. Such changes as shorter hours of work, it was argued, would be detrimental to the commercial basis of manu-facturing[8] and would impinge negatively on the economy of the family because shorter hours and restrictions on women working would diminish family earnings.

The early period provided important precedents. During this time ideas had gradually developed, even if 'cautiously and slowly',[9] that the State would regulate industry to protect the workforce from some of the excesses of production. As Ashley informed the House of Commons in 1844, 'The State has an interest and a right to watch over and provide for the moral and physical well-being of her people.'[10] In fact the Factory Act 1833, which introduced factory inspectors, marked the 'beginning of economic regulation as we know it'.[11] The principle that such regulation should be applied selectively to those classes of person – women, young people and children – who were physically vulnerable and politically dependent was gradually accepted. Such groups required others to 'protect' their interests, at the outset enshrining women's political dependence on men. What was already clear, or at least strongly signalled in the debates about factory reform from the 1830s onwards, were the potential conflicts of interest between capital and labour, between bourgeois and working-class moralities, between women and men and between the separate spheres of work and home. The contradictions were also beginning to show. A debate was developing about work-related ill-health. Was it occupational 'disease' or the steady undermining of health, brought about by long hours in poor working conditions? In a view offered by one opponent of the Ten Hours Bill:

> The only thing which makes factory labour trying, even to delicate chil-dren, is that they are confined for long hours and deprived of fresh air; this makes them pale and reduces their vigour, but it *rarely brings on disease.*[12] (my emphasis)

By the beginning of the period, the principle of 'protective' legislation as one with applicability to women had been further entrenched by measures to limit women's hours of labour in exclusions from night-work and in the length of the working day in the textile industry. There had also been limited measures for these groups in certain 'dangerous' industries. The principle was still 'contested' and from the mid-nineteenth century, feminist activism, with its central concerns around women's political and economic dependence, sought to defeat any attempts to intervene in women's work in ways that would restrict their participation. Calls for intervention occurred within the male-dominated trade-union movement, within political organ-izations and within the 'State' itself through officials such as medical officers of health at the Local Government Board and in Parliament. Resistance on the part of women activists targeted all these.

I return to political issues of activism and resistance later in this conclusion. Here I consider 'protective' legislation as health and safety legislation. Within this framework the analysis has raised a number of problems: the appropriateness of the model of prevention and control pursued within the legislation and the legislative and regulatory apparatus of factory inspection as a strategy whatever the content. In the context of considering factory reform by means of legislation, the nature of support for and opposition to it poses a particular paradox. It suggests that the expressed aim of reducing the threats to the health of workers – and especially women workers – was not, in fact, the primary motive of the 'reformers'.

Any health and safety legislation might be expected to have perceived benefits for all workers. Restriction or exclusion of particular people from work is therefore not a measure to improve conditions and reduce risk. Feminists often pointed to the illogicality of this position, when they attacked measures that targeted women, rather than improving conditions for everyone. Support within male trade unions for legislation that applied to women might then be, as many women suggested at the time, because of their own interests not as workers but as men. Accusations were made about sexual antagonism and a fear of competition.[13] There is also another interpretation of men's motives, however. This has suggested that their support for 'protective' legislation was to secure some improvement in conditions for themselves in recognition that State intervention in men's labour would prove more difficult. This view was also expressed by contemporary commentators, and later analyses have reiterated the phrase of 'behind women's petticoats'[14] as an indication of this intention.

Aside from the difficulty of establishing with any certainty that certain motives or intentions underpinned men's support for factory legislation, the extent to which they benefited in terms of health and safety was strictly limited. Their own hours were reduced only in industries where they worked alongside or with women and where there was some interdependence of gendered work processes. In textiles, when women's work was shortened on Saturdays to allow time for cleaning (women's work), a high number of accidents occurred to women, including scalping, because shafting was still in use to drive the men's machines.[15] In many other industries, neither restrictions on hours or night-work prevented long working hours either for women or men. Hours remained one of the most enduring problems of working conditions, one that directly impinged on other identified problems and hazards because it resulted in long exposure. These limited health gains may have led feminists to suspect that men's true motives lay elsewhere.

There were certainly flaws in the preventive approach that was pursued with considerable consistency, perhaps surprisingly. There was an increased emphasis on the value of empirical data as a support for the development of social policy. There was also mounting evidence that the strategy was not, in many cases, reducing the measurable indices of ill-health. Constant enquiries were initiated by the State, supported by the reports of its own inspectorate. These suggested there were inadequacies in the content of legislation as well as in its scope. This failure in approach was most evident in relation to the designated 'dangerous trades', where there was a clear alternative legislative remedy: a prohibition on the use of a product or processes which used it in manufacturing. This alternative was certainly demanded. Medical and scientific evidence, factory inspectors, political activists and political practice in other countries with respect to some industries (for example, match-making) all pointed to prohibition as a single remedy at least for industrial poisoning. Despite the pressure, prohibition was instituted legally in many cases only after 1914.[16]

The alternative strategy to prohibition was a 'sanitary' model of prevention. Apart from working hours, which were only minimally reduced and only in selected and limited work arenas, the main focus of regulation was concerned with the working environment and with controls on workers themselves, including surveillance of their 'fitness' for work. Given the framework of 'protective' legislation, women were considered vulnerable to such conditions and they were to be more often subject to such requirements (although increasingly men were also included). In some cases regulation of the environment, as in machine-guarding, was directly targeted at men, leaving women at risk. An environmentally oriented preventive strategy might well be seen in a positive light. In the nineteenth and early-twentieth centuries, as well as in the present context, analyses have pointed to the importance of broad-based sanitary or environmental health measures in securing improved health status,[17] even if such approaches also have their limitations. So why do I consider it to have largely failed in the specific context of factory legislation and occupational ill-health?

Some writers have argued that the main weakness of the sanitary model of prevention in relation to occupational ill-health in nineteenth-century Britain was that it hindered the development of occupational medicine and the understanding of diseases caused by work. Hence Lee's comment that occupational medicine was 'stillborn' in the era of public health[18] and Wohl's belief that identification with public health lost occupational medicine the opportunity for the higher status being acquired by clinical medicine and mitigated against the acquisition of expertise about industrial disease.[19] These arguments essentially reflect an unquestioning assumption about the importance of developing clinical knowledge about disease to a reduction in its incidence.

My argument is a different one. It is not about the superiority of either a clinical or a public-health approach to the problem of occupational ill-health, since arguably both can make a contribution to prevention. Rather the failure in this case was in relation to the specific measures taken toward the problems of the working environment despite an adherence to a sanitary model. These flaws were because it was limited to low-cost measures that targeted a small range of problems. These were primarily the increasing regulation of the air by requiring increased (but often primitive) ventilation and standards of cubic space per worker; and by improvements in the cleanliness of workrooms, especially where there were dusty work processes. There were also requirements about the provision of sanitary and washing facilities. Thus, despite a recognition that there were problems with the working environment, the approach was not to change the environment itself, but to protect workers from its effects. They were required to wear protective clothing, including respirators, to wash before eating, to wash or bath before returning home. Since dangerous substances were not to be excluded from that environment, then in some cases it was considered necessary to exclude women workers from them.

The prohibition of women from some processes in lead manufacture and the Potteries was one extreme form of preventive strategy. Less extreme was the increased use of medical inspection to monitor health status with the possibility that women would be suspended or excluded from work. I have also highlighted how this approach to regulation was often defended on the ground that such measures would be effective if it were not for a failure on the part of workers. They were accused of either neglecting to take care of themselves outside work, so that they brought a physical 'susceptibility' to the workplace; or that they ignored those regulations that were intended for their benefit. The prominence of these ideas in accounting for the failure of legislative remedy served to deflect attention away from its own intrinsic weakness and to undermine any intent that such legislation was a means of ensuring some collective responsibility for securing good working conditions. As feminist activists at the time were constantly to note, the approach sought to 'muzzle the worker and not the process'.[20] However, despite the weak approach the content of the legislation reveals, some minimal benefit from it would probably have been derived.

Explanations of the failure of the content of the 'sanitary model' were exacerbated by issues about its scope and application. The legislation focused on only a small number of the underlying causes of ill-health to be found in the working environment. But many problems that women experienced as damaging to their health and wellbeing and to which medical experts and factory inspectors drew attention were not included within the legislation. There were also industries where similar problems to those that were regulated existed but which were not included. Within the 'dangerous trades', there were the examples of lack of control over dusts in asbestos-spinning and in jute, linen and flax-spinning. In 1892, 115 operatives between the ages of 15 and 29 in the Belfast mills died of phthisis. Inspectors noted that if you started work at 18 you were likely to be dead by 30.[21] Hours of work regulation excluded many areas of women's work allowing for exceptions and exemptions. Adequate lighting, seating, extremes of hot and cold temperatures, wet floors (and thereby clothes) and the lifting of heavy weights are all examples of observed and experienced problems that largely remained outside regulation.

Issues of scope and application overlap. As health and safety legislation, factory legislation was further hampered by its application to factories and workshops and factory inspectorate powers only to those areas encompassed by legislation. Working conditions that could and did undermine women's health were outside both factory and workshop sectors of employment. There was some extension in relation to non-industrial employment such as shop-work and a concern with industrial employment drew attention to other environments, such as domestic workshops and homework. These aside, for many groups of working women what few benefits, if any, might have been gained from legislation were denied them. Chapter 4 documented the extent of poor working conditions in many non-industrial but mainly working-class women's work and in white-blouse and new 'professional' areas of work that provided opportunities for middle-class women. Conditions here were frequently little better than those in factories and even when they were, reform was still much-needed. It was left to women's organizations and the gradual growth of trade unionism to highlight such concerns and to seek their redress, although the latter often focused on pay to a neglect of working conditions.[22]

A number of other causes of failure in terms of scope and application have been highlighted. The linguistic framing of legislative regulation allowed for considerable variations in interpretation and for matters of transgression to be open to dispute: expressions such as 'where reasonably practicable' or 'normally', for example. Enforcement suffered from inadequate resources to meet the requirements of inspection and prosecution. Women inspectors were only able to deal with a small proportion of the abuses that occurred and, without the help of women's labour organizations who also took on the role of channelling possible problems and complaints to the inspectorate, it would have been much less. Despite considerable work overload for inspectors, the proportion of women receiving benefit was probably small.[23] The work of the women's inspectorate also revealed the difficulties of achieving change through the mechanism of the law, when those responsible for its local administration were not free from political favour. Such political interests operated within local administrative authorities who were charged with certain obligations under the legislation. This applied to local sanitary authorities who had a number of responsibilities with respect to sanitary conditions and the inspection of workshops. At the end of a process from detection to prosecution, probably only a small number of offences were dealt with – and even if they were, it was no guarantee that improvements would have been the result.

'Protective' Legislation – Intentions and Consequences

If factory reform and the regulation of working conditions through the vehicle of 'protective' legislation was intended to have a major influence on disease prevention and thence the improvement of workers' health, it failed. Another aim of legislation was to return women to the domestic domain and to preserve patriarchal social relations at work and at home. Was this aspect of the legislation any more successful?

If the impact of paid employment in terms of its social consequences was of the order claimed by many 'reformers' of the industrial system as well as 'antagonists' of women's work then, logically, we might have expected the exclusion of women to have been pursued with some vigour and to have been implemented more widely. There were certainly exclusions, at least with respect to the employment of married women in some localities and in particular fields of employment such as the civil service, but these were not legislatively required. Exclusion was also a possible preventive health remedy, but in many cases the marriage bar was not based on such arguments. There were demands for exclusion from some quarters and consideration given to it within State-initiated enquiry into working conditions in the context of expressed 'ideals' about the undesirability of women working.

The extent to which the State adopted this approach was limited: where it did so, it was more evidently related to health risks. Even when such regulations were introduced which either prohibited directly, or allowed for temporary or permanent exclusion on grounds of fitness or signs of illness, the actual impact on women's participation in paid work seems to have been minimal. Some authors[24] have argued there was a decline in the proportion of married women working before the 1880s but not in the next four decades, when arguably the debate was more vociferous and intervention greater. While it may have made it more difficult for women to be employed in certain industries, there were usually, depending on local labour markets, other kinds of work to be found including charing, casual work and home-work. Thus overall participation rates changed little, either among married or single women,[25] although it did structure the kinds of access women may have had to certain types of work and to higher pay. Bowley's Commission of Inquiry for the British Association for the Advancement of Science concluded that the economic effects of the Factory Acts were minimal. He argued that 'the line of demarcation between men's and women's work is in a great majority of cases rigidly fixed by physical suitability, by relative cheapness or by custom'.[26]

The fact that prohibition or the exclusion of women was not accepted as a legislative remedy can be easily explained. The use of health-based arguments about the impact of working conditions, in part, meant that if these conditions or their effects could be remedied by other means then there was no need for more drastic measures. By itself, however, this would not have swayed those for whom working conditions were not the issue. More importantly, the very ideal on which prohibitionist arguments rested – the preservation and sanctity of family life – could also be used by their opponents. Furthermore, given the growing rationale for an interventionist State to protect collective health and welfare, these arguments were difficult to ignore. Again and again evidence was presented that showed the economic realities of working-class family life to be so impoverished that, however meagre, the income earned by women was essential to survival. 'Ideals' of a male breadwinner, earning a wage sufficient to support a family, were far from being achievable. Male unemployment was high, casual labour common, and men's wages low. In 1911 Bowley estimated that 2.5 million adult men earned less than 25s a week while working full-time.[27] Eleanor Rathbone's study of pre-First World War wage levels estimated that 74 per cent of men earned less than 35s a week, and 32 per cent less than 25s when in full work, both she regarded as subsistence.[28] In her later attack on the concept of 'the family wage' she argued there was no guarantee that whatever a man earned, he would adequately provide for his wife and children. Barrett and McIntosh argue similarly that historically it did not raise living stand-ards for the working class as a whole, nor did it prevent competition from women, resulting in division between working-class men and women.[29] Further, as many women campaigners were to document, households without men, or where women were required to support their paternal families, were not uncommon. It was often the case that those people who argued in favour of prohibition, would at one and the same time express concerns about the impact on families arising from a loss of women's income, including male unionists. Such views were probably related to an increasing exposure to, and debates about, poverty from the 1880s.[30] As the example of 'sweated' work indicated, questions of poverty and working conditions became interlinked, and local and central State responsibilities for amelioration of poverty were central to evolving ideas of controls on capitalist industrial enterprise as well as State formation and regulation.[31]

There were also powerful interests opposed to interference in economic life, who constantly attempted to thwart any legislative controls on their activities even on health grounds. Despite some acceptance that the consequences of *laissez-faire* in economic life now necessitated limited controls, industrialists and employers still resisted attempts to interfere with labour supply, productive processes and social relations. Interference was seen as undermining the (fair) competitive rationality of the market, either between firms within Britain or in the wider international marketplace. Women provided an important source of cheap labour, but where gender-segregated work was well-established, with specific areas delineated as 'women's work', intervention would have a major impact on production and profitability. Employers often disagreed with the State and they were often 'successful' in defeating or undermining regulation.

It might be argued, therefore, that these attempts are indicative of their bourgeois class interests. However, as Marxist scholars have noted, capitalist employers also have other interests in women which might be consistent with their removal from the workplace. In drawing a distinction between the productive power of men and the reproduction of labour power, where women ensure the health of the current and future work force, capitalist interests become interests shared with other men. Bourgeois class values had strong views about the nature of the working-class family that supported the 'separate spheres' ideology. The contradiction between the requirement for women workers within industrial and other work arenas and support for healthy mothers of the new generation which required women's confinement to the domestic sphere were clearly evident in the approaches taken by many individual employers and manufacturers and in the State's prevarication over the prohibition of women from work. In fact, those regulations instituted under 'protective' legislation required some changes to manufacturing conditions and both this expenditure and the increased regulation and surveillance of the workforce incurred employers' costs, in some cases, especially in small firms, impacting on economic viability. But for most industrialists these costs were small, as were those for contravention (low levels of prosecution and fines for the guilty, for example). In all, legislation had little impact on the recruitment and patterns of women's employment in regulated industries, and left untouched many areas of production outside regulation.

I suggest that despite a more sustained attack on the problems created by industrial capitalism and the basis this provided for a development of a State welfare system, there was limited intervention in capitalist production and social relations. However, rather than accepting this as evidence of class domination in State formation, it can be equally, if not more persuasively, seen as a result of men's interests and the exercise of male power. While prohibition seems more clearly to be an assertion of male interests, these might also be equally served by a perpetuation of capitalist social relations in which men's social power over women was confirmed by their position within the workplace and in relation to the family and domestic domain. The role of the State and factory legislation can be understood as patriarchal in these terms. Equally, the failure of 'protective' legislation to reduce women's participation did not mean that sexual antagonism was not present or that men's motives were not to reduce that participation. Motives or objectives are not always realized in particular outcomes. But there are problems with any idea that male opposition was universal, as some studies in particular industries, such as coal mining,[32] or in different localities[33] have indicated. If women at work *per se* were the issue, then why were men's campaigns only targeted at factories and workshops? Why not target all areas of women's employment, including shop-work and domestic service which shared similar poor conditions?

There are two possible explanations: first, there was already an attack on the industrial system which lay outside the specific issue of women's employment in it. Thus it was not difficult to graft on this particular grievance especially as the quality of domestic labour came under scrutiny. Second, men's opposition to women's employment was much more visible in those industries where there had not been a tradition of women working and where there was a perceived threat to men's jobs and pay levels. Neither shop-work or domestic service provided such a competitive threat. There were some non-industrial employments where such male hostility to women was visible, such as clerical work. Here anti-women sentiments justified sexual segregation and low pay in the same way that feared competition operated within the industrial sector.

Capitalism and Patriarchy: Men's Interests and the Subordination of Women

At the heart of feminist debate about women's oppression has been the theorized relation of it to capitalism and patriarchy. It has been in relation to women's participation in the paid labour market that such debates have been so clearly articulated. These debates, particularly within Marxist Feminism, have centred around the extent to which gender subordination is integral to capitalist production or is independent of it.[34] Some have considered that a 'dual system' of capitalism and patriarchy have existed relatively independently of each other while both exerting an influence,[35] whereas others argue it is important to consider capitalism and patriarchy as a single system which mutually benefit each other.[36] An important aspect of feminist analysis whatever view of this relationship they hold, has been to articulate the relation, if any, between the extent to which oppression is located at the level of ideology, and the relative importance of material practices and institutional structures in realizing gendered institutions, social relations, experiences and subjectivity which disadvantage women. In this section some of these issues are addressed in relation to the preceding research analysis.

One of the rationales for examining the discourses around women's participation in the paid labour market, and women's role within the family and domestic division of labour was because I believed that ideological constructions of women, men and the relations of gender, are important in understanding the oppression of women. At the same time I agree with Barrett,[37] that it is important to assess how such representations are linked to various social practices and interests as it is here that oppression is effected. At the same time, if ideology is essentially concerned with meaning construction, then it does not necessarily have a direct relationship to material practices, otherwise there would be no possibility for a politics and practice of opposition. Brenner and Ramos[38] are critical of Barrett's arguments for the degree of autonomy she grants ideology at the level of culture and the deterministic role of gender ideology in relation to the capitalist division of labour. They are concerned with understanding ideology as it pertains to 'real conditions of existence'. That raises the problematic issue of the relation of ideology, or discursive practices, to experience. It is probably more important to recognize that gender can be constituted and operate ideologically, that is as a symbolic system, but the precise way in which such meanings of gender become the basis for structured inequality requires scrutiny of particular social practices.[39]

In this study, the ideology of 'separate spheres', the assertion of paid work as belonging to men, and unpaid domestic work as the domain of women, or between productive and reproductive work, was constantly visible. Furthermore, it evidently rested on a biological and social constitution of 'femininity' and 'masculinity' as a basis for that differential eligibility. The ideology provided a normative justification for intervention by the State in both the paid labour market and in the family household or domestic economy, and it largely did so through an emphasis on the maintenance of the family and the different obligations of men and women as maintainers of it. Thus a number of other ideological conceptions and discursive rhetoric were interlinked, for example, the 'family wage' which suggested that men's work and the wages received for production should be sufficient to provide for their families, and 'maternalism' which rhetorically emphasized women's particular responsibilities for the duties and care of children. Mothering and breadwinning were oppositional constructs. According to Rose,[40] this ideology accounted for the high numbers of homeworkers in Britain, but although homework might have resolved this contradiction for women, it was still disruptive to domestic routines.

Throughout the period there are a number of examples of how these ideological beliefs influenced further constitutions of gender difference. For example, in the face of clinical and statistical evidence (however imperfect) on industrial poisoning, doctors, state officials and campaigners continued to assert the special susceptibility of women, drawing on the same biological factors which were thought to determine women's general unsuitability for paid work. More specifically, lead poisoning came to be seen as a risk to reproduction, with reproductive risks defined as sex-specific. A further consequence of utilizing biological factors as a basis for social differences between men and women was the neglect of those material factors which impinged more dramatically on women's health and domestic responsibilities.[41] In the continuing debates about infant mortality and the national health, the idea that a 'failure of mothering', either through lack of skill or knowledge, or through being in paid work, continued to hold sway despite evidence of environmental factors and infectious disease as causes of infant deaths.[42]

The pervasive nature of such ideologies was also evident in oppositional discourses and political practices. While different meanings might be attributed to the consequences of the ideology, and experienced realities tempered generalization, the acceptance of a fundamental premise was widespread. Feminist campaigners for suffrage, work opportunities, and on both sides of the 'protective legislation' debate, while emphasizing the needs of different women and the practical realities in their lives, still gave support to the 'ideal' of women providing full-time care for the family. Feminists supported 'minimum wage legislation' on the grounds that it would make it less necessary for women to work as well as remedying 'sweated' labour. Even if the legitimacy of women's right to work was accepted, such claims were often on the basis of gender difference, emphasizing that the attributes and skills women possessed for 'motherhood' could be successfully utilized in paid work. Areas of professional employment, including that of factory inspection itself, drew on such ideological constructions of 'femininity'.

Despite the importance of such ideological constructions of gender difference, it is evident that social practice did not necessarily follow. The failure to remove women from the labour market, at least in terms of overall participation levels was a clear example. It did, however, often impinge on individual women's decisions not to work, and their experience of work as an 'economic necessity' rather than a positive opportunity. There is also evidence here that while prohibition was not a practical possibility, ideological frameworks were preserved by alternative solutions. In this case 'protectionism' served the purpose, and enabled the State to be seen as exercising its humane responsibility. Male power was left intact in a 'protective strategy'.

This makes us aware of how conflicts and contradictions occur both ideologically and in the practical pursuit of interests. An important aspect of Walby's argument that patriarchy has historically specific forms,[43] is her assertion that in 'protective legislation' and in trade unionist strategies, there are evident contradictions between patriarchy and capitalism.[44] She argues that employers' use of women as cheap labour and as a 'docile' workforce, resulted in women receiving wages in their own right for long hours away from home, with less time to devote to unpaid domestic labour. This, she suggests, would have undermined an important source of patriarchal power, and so factory legislation can be seen as an attempt to reassert that control. However, there are other ways of viewing this possible relationship and its contradictions, such as the interest of capitalist men in women's domestic labour in order to secure the reproduction of labour power, while at the same time wishing to resist men's demands for higher wages on the grounds of providing for all the family. Given the capitalist drive to accumulate, there would be an inevitable pull of the labour power of women into work, yet this did not actually occur.[45] Both Barrett[46] and Walby argue that 'protective legislation' played an important part in the developing sexual division of labour under capitalism, whereas I would argue it was a necessary precondition for being able to pursue sex-specific legislation, and that it was this particular form of capitalist social relations which ensured patriarchal control was maintained at work as well as in the domestic sphere. The very basis of job segregation where women were confined to low status, low paid and sex-typed work, was their different relation to domestic and paid work arenas.

This research lends support to those feminists who argue that patriarchy may be viewed as a single process encompassing economic and familial relations. It has demonstrated that ideologically, and at the level of material practice, power inequality on the basis of gender was the basis for economic organization, familial relationships and State intervention. I concur with Lown's view that 'the need to distinguish economy and family' is irrelevant. As she argues:

> The constant reification of capitalism obscures the historical reality of both capitalists and workers as gendered beings with different interests and stakes in the material features of employment and marital arrangements.[47]

In her study of Courtaulds, Lown[48] demonstrates how the management of the labour market occurred through particular management and employment practices. As an example of 'paternalism', which was often associated with a more humane and community-welfare form of business practice, Courtaulds exemplified how paternalism was simultaneously a form of class and patriarchal control. Male interests and an imposition of male authority within the workplace, reproduced bourgeois family values and the traditional class-based hierarchies of authority. The consequence of these ideals was often a strict physical segregation of men and women and the operation of the marriage bar. Equally, it must be emphasized that concerns about women's work and family responsibilities were related to controls over their sexuality. The evident stress on moral degradation, the threats to 'femininity' and the links made between physical status and maternity, were at the core of ideas about their unsuitability for work and work for them. This in turn justified male initiated practices to restrict work opportunities.

Brenner and Ramos[49] ask feminists to think again about the importance of biological differences as they directly impinge on gender inequality, not in a reductionist way, but because biologically based roles shaped what was possible for women in terms of participation in paid work. Women's assignment to reproduction and a consequent marginality in the paid labour market, they argue, preceded 'protective legislation' and trade unionist calls for restriction. It was not just gender ideology which devalued women in ways realized within the sexual division of labour. It was that maternity and childrearing were duties they performed, and at this time, given the material circumstances of family life, they had little alternative. This, they suggest, led women to seek work which fitted with their family responsibilities, and for this work to become identified with women and thus attract low pay. It is their view that even changes in fertility control, resource distribution, and work opportunities has not changed the importance of this aspect of women's lives in their continuing subordination. It can be argued that such biologically-based roles were, in fact, in their material form a consequence of gender ideologies, and the unequal distribution of power between men and women. It was not that it could be otherwise, that women would be the bearers of children, but it is particular gendered social formations and relations that constitute how this will then become part of women's lived experience.

In as much as capitalism allowed for a distinction between productive and non-productive labour, then it provided patriarchy with a material basis, and it was to achieve its material form through job segregation and gender hierarchies at work. It is contended that the idea of consequential material benefit has led to alternative interpretations of whether men's opposition to women's work, and the power and privilege they exercised in this domain, represented class or patriarchal interests or both. Arguing that a 'naturalised' division of labour, as an essential organizing basis for capitalist productive relations, and for men's opposition to women's work, as Hartmann[50] claims, does not preclude the possibility that men would benefit materially. Humphries[51] asserted that this material benefit needs to be seen in class-terms. Men's opposition to women's work was essentially a struggle with capitalists to secure the 'family wage'. It was not a gain for themselves as men, but improved conditions for the working-class household. This view has been disputed by later analysts such as Barrett and McIntosh[52] because it did not necessarily 'free' women to provide use-value in the home, or men to secure power over labour supply. This divided the working-class and undermined its political strength.

It is important not to ignore the class dimension that was a factor in men's opposition. Men were not particularly secure in their employment either, and there were constant attempts to drive down wages. Competition was an important economic reality which undermined men's position in employment and in the family, their masculine identity and their power. Gray,[53] Rose[54] and Valdverde[55] have argued that the aspiration to 'respectability' as a core component of a working-class masculine identity required a life style which emphasized women's domesticity. In such circumstances, women were sometimes accused of assisting capitalist men and undermining male workers' bargaining position.[56] To this extent men's struggles over wages and employment might be a class struggle, but it was articulated through the gendered ideology of 'separate spheres' of the family and maternalism. It is also essential not to over-emphasize the extent to which the neglect of domestic responsibilities was the main focus of opposition to women's participation in paid work. There was a considerable body of opinion that was concerned about the impact on men's responsibilities as 'breadwinners'. An additional threat to the patriarchal form of the working-class family was that men might be encouraged to stop work altogether. Evidence to the Committee on Physical Deterioration[57] frequently raised the possibility that men had learned to be idle.

While there may have been some support among men and trade unionists for women's right to work and involving them in their own industrial struggles, these were, in my view, exceptions rather then the rule. It seems that men did not consider it appropriate to incorporate women into their political organizations. Even when some trade unions did so, women had few opportunities for participation or a share in men's claims, if these aspects were indeed a consequence of a shared class-consciousness. Rather, it must be concluded that what might seem to be class-based labour struggles were first and foremostly struggles to secure men's advantage in the labour market. Limiting women's participation and confining it to sexually-segregated processes was in the interests of both capitalists and working-class men. There was material benefit to capitalism, and both benefited as men.

The State: Toward a Feminist Analysis

I have argued earlier that the emerging State in late nineteenth century Britain has been attributed with a particular relation to capitalist and patriarchal interests. State intervention in the form of the Factory Acts, with their increasing enshrinement of the 'protective' principle, was significant in shaping patriarchal relations. Over and above men's direct representations through the political process, the ways in which the State and the law shape gender inequality and preserve male domination requires scrutiny. Much traditional analysis of the State has either adopted the early Marxist approach, in which the state functioned as an instrument of the economic interests of the dominant class, to one which suggested that the State also had relative autonomy and independence from class interests. This provides a useful starting point for considering how, as feminists, we can conceptualize State power. Ideas of autonomy, which suggest that the State has interests of its own independently of class, gender or race, bring us to a consideration of the extent which such claims have resulted in a perception of the State as independent of interests, as somehow neutral and objective, above interests as it were. If this were so then it might be difficult to argue either that State power shapes the social relations of male domination and women's subordination, or that it offers women possibilities of obtaining redress as citizens who are deprived of equal rights.

This possible paradox of women's relation to State action and their political engagement with it, which has been founded on more contemporary issues, was evident during the late-nineteenth century. Many feminists and socialists took a view that 'protective legislation' was a necessary form of State action to provide redress for the particular grievances of women against both capitalist exploitation and their unequal position in labour organizations and industrial employments; and in the State's duties by these means to a broader collective set of rights – the national interest. More recently, feminists have sought to secure other rights through the law around abortion, domestic violence, rape, property and a broad range of 'equal rights'. In all these examples, it can be argued that both gender difference and a gender hierarchy have been maintained. It is this possibility of 'everything and nothing' that MacKinnon[58] argues has left feminism with a 'schizoid' posture toward the State. In her view we have failed to ask two crucial questions: what role has the State played in sexual politics and what is the State 'from a woman's point of view?'. While it is not evident to me that MacKinnon provides an answer to this question, she does provide a necessary deconstruction of views of the State which have obscured our ability to analyze its maleness.

It can be argued that 'protective legislation' provides a more explicit example of the ways in which the State and law perpetuate male dominance. Catherine MacKinnon's[59] analysis is informative in understanding the ways in which the social power of men is exercized, and gender inequality perpetuated and legitimated through the law and the 'liberal' State. An important feature of this process, she argues, is that the idea of the State and the law as neutral, abstract and to some extent above everyday interests, serves to obscure that there are values and standards represented in law. The neutrality principle is taken-for-granted, as the way things are, rather than as institutional expressions of male dominance. An important aspect of MacKinnon's argument that has direct relevance here is that the sex-specific framing of legislation may be less important than the way in which any law works in practice. In the case of 'protective legislation', I have argued that it did fail to achieve those explicit aims of 'protecting' women from working conditions, and the less directly expressed intention of returning women to the domestic domain as the primary place of work. However, it did succeed in preserving the ontological conditions of gender difference, and the legitimacy of male social power that denied women any entitlement to equal rights.

Laws and public policy also 'construct and authorise particular ways of thinking about social problems'.[60] They are forms of discursive practice which, as Foucault[61] emphasized, served to create new 'subjects', new legal identities. In this way 'working women' acquired a particular status through factory legislation and thus came under increasing scrutiny and surveillance. It is in this way that social power is also exercised, allowing for particular interpretations and regulations to be imposed as in this case, on one gender. Coercion is thus effected symbolically as well as by legal restriction. The extension of 'working women' into 'working mothers' extended these coercive possibilities. An important aspect of 'protective legislation', as Levine[62] argues, was that its rhetoric served to mask the 'real beneficiaries' – men.

What was upheld in the case of factory laws was men's rights as producers, and in the case of prostitution, legislation protected their rights as consumers. It is Levine's contention that both cases presented 'a unified meaning of gender' enacted in discursive sexual differentiation. Throughout the analysis there have been examples of such a consequence: the gendered constitution of types of work and hierarchies of status and pay within the workplace which legislation reinforced. It also reinforced women's subordinate role within the family, as workers who should maintain the domestic economy and the health and care of men and children, and suggested they should not occupy positions in the paid labour market at all. Legislation limited participation through medical surveillance, restrictions on dangerous processes and hours of work. It legitimated institutional and local employment practices that excluded married women from employment through marriage bars. More important than any legally enshrined inequality was the legitimacy given to a wider social discourse that constituted the attributes and aptitudes of men and women, the social and personal identities of masculinity and womanhood, and their relative places within the social world.

While MacKinnon has laid stress on the law as an epistemological representation of ontological gender differences and inequality, it seems important to extend such possibilities to discourses around the law as much as those principles which it eventually came to embody. Thus, it may be that the content, scope and failure of factory legislation to achieve either health gains or a relocation of women out of the workplace was less important in perpetuating women's disadvantage than the opportunities it gave for representations of relations between women and men in terms of male definitions, allowing patriarchal control to be constituted and reconstituted.

Thus while State action was in many respects minimal in terms of its actual intrusion into the world of work, or the private realm of sexual activity, it increasingly provided a focus for definitions of normative patterns of gendered behaviour. It was helped, as Levine[63] notes, by the increasing use of professional experts. In my examination of the role of the medical profession in relation to factory legislation and women's work, I argued that their involvement was more important in confirming the social dimensions of legislation rather than in articulating its role in relation to occupational ill-health.

In liberal conceptions of the State, claims to neutrality and objectivity are central. This fails to acknowledge the extent to which, if it reflects society, it must inevitably reinforce existing distributions of power and thus gender-based stratification. At the same time, it is important to incorporate an appreciation of how the State frames these power relations through the content and practice of the law, and equally through non-intervention or interference. Belief in the desirability of freedom from restraint/constraint was a still powerful political philosophy in late Victorian Britain. Despite encroachments, which an evolving state form and defined obligations were making, the *status quo* largely remained intact. Just as voluntary codes or self-policing are currently widely used as mechanisms to legitimate non-interference, so from the turn of the century, voluntarism, self-help and the preservation of local political autonomy offered a compromise between action and non-interference.[64] It must be doubted that whatever 'rights' were ostensibly to be gained for women through 'protective legislation' were minimal and that they confirmed women's status as 'unfree'. Factory legislation did not protect their health from the dangers of work, nor did it secure their right to work, or equal rights at work, in fact the opposite was true. Even if the content of the law had been more effective it would not necessarily have reduced substantial inequality across the social system. 'Protective legislation' did not prevent men from expressing hostility to women in the workplace, from instituting policies which denied them access to certain jobs, from acquiring skills, status and higher pay, or from subjecting women workers to health risks and dangers. 'Protective legislation' confirmed women's social and political dependence on men. The State and the law are not then autonomous or neutral of sex, they are patriarchal-literally the rule of men.

Feminist Politics and Women's Resistance

The period examined for this study provides a fruitful source of material for an analysis of forms of political activism among women and the degree to which there is evidence of a solidarity between women. The idea of resistance is important in recognizing the structural limitations of women's position and power, and that despite them women were historical actors who engaged in struggles against such inequalities and formulated their own forms of politics. Any analysis of 'first wave' feminism must appreciate its complexity as Walby[65] has rightly stressed, there will be within it perceived and expressed antagonisms and different political priorities and forms of strategic action. This required an acceptance of conflict between women, and a willingness to appreciate that even so, there was a commitment as women to women – a gendered identity as a basis for their feminisms. Women's work as a major focus of 'first wave' feminism, and the issue of 'protective legislation' more particularly, resulted in divisions between women organizationally that was expressed vocally but did not preclude a gender-based politics.[66]

Although it can be argued that patriarchal social relations were an important feature of the paid labour market, this did not necessarily deny women forms of authority or power. On the contrary, physical and social segregation of women and men allowed women to experience work environments free from male power, including such oppressive practices as sexual harassment, and to have other women supervise their work. This was certainly true of women factory inspectors themselves. They fiercely guarded attempts to restructure their working arrangements where this would threaten their autonomy and control, including the supervision and training of 'juniors'.[67] As new areas of clerical and 'professional' employment opened up for women there were other examples of developing autonomy and opportunities for management such as in nursing and teaching, however limited by today's standards, and dependent on already existing sexual divisions. In addition, it is suggested that teaching, where some women and men who both worked as teachers and married, provided an opportunity for marriages to develop toward a more 'companionate' model[68] that some feminists espoused.[69]

Although working conditions could be poor in occupations which both middle and working-class women might enter, and male power ubiquitous in its variety, women were able to achieve a new status and identity. As such, 'working women' was a much more salient category of feminist politics, and one which first and foremost provided for a unity around gender, rather than issues of class.[70] A further source of different interests, and one which has received relatively less attention, was women's marital status. It was evident that in some of the campaigns around 'protective legislation' single women, the majority of those at work, were often invisible as women workers, especially by those who laid greatest emphasis on family life. While feminist activists were both single and married, and pursued issues of concern to both, they were often constrained to respond to the terms of the debate in terms of other interest groups. However, class divisions were a major determinant of different experiences and opportunities for women, and these cross-cut the experiences of married, single and widowed/divorced women. It is also important not to dismiss the role of class-based values and life-styles in creating some difficulties for feminist politics.

While factory employments were less likely to offer the same opportunities for gender-based politics, they did provide for a kind of social life and forms of social relationships between women. For example, there were casual and even peripatetic groups of women, who formed generational communities of workers, such as those in fish curing and packing in Scotland, or the 'dustwomen' of London.[71] Without these it is hard to envisage how any spontaneous protests, including the many strikes by women workers, would have occurred, such as those in the Dundee jute industry.[72] There is some evidence also from working-class women that a gender identity was realized. It was not just women inspectors who claimed that women preferred to speak to other women about their grievances, there was evidence to support this from women themselves. A distance between middle-class activists and working-class women should not be taken as evidence either of the failure of feminism to create a gender-based political agenda, or of working-class women to resist at more local levels. By looking at such diversity of working women's experience it has also been possible to identify working-class women who took a significant part in suffragist political struggle.[73] There has to be some recognition of the pragmatic limits to a movement which could have encompassed women across the classes.

There was likely to be mixed perceptions of both factory regulation and other forms of State intervention by working women themselves. Testimony suggests factory regulation may have been less intrusive into working-class family life than other kinds of State intervention such as compulsory education for children. In terms of the dictates of family economy, restrictions on the work of children might have had a greater effect in that it both reduced their contribution to the family's income and made women's own labour force participation more difficult since they were often a source of unpaid child care.[74] As early twentieth century policy interventions around maternal and child welfare, also emphasized the 'failure' of household management and child-rearing practices, 'expert' interference, as it was often seen,[75] ignored many positive features of family life. There is no doubt that poverty and poor living environments were a reality for many women,[76] but families were essential sources of affection and support.[77]

Given these claims for the achievements of women's activism, there were at the same time costs of the approaches taken. The feminist historian has some difficulty in assessing the relative importance of the costs versus the achievements in relation to the specific area of women's work and lives. Throughout the book, I have taken the position, as have some other feminist scholars[78], that undoubtedly in many cases these efforts reinforced gender divisions, that patriarchal authority remained intact, and women's status was confirmed as less than equal. The sexual segregation of employment, which I argued provided opportunities for women, at the same time confirmed their lesser eligibility to paid work and to a living wage, let alone equal monetary rewards for similar work.

Ideals that framed women's participation in different areas of the public domain, including paid work, reflected the widespread acceptance of moral virtue as an essential defining quality of womanhood. Those middle-class activists who had equal rights aspirations for wider employment opportunities and improvements in conditions, constantly drew on discursive representations of 'virtue', 'respectability' and women's unique qualities that could bring new dimensions to work. These frequently harnessed those humanitarian sentiments which emphasized the 'morally good' progressive notions which had been prominent in reformers demands for factory regulation itself. Here the idealization of family life was integral to such notions of progress, and thus in engaging with factory reform as moral reform, it was the case that feminists also supported a view of family life that preserved its patriarchal structure and social relations. Many feminists shared a view of factory reform, through both the regulation of conditions and women's participation, as a necessary strategy for the physical and social health of the community and the nation.

Although feminists worked within and promoted values that were part of mainstream society, and which both explicitly and implicitly reinforced the patriarchal family and ideas of separate spheres, there was also a recasting of these. Forms of female organization, although not able to escape forms of male control or at least patronage, allowed some alternatives to be considered. For example, women's periodicals were often financed by men, but this did not prevent women writing in them from challenging male perspectives. Alliances had to be made with philanthropist manufacturers to push forward the campaigns on 'sweated labour'. Networks, including men friends (often as parliamentary spokespeople) were often the only vehicle for protecting hard-won victories, as in the case of maintaining the separate branch of the women's inspectorate. Despite the political necessity of some 'dependence' on men supporters, ideals of women's autonomy and women's concerns for women's issues were not necessarily compromised.

Talking about Women

It is important not to leave a book such as this without some acknowledgement of recent feminist theoretical concerns with the category 'woman' and 'women', or to how we can come to theorize gender difference. In leaving this to the final word, I do not wish to imply that it is a mere epistemological afterthought. It is an important issue for any feminist to address. It raises questions of validity about the analysis I have made, which claims to provide evidence of a number of aspects of women's experience as well as how discursive representations may be related to material practices in the period 1880–1914. Joan Scott[79] has stressed the importance of historical scholarship being alert to appropriating categories of analysis that were not analytic but rather a linguistic or rhetorical category of political struggle. From her concerns with the category of 'class' to the neglect of gender within labour history, she has subsequently developed her concerns about 'gender'.[80] In doing so her argument also goes beyond the view that an uncritical borrowing of categories is unhelpful to theoretical analysis to one which suggests what the core theoretical problems should be for feminist history.

In part, the issues are concerned with the same problem. Denise Riley[81] has argued that the category 'women', so central to feminism, as a discursively constructed category is subject to instability and change, not least because any category so constructed is relational. The category women will require the category men, for example, and it is important to understand how that naming occurs and in what contexts. But Riley has not been alone in wanting to deconstruct the category because of issues arising out of its use within Feminism, to indicate a common oppression. From the 1980s there has been repeated questioning of a shared political alignment on the basis of gender, to the exclusion of differences in power, resources and other oppressive relationships that women are party to, such as those of class, race, heterosexuality and able-bodiedness.[82] It is important not to attend to such differences ritualistically[83], but to consider how other patterns of differentiation will inevitably be effected alongside those of gender, and to eschew any 'essentialism' beneath the use of the category women. I have tried to ensure that while I talk about women, that I am also talking about different women. I have recognized that there was often a discursive construction of women that produced or impacted on their lives in both different and yet similar ways. Finally, in examining feminism within a particular historical context, it is evident that difference is constituted by and for women, as much as it is by those who use it to justify their subordination.

'Deconstructionism' of the category 'women' is part of what has been categorized as the 'linguistic turn', a characterization of what might be called a 'post-structuralist' feminist history, which takes representations to be the subject of study.[84] Joan Scott[85] has been at the forefront of developing these ideas. She takes the relationship between representations, or discursive constructions, and a retrievable historical reality, or what might be termed 'experience' as problematic. She challenges the authority of experience as evidence or as a source of explanation. Experience, she argues, is a linguistic event, that is language actually produces experience.[86] Ideas of human agency are then seen as meanings (interpretations) which are dependent on available discourses of the time. She is right to emphasize the difficulties with ideas of agency as autonomous, as resting in individual forms of resistance for example, and for these somehow to be outside of discursive constitutions of difference. Equally, I am uncertain that she does not give an over-deterministic role to discursive constitution, as imposing upon, and a precedent for, social formation. For example, she argues that a preoccupation with the sexual division of labour shaped the productive relations of industrial development, rather than being caused by them. These relations, I have argued, also gave patriarchal values within discourse a material basis.

As I have implied earlier in this chapter, as sites through which social power is exercized, discourses are the stuff of human agency. But they are also contested and subject to challenge, transformed and reformulated, and this has some actual basis in broader discursive domains, in historical conditions and contexts, and in the ways in which people lived and interpreted their everyday lives. There is a mutuality between text and context. There will be experiences that will destabilize particular discourses, as the increasing participation of women in the labour market did, and so in turn required some re-working of the discursive boundaries of 'separate spheres' ideology, as it did men's day to day relations to women. Equally, the construction of female bodies as particularly susceptible to some industrial diseases required modification when not all women succumbed and when men were also evidently being poisoned. To say this, is not to dispute the notion that there are difficulties with the 'essentialism' and 'empiricism' of assuming some actual reality that is knowable outside of language and texts, but it is to accept that there are discourses through which we may come to know women, and be able to talk about women, even when the historical record has already constituted them as 'different' or 'other'. In women's own discourses there are theorized categories of women too.[87] The difficulty Scott's position has raised for many feminists has been their suspicion that having spent their early years recovering the subject women from the invisibility of the historical record,[88] that such a reformulation will again exclude. More importantly, feminism makes an important connection between women's experience of disadvantage and powerlessness to the growth of a feminist consciousness – a particular identity as subject women to feminist politics. This has led some to argue[89] that her position undermines gender as power domination, obscures inequality and the possibilities for political struggle.

Of course there must be a critical reflexivity in our use of all sources that we take as our data and what we interpret that data to be about, but that is a problem of analyses of discourse. I wonder at Scott's insistence, that women as active agents, is simply a wish rather than historical reality, an accusation she makes about Gordon's reading of her data. Gordon, argues the discourse must be seen to co-exist with 'real family oppression'.[90] Women might frame these problems and act in ways that are discursively effected, but they were still problems to be acted upon. While Scott's work raises the importance of theorizing linguistic signification in the production of power and inequality as the basis for feminist politics, then it must also reveal gender, not just as constituted difference, but as forms of material practice. In the period 1880–1914 women's bodies, women's work and women's responsibilities within the domestic domain and in family-based households were all represented in discourses around their participation in the paid labour market and the dangers of that work to their own and others' health. All these aspects constructed women as different and as citizens 'not free', less eligible and more vulnerable. Their constructed identities confirmed their material disadvantages and preserved male power and privileges, which were in turn maintained as well as reconstituted within discourse. For the women (and the men) examined in this study, these constructions obscured the fact that it was the material conditions of life and work which resulted in both men and women getting sick, so that disease, disablement and death were too often part of people's everyday experience.

Notes

1 See Branca (1977) *Silent Sisterhood*.
2 Dyhouse (1989) *Feminism and the Family*.
3 The use of the term 'servants' here is interesting, as it was constantly used by their supporters and themselves. It may well have been purely a reflection of the fact they were civil servants, but equally it signified the limited scope they had outside their State-defined role. However, they were not always compliant employees.
4 See Langan and Schwartz (Eds) (1986) *Crises in the British State 1880–1930* for examples and analysis of such changes.
5 Mockett (1988) 'A danger to the State' discusses the debates around women's labour in factories in the 1830s and 1840s.
6 Gray (1991) 'Medical men, industrial labour and the State in Britain'.
7 Hutchins and Harrison (1903) *A History of Factory Legislation*.
8 Hutchins and Harrison (1903) ibid.
9 Ibid., characterizes the nineteenth-century development of legislation in these terms.

10 *Hansard*, 15 March 1844.

11 Marvel (1977) 'Factory regulation: a reinterpretation of early English experience' p.380.

12 Baines, cited from Hutchins and Harrison (1903) *A History of Cotton Manufacture* p.90.

13 See Lewis and Davies (1991) 'Protective legislation in Britain 1870–1990'; Rose (1988) 'Gender antagonism and class conflict'.

14 Webb and Webb (1911) *A History of Trade Unionism*. Rose Squire expressed a similar view in her autobiography (1927), as did Hewitt (1958). See also Strachey (1978) *The Cause* on first wave feminism.

15 Harrison (1993) 'Are accidents gender neutral?'.

16 White or yellow phosphorous was the exception. It was finally banned in 1910. Some changes occurred without awaiting legislation.

17 See the emphasis on material factors in reports on health inequalities such as Whitehead (1986) *The Health Divide*; Doyal (1979) *The Political Economy of Ill-health*.

18 Lee (1964) 'Robert Baker: the first doctor in the Factory Department'.

19 Wohl (1983) *Endangered Lives* makes this argument in the chapter on 'The canker of industrial disease'.

20 A number of feminist critics writing on many occasions to the ER used this or equivalent expressions, as did Gertrude Tuckwell in her separate Memorandum opposing the findings of other members of the 1910 Report on the Inquiry into the Potteries, on the grounds 'a definite alternative exists by imposing limitations on the use of material instead of on classes of worker', PP XXIX, p.223. This quote is from Nash (1897) p.10.

21 *Annual Report for 1898*, PP XII, p.171.

22 A overview of this early activism is provided in Holcombe (1973) *Victorian Ladies at Work*.

23 This argument is made by Jones (1988) 'Women as health workers'.

24 Hewitt (1958) *Wives and Mothers in British Industry*.

25 Hakim (1979) *Occupational Segregation*; Lewis (1984) *Women in England 1870–1950*.

26 Cited in Rose (1992) *Limited Livelihoods* p.75.

27 Thane (1982) *Foundations of the Welfare State* p.53.

28 Rathbone (1924) *The Disinherited Family* pp.16–17.

29 Barrett and McIntosh (1980) 'The "family wage": some problems for socialists and feminists', pp.66–7.

30 Hennock (1976) 'Poverty and social theory in England'.

31 Such arguments are particularly evident in the works of Sidney and Beatrice Webb around the Factory Acts.

32 John (1981) in her letter to *Feminist Review* takes issue with Jane Humphries on this point.

33 See Rose (1992) in particular her discussion of case-studies of different industries and localities.

34 This debate is most clearly evident in Barrett (1988) *Women's Oppression Today*.

35 'Dual systems' theory is most often associated with the work of Hartmann. See Hartmann (1976 and 1979).

36 See Lown (1990) *Women and Industrialisation*.

37 Barrett (1988) *Women's Oppression Today*.

38 Brenner and Ramos (1984) 'Rethinking women's oppression'.

39 Rose (1992) places particular emphasis on gender as a symbolic system that is embedded

in representations and social practices, so that both are sites where the meaning of gender is evident and negotiable. Barrett (1988), while emphasizing a relation to material practice, distinguishes ideology as mental rather than material and as operating within a cultural domain. Struggles over the meaning of gender, important as these are, therefore occur at the level of consciousness and cultural practice.

40 Rose (1992) *Limited Livelihoods* p.99.
41 Harrison (1995b) 'Women's health', for a fuller summary of these arguments.
42 See Dyhouse (1978) 'Working-class mothers and infant mortality' for a summary of this debate; Davin (1978) 'Imperialism and motherhood', for how policy and practice developed in accordance with an 'ideology of motherhood'.
43 Walby (1990a) 'From private to public patriarchy', and reiterated in her (1990b) *Theorising Patriarchy.*
44 Walby (1986) *Patriarchy at Work* especially p.41.
45 See Brenner and Ramos (1984) for a more extended argument about this particular contradiction.
46 Barrett (1988); Walby (1986).
47 Lown (1983) 'Not so much a factory, more a form of patriarchy', p.36.
48 Lown (1990) *Women and Industrialisation.*
49 Brenner and Ramos (1984) 'Rethinking women's oppression'.
50 Hartmann (1976) 'Capitalism, patriarchy and job segregation by sex'.
51 Humphries (1977) 'Class struggle and the persistence of the working class family'.
52 Barrett and McIntosh (1980) 'The "family wage" ', pp.59–66 provides a detailed analysis of their objections.
53 Gray (1987a) 'The language of factory reform'.
54 Rose (1992) *Limited Livelihoods.*
55 Valdaverde (1988) 'Giving the female a domestic turn'.
56 See Rose (1992) analysis of Kidderminster carpet-weaving.
57 PP XXXII (1904).
58 MacKinnon (1989) *Toward a Feminist Theory of the State* p.160.
59 MacKinnon (1989) *Toward a Feminist Theory of the State.*
60 Rose (1992) *Limited Livelihoods* p.50.
61 Foucault (1979) *Discipline and Punish.*
62 Levine (1993) 'Consistent contradictions', p.21.
63 Levine (1993) 'Consistent contradictions'. See also Chapter 6.
64 Thane (1982) *Foundations of the Welfare State.* See also Wohl's discussion of such compromises in relation to public health in his *Endangered Lives* Chapters 6 and 7.
65 Walby (1990a) 'From private to public patriarchy', p.97.
66 Feurer (1988) 'The meaning of "sisterhood" ', implies that such divisions undermined gender as a basis for alliances. Although such divisions were important, it is essential not to equate such political differences as necessarily undermining the idea of the 'women's movement' *per se.*
67 Martindale (1944a) described this as a particularly rewarding aspect, facilitated by a lessening of their peripatetic duties.
68 Copelman (1986) 'A new comradeship between men and women'.
69 See Bland (1995) *Banishing the Beast: English Feminism and Sexual Morality* Chapter IV for an overview of marriage during the 1885–1914 period; Dyhouse (1989) *Feminism and the Family in England.*
70 Swindells (1985) *Victorian Writing and Working Women* argues that such identifications are visible in written textual forms including those produced by women themselves.

71 These women lived together as well as worked together as they moved around the fishing ports, described in a number of reports by the women's inspectorate; for the latter see Hobhouse (1900) 'Dustwomen'.

72 Gordon (1987) 'Women, work and collective action'.

73 Liddington and Norris (1978) *One Hand Tied Behind Us.*

74 Lewis (1986c) 'The working-class mother and State intervention'.

75 Thane (1982) *Foundations of the Welfare State* p.62.

76 Social investigation into the working-class family by women provides ample evidence of this and its consequences for women. See Davies (1915) *Maternity*; Reeves (1914) *Round about a Pound a Week*; Chinn (1988) *They Worked All their Lives.*

77 Roberts (1984) *A Woman's Place*; Ross (1986) 'Labour and love: London's working-class families'.

78 Mappen (1986) 'Strategists for change'; Dyhouse (1989) *Feminism and the Family in England*; Levine (1988) *Victorian Feminism.* Many writers accept this contradiction in feminist politics.

79 Scott (1976) 'On language, gender and working-class history'.

80 Scott (1988) *Gender and the Politics of History.*

81 Riley (1988) *Am I that Name: Feminism and the Category 'Women' in Feminist History.*

82 See especially Anthias and Yuval-Davis (1983) 'Contemporary feminism – gender, ethnic and class divisions'; Ramazanoglu (1989) *Feminism and the Contradictions of Oppression.*

83 Stanley (1990) makes the point that this can happen and argues it is important to look at actual power dimensions embedded in difference.

84 See Canning (1994) 'Feminist history after the linguistic turn'.

85 Especially in her collected essays (1988) *Gender and the Politics of History.*

86 See also the work of Dorothy Smith (1985) on documents as reality constructions in her *The Everyday World as Problematic* and in her edited works (1990) *Talk, Facts and Femininity.*

87 Stanley (1990) makes this point about her reading of Hannah Cullwick's diaries in 'Recovering Women in history from feminist deconstructionism'.

88 For a recent overview of issues of invisibility in feminist history see Kleinberg (Ed.) (1988) *Retrieving Women's History.*

89 See especially Gordon (1988) in her review and debate with Scott (1990) in *Signs.*

90 See the review by Scott of Gordon's *Heroes of their Own Lives* and Gordon's reply in *Signs* (1990) pp.848–60.

Appendix

Chronology of the Women's Inspectorate Personnel 1893–1921

Taken from the Annual Reports of the Women's Inspectorate

1893   Miss Mary Muirhead Paterson, clerk and précis writer, Royal Commission on Labour, appointed.
Miss May Abraham, assistant commissioner, Royal Commission on Labour, appointed.

1894   Miss Lucy Deane, sanitary inspector, Kensington and Chelsea, appointed. Miss Adelaide Anderson, clerk and précis writer, Royal Commission on Labour, appointed.

1895   Miss Rose Squire, sanitary inspector, Kensington and Chelsea, appointed in December.

1896   Miss May Abraham becomes superintending inspector.

1897   May Abraham marries Harold Tennant and retires under pressure. Remains on the Committee for the Dangerous Trades. Miss Adelaide Anderson becomes principal lady inspector. Miss Anna Tracey, clerk to the Royal Commission on Labour, appointed.

1898   Departmental enquiry on the organization of staff.
Miss Emily Sadler, private secretary, appointed.

1899   Miss M. Vines, sanitary inspector, appointed.

1900   No additions.

1901   Miss G. Hodgson appointed and lasted two weeks. Miss Deane sent to South Africa. Miss Hilda Martindale appointed temporarily.

1902   Miss Hilda Martindale's appointment made permanent, previously inspector of Children's Boarded Homes for Dr Barnados. Miss Lucy Deane returned.

1903   Misses Paterson, Deane and Squire all promoted to senior grade.

1904   Temporary appointments of Miss Emily Jane Slocock and Miss Mildred Power (Miss Deane ill).

1905   Miss Emily Jane Slocock, clerk to principal lady inspector, Miss Mildred Olive Power, assistant bacteriologist to the Royal Commission on Sewage Disposal, made permanent.

1906   Miss Mary Paterson, acting principal. Miss Irene Whitworth BSc, sanitary inspector, Miss Isobel Meiklejohn MA, lecturer in hygiene, both candidates in competitive examinations, appointed.

1907   Miss Lovibond and Miss Newton appointed temporarily, then made permanent.

Additional 5–12 posts now seem to be available. Miss Squire returns from Royal Commission on the Poor Law. Miss Lucy Deane on sick leave.

1908   Miss Lucy Deane retires on health grounds. Miss Power is transferred to the Local Government Board, Misses Tracey, Sadler and Martindale promoted to senior. Miss Paterson, deputy principal Southern Division. New divisional structure, Miss Squire to Manchester, Miss Martindale to Belfast, Miss Vines to Glasgow, Miss Sadler to Birmingham. Miss A.J. Perry, Miss H.C. Escreet and Miss L.M. Pearson appointed.

1909   Miss Newton (Currelly) married, having just completed two years' probation, Miss F.I. Taylor, Miss A.M. Ahrons, Miss A.M. Young appointed.

1910   Miss Vines promoted to senior. Miss Whitlock, MB, BS, DPH, first medically qualified woman inspector, appointed. Industrial health specialist.

1911   Resignation of Miss Mary Paterson, appointed Scottish Insurance Commissioner.

1912   Shortage of staff, transfers, retirements and promotions, only 14 of 17 posts filled. Miss Squire becomes deputy principal, Miss Slocock is promoted, Miss Florence Lovibond resigns on marriage, Miss A.M. Taylor retires and Miss D.C. Lindsay BSc and Miss E.F. Stevenson MA BSC appointed.

1913   No shortage, 19 staff, Miss Constance Smith, Lady Margaret Hall, legal training, previously in Labour Exchange, appointed.

1914   Miss Squire gives evidence to the Departmental Committee on Lighting. Miss Whitlock transferred to Industrial and Reformatory Schools. Miss Keeley and Miss Anne Smith appointed.

1915   No figures; Miss Lennard mentioned. Staff increased by 50 per cent, both temporary paid and four unpaid.

1916   No information on staffing in short annual report.

1917   Mention of Miss McLeod, Mrs Shaw, Miss Sanderson, but no figures.

1918   Two inspectors lent to other government departments, one Miss Squire. Miss O.L. MacDonald, a temporary inspector, died, three retirements, Mrs Mumby, Miss Whitworth and Miss Tracey. Miss M.C. Anderson, Miss Pease temporary staff.

1919   New names mentioned: Miss Coombes, Miss Gwynne, Miss Dunch, Miss Andrew and Miss Hastings.

1920   Miss Footner and Mrs Bridge, Miss Cave retired. Miss A.R. Ewart and Miss A.D.E. Dunch permanent appointments, mentions Miss Messiter and Miss Mellor.

Note: This information is not complete. The routine reporting of staffing matters seems to have been highly variable.

Selected Biographical Details of Prominent Inspectors

May Abraham (1869–1946)

Daughter of a distinguished member of the Irish bar who lost family fortune. May came to London, worked for Lady Dilke, (Women's Trade Union League) and with

Sir Charles Dilke, a prominent campaigner on industrial conditions, especially for women. Shared house with Gertrude Tuckwell (Sir Charles Dilke's niece), later to become secretary and president of Women's Trade Union League. In 1892 May was appointed as one of four lady assistant commissioners, Royal Commission on Labour. In 1893 appointed to WFI and became principal inspector. Resigned on marriage to Harold Tennant MP in 1897. Member Dangerous Trades Committee. Chair Industrial Law Indemnity Fund and Industrial Law Committee. Director Women's Department of National Service, then chief adviser to Women's Welfare Labour Regulation Department. Active member Central Committee on Women's Employment 1914–18. Member Royal Commission on Divorce, National Association for the Prevention of Tuberculosis, chair of the Maternal Health Committee and governor of Bedford College.

Lucy Deane (c. 1860–1950)

Middle-class 'leisured' background. Trained at the National Health Society and Chelsea Infirmary, working as nursing sister. Appointed sanitary inspector, Kensington Vestry, and WFI in 1894. Study of Boer War concentration camps 1901. Left Factory Department in 1906, married Major Streatfield in 1911. In 1912 appointed to Royal Commission on the Civil Service. Chief woman organizer of outdoor staff for National Health Insurance. Member of War Office Appeals Committee. Member National Union Women's Suffrage Societies.

Adelaide Anderson (1863–1936)

Studied German and French. Attended Queen's College, Harley Street, then Girton College, Cambridge. Second class honours. in Moral Sciences (1887). Initially coached young women for exams and lectured for Women's Cooperative Guild. Appointed to staff of Royal Commission on Labour in 1892, then to WFI in 1894. Promoted to principal in 1897, retired in 1921. Member of the Commission on Child Labour. Investigator for the Shanghai Municipal Council on industrial conditions and child labour. Awarded MBE and CBE.

Rose Squire (1861–1938)

Daughter of Harley Street doctor, educated at home. At 32 needed to earn livelihood. In 1893 gained the Diploma of National Health Society and in 1894 Sanitary Inspector's Certificate. In 1893 sanitary inspector, Kensington Vestry, then in 1894 joined the inspectorate. Special investigator Commission on Poor Law 1906–7. From 1912 to 1921 Deputy Principal, Lady Inspector. Health of Munitions Workers Committee 1915–17. Director of Women's Welfare at the Ministry of Munitions 1918–19. Director of Women's Training Ministry of Labour 1919–20 Home Office. Awarded OBE. Retired in 1926.

Hilda Martindale (1875–1952)

Came from radical family. Sister Louisa became one of the first women doctors. Studied at Royal Holloway College; determined to be a social worker with children. No training available. Devised her own, then became an associate of Royal Sanitary Institute and undertook a new course in hygiene and public health. Inspector for Dr Barnardos boarding-out scheme and first woman on their Board. After a world trip in 1900 she joined the inspectorate in 1901. In 1916 was member of a committee to enquire into excessive drinking among women in Birmingham. Senior lady inspector, superintending inspector and in 1925 deputy chief inspector of factories. In 1933 she became director of women establishments in the Treasury. Retired in 1937. Awarded the CBE.

Bibliography

Parliamentary Papers

Annual Reports of Her/His Majesty's Chief Inspector of Factories and Workshops 1880–1914; and of Her/His Majesty's Women Inspectors of Factories 1893–1914; and Chief Medical Inspector for Factories and Workshops, 1898–1916.

Commissioners' Report on the Working of the Factory and Workshops Acts – with a view to Consolidation and Ammendment, Vol. I Report, PP XXIX, 1 1876; *Vol. II Minutes of Evidence*, PP XXX, 1 1876.

Copy of Communications addressed to the Secretary of State on the subject of Lead Poisoning with a Report by Alexander Redgrave, Her Majesty's Chief Inspector of Factories upon the same Subject, PP XVIII, 1883.

First Report of the Departmental Committee Appointed to Inquire into the Ventilation of Factories and Workshops 1902, PP XII, 1902.

First Report of the Departmental Committee on Lighting in Factories in Workshops, PP XXI, 1914–16.

Fourth and Sixth Reports of the Medical Officer of Health to the Privy Council, Local Government Board, PP XXVII, 1862, PP XXVIII, 1864.

Report of Alexander Redgrave Esq, Her Majesty's Chief Inspector of Factories upon the Precautions which can be enforced under the Factory Act, and as to the Need for Further Powers for the Protection of People Employed in White Lead Work, PP XVIII, 1882.

Reports of the Select Committee of the House of Lords on the Metropolitan Hospitals, Provident and Other Public Dispensaries and Charitable Institutions for the Sick Poor, PP XVI, 1890; PP XIII, 1892.

Reports of the Select Committee of the House of Lords on the Sweating System: First Report, 1888, PP XX; 1889, PP IV; *Fifth Report*, 1890, PP XVII.

Report of the Departmental Committee on the Various Lead Industries, PP XVII, 1893–4, referred to as *The White Lead Committee*.

Report To Her Majesty's Principal Secretary of State for the Home Department on Lucifer Match Works by the Chemical Works Committee of Inquiry, PP XVII, 1893–4.

Report of Her Majesty's Principal Secretary of State for the Home Department on Conditions of Labour in the Potteries, and the Injurious Effects upon the Health of the Workpeople and the Proposed Remedies (Also known as the *Potteries Committee of Inquiry*), PP XVII, 1893–4.

Reports of the Departmental Committee to Inquire and Report upon the Miscellaneous Dangerous Trades, PP XXX, 1896; PP XVII, 1897; PP XII, 1899.

Report of the Committee to Inquire into the Working of Cotton Cloth Factories Act 1889, PP XVII, 1897.

Report to the Secretary of State for the Home Department on the Visit to Match Factories in France by Thomas Oliver, PP XIV, 1898.

Report to the Principal Secretary of State for the Home Department on the Employment of Compounds of Lead in the Manufacture of Pottery, their Influence on the Health of the Workpeople, with Suggestions as to the Means which Might be Adopted to Counteract their Evil Effects, PP XII, 1899 (referred to as the *Thorpe/Oliver Report*).

Reports to the Secretary of State for the Home Department on the use of Phosphorous in the Manufacture of Lucifer Matches, by Professor T. Thorpe, Dr T. Oliver, and Dr G. Cunningham, PP XII, 1899.

Report of the Select Committee of the House of Lords on the Early Closing of Shops, PP VI, 1901.

Report of the Interdepartmental Committee on Physical Deterioration and *Minutes of Evidence*, PP XXXII, 1904.

Report upon the Conditions of Work in Flax and Linen Mills as Affecting the Health of Operatives Employed Therein, PP X, 1904.

Report to the Secretary of State for the Home Department by H.H.S. Cunnynghame Esq, Assistant Under Secretary of State, and B.A. Whitelegge Esq, His Majesty's Chief Inspector of Factories on the Match Factory of Messrs Moreland and Sons, Gloucester, with reference to a recent fatal case of Phosphorous Necrosis, PP X, 1907.

Not Only the 'Dangerous Trades'

Report of the Departmental Committee on the Truck Acts, PP LIX, 1908.

Report of the Select Committee on Homework, PP VIII, 1908.

Report of Judge Ruegg KC on the Application of the Factory and Workshops Act of 1910 to Florists Workshops, PP XXI, 1909.

Report on Conditions under which Bronzing is Carried on in Factories and Workshops, Messrs E.L. Collis, W.S. Smith and Miss R.E. Squire, PP X, 1910.

Report on Conditions and Hours in Typewriting Offices (1910), PP XXII, 1911.

Report of the Departmental Committee Appointed to Inquire into the Dangers Attendant on the Use of Lead, and the Danger or Injury to Health Arising from Dust and other Causes in the Manufacture of Earthenware and China and the Processes Incidental Thereto in the Making of Lithographic Transfers, PP XXIX, 1910.

Report of Judge Ruegg KC on Draft Regulations for the Manufacture and Decoration of Pottery and any Process Incidental Thereto, PP XXVI, 1912–13.

Report on Regulations in the Potteries by Inspectors Pendock and Werner, PP LXXI, 1914.

Royal Commission on Labour. *Conditions of Work in Various Industries in England, Wales, Scotland and Ireland. Reports on the Conditions of Women and Girls*, PP XXXVII, 1893–4.

Primary Sources: Books/Periodicals/Articles/Pamphlets/Tracts

ABRAHAM, M. (1897) *The Law Relating to Factories and Workshops*, London, Eyre and Spottiswoode.

ANDERSON, A. (1900) *Legislation Affecting the Conditions of Employment in Homework and Domestic Industries in England*, London, Industrial Law Committee.

ANDERSON, A.M. (1922) *Women in the Factory: An Administrative Adventure 1893–1921*, London, John Murray.

ANON. (1902) *Life in the Laundry*, Fabian Tract No. 112, London, The Fabian Society.

ARLIDGE, T. (1892) *The Hygiene, Diseases and Mortality of Occupations*, London, Percival.

BATESON, M. (1895) *Professional Women Upon Their Professions: Conversations Recorded by Margaret Bateson*, London, Horace Cox.

BEETON, I. (1863) *Mrs Beeton's Book of Household Management*, 2nd edn, London, S.O. Beeton.

BELL, LADY F. (1907) *At the Works: A study of a Manufacturing Town*, London, Edward Arnold. (Reprinted, Newton Abbot, David and Charles, 1969.)

BLACK, C. (1889) 'The organisation of working women', *The Fortnightly Review*, **46**, pp.695–7.

BLACK, C. (1891) 'Matchbox making in the home', *English Illustrated Magazine*, August, p.629.

BLACK, C. (1902) 'Some current objections to factory legislation for women', in WEBB, MRS S. (Ed.) *The Case for the Factory Acts*, London, Grant Richards.

BLACK, C. (1907) *Sweated Industry and the Minimum Wage*, London, Duckworth.

BONDFIELD, M. (1899) 'Conditions under which shop assistants work', *Economics Journal*, **9**, pp.277–86.

BOOTH, C. (1888) 'Conditions and occupations of the people of East London and Hackney', *Journal of the Royal Statistical Association*, **LI**, pp.276–339.

BOOTH, C. (1905) *Life and Labour of the People of London*, London: Macmillan.

BOUCHERETT, J. and BLACKBURN, H. (1896) *The Condition of Working Women and the Factory Acts*, London, Elliot Stock.

BRADBY, B. and BLACK, A. (1899) 'Women compositors and the Factory Acts', *Economics Journal*, **9**, pp.261–6.

BRITISH ASSOCIATION FOR THE ADVANCEMENT OF SCIENCE (1903) *Women's Labour, Report of the Committee Apointed to Investigate the Economic Effect of Legislation regulating Women's Labour* (drawn up by A.L. BOWLEY, secretary).

BRITISH MEDICAL JOURNAL.

BROWNLOW, JANE M.E. (1896) 'Women and Factory Legislation', paper read at the London Conference of The Women's Emancipation Union, 14 October, 1896.

BULLEY, A.M. and WHITLEY, M. (1894) *Women's Work*, London, Methuen.

BURDETT, H.C. (1890) *Nurses' Food, Work and Recreation*, The Hospitals Association, Pamphlet No. 13, London, Whiting.

BUTLER, C.V. (1916) *Domestic Service: An Enquiry by the Women's Industrial Council*, London, G. Bell and Sons.

BUTLER, J. *et al.* (1874) *Legislative Restrictions on the Industry of Women considered from a Women's Point of View*, London, Matthews and Sons.

CADBURY, E., MATHESON, M.C. and SHANN, G. (1906) *Women's Work and Wages: A Phase of Life in an Industrial City*, London, T. Fisher Unwin.

CADBURY, E., and SHANN, G. (1907) *Sweating*, Social Service Handbooks No. V, London, Headley Bros.

COLLET, C. (1891) 'Women's work in Leeds', *Economic Journal*, **1** (3), pp.460–73.

COLLET, C. (1896) 'Report by Miss Collet on the statistics of employment of women and girls in England and Wales', *Bulletin of the Department of Labour*, **1**, November 1895–6, No. 1.

COLLET, C. (1898) 'The collection and utilisation of official statistics bearing on the extent and effects of the industrial employment of women', *Journal of the Royal Statistical Society*, June, pp.219–61.

COLLET, C.E. (1902) *Educated Working Women: Essays on the Economic Position of Women Workers in the Middle Classes*, London: P.S. King and Son.

COLLET, C.E. (1911) *Women in Industry*, London, Women's Printing Society.

DAVIES, M.L. (1915) *Maternity: Letters from Working Women*, London, G. Bell and Sons. (Reprinted by Virago, 1978.)

DEARDON, W.P. (1923) 'What medical science can do for industry', *Association of Certivfying Factory Surgeons, Health and Industry Series*, No. 1. British Library of Political and Economic Science (BLPES).

DILKE, SIR C. (1896) 'Shop life: verbatim report of an important speech delivered to conference at the Memorial Hall Caridff on December 8th 1896', *The Shop Assistant*, Pamphlet No. 1, Cardiff.

DILKE, LADY E.F.S. (1895) *The Industrial Position of Women*, London, WTUL and Twentieth Century Press.

DRAKE, B. (1920) *Women in Trade Unions*, London, Allen and Unwin. (Reprinted by Virago, 1984.)

ENGLISH WOMAN'S JOURNAL.

ENGLISHWOMAN'S REVIEW.

FORD, I.O. (1902) 'Women as factory inspectors and certifying surgeons', *Women's Cooperative Guild Investigative Papers*, **1V**.

FOX, S. (1899) 'Factory and Workshops Bill', *Economics Journal*, **9**, June.

FOX, S. and BLACK, C. (1894) *The Truck Acts: What They Do and What They Ought to Do*, Issued by the Women's Trade Union Association, London, George Reynolds.

GILPIN, F. (Ed.) (1923) *Scenes from Hospital Life: Being the letters of a Probationer Nurse*, London, Dranes.

HAMILTON, A. (1912) 'Lead poisoning in potteries, tile works and procelain, enamel, and sanitary ware factories', *Bulletin of the US Bureau of Labour*, Department of Commerce and Labour, House Documents, **93** (104).

HANSARD.

HARRISON, A. (1904) *Women's Industries in Liverpool: An Enquiry into the Economic Effects of Legislation Regulating the Labour of Women*, Liverpool, University Press of Liverpool, Williams and Norgate.

HOBHOUSE, W. (1900) 'Dustwomen', *Economics Journal*, **10**, pp.411–20.

HUTCHINS, B. (1902) 'The historical development of the Factory Acts', in WEBB, MRS S. (Ed.) *The Case for the Factory Acts*, London, Grant Richards.

HUTCHINS, B.L. (1907) 'Homework and sweating: the causes and the remedies', *Fabian Tract*, No. 130.

HUTCHINS, B.L. (1909) 'Statistics of women's life and employment', read before the Royal Statistical Society 16 March 1909, *Journal of the Royal Statistical Society*, **LXXII**, Part II.

HUTCHINS, B. (1915) *Women in Modern Industry*, London: G. Bell and Sons.

HUTCHINS, B. and HARRISON, A. (1903) *A History of Factory Legislation*, London, Frank Cass. First Edition 1903, Third Edition 1966.

JEUNE, LADY (1893) *Paid Employment for Women*, London: A.D. Innes.

JOHNSTON, M.E. (1902a) 'The case against hospital nurses', *Nineteenth Century and After*, **51**, pp.595–603. Replies from HOLLAND, S. 'The case for hospital nurses', pp.770–9 and STEWART, I. pp.780–4.

JOHNSTON, M.E. (1902b) 'The question of modern trained nurses', *Nineteenth Cen-*

tury and After, **51**, pp.966–71, with replies by RAE, L. pp.972–4, and WARDE, E. pp.975–9.

JOINT COMMITTEE ON THE EMPLOYMENT OF BARMAIDS (1900) *The Barmaid Problem*, London, James Wakenam.

JONES, DR H. (1894) 'The perils and protection of infant life', *Journal of the Royal Statistical Society*, **LVII**, pp.1–98.

KNIGHTLEY, L.M. (1901) 'Women as homeworkers', *Nineteenth Century and After*, **L**.

LAURIE, A.R. (1895) 'The medical profession and the unhealthy trades', lecture given at St Mary's Medical School, *British Medical Journal*, 5 October, p.833.

LONSDALE, M. (1880) 'The Present Crisis at Guy's Hospital', *The Nineteenth Century*, vol. 7, pp.667–84 and replies by GULL, W., pp.884–9.

MACDONALD, J.R. (Ed.) (1902) *Women in the Printing Trades*, London: P.S. King. (Reprinted London, Garland, 1980.)

MACDONALD, MRS J.R. (1906) *Interim Report of an Inquiry by the Investigating Committee: Home Industries of Women in London*, London, Women's Industrial Council.

MARKHAM, V. (1949) *May Tennant: A Portrait*, London, The Falcon Press.

MALLETT, C. (1893) 'Dangerous trades for women', *The Humanitarian League*, No. 9, London, William Reeves.

MALLON, J.J. (1915) 'Women's wages in the census of 1906', in HUTCHINS, B. *Women in Industry*, London, G. Bell and Sons.

MARCH-PHILLIPS, E. (1902) 'The evils of homework for women', *Women's Cooperative Guild Investigative Papers III*, Manchester.

MARTIN, A. (1911) *The Married Working Woman*, London, National Union of Women's Suffrage Societies.

MARTIN, A. (1913) *The Mother and Social Reform*, London, The National Union of Women's Suffrage Societies.

MARTINDALE, H. (1938) *Women Servants of the State, 1870–1930*, London, George Allen and Unwin.

MARTINDALE, H. (1944a) *From One Generation to Another 1839–1944*, London, George Allen and Unwin.

MARTINDALE, H. (1944b) *Some Victorian Portraits and others*, London, George Allen and Unwin.

MORLEY, E.J. (Ed.) (1914) *Women Workers in Seven Professions: A Survey of their Economic Conditions and Prospects*, London, Routledge and Sons for the Fabian Women's Group.

NASH, R. (1897) *Public Health Laws: The Law Relating to Health in Factories and Workshops*, London, Women's Cooperative Guild.

NEWMAN, G. (1906) *Infant Mortality: A Social Problem*, London, Methuen.

NEWMAN, G. (1907) *The Health of the State*, Social Service Handbooks No. 2, London, Headley Bros.

OAKSHOTT, G. (1900) 'Women in the cigar trade in London: an enquiry by the Women's Industrial Council', *Economics Journal*, **X**, pp.562–6.

OGLE-MOORE, H. and HARE, E. (1896) 'Report to SPEW on work of women in white lead trade', in BOUCHERETT, J. and BLACKBURN, H. (Eds) *The Conditions of Working Women and the Facgtory Acts*, London, Elliot Stock.

OLIVER, T. (Ed.) (1902) *The Dangerous Trades: The History, Social and Legal Aspects of Industrial Occupations Affecting Health by a Number of Experts*, London, John Murray.

OLIVER, T. (1906) *Maladies Caused by the Air we Breathe Inside and Outside the Home*, The Haben Lectures for 1905, London, Balliere, Tindall and Cox.

OLIVER, T. (1914) *Lead Poisoning: From the Industrial, Medical and Social Points of View*, London, H.K. Lewis.

O'NEILL, H.C. and BARNETT, E.A. (1888) *Our Nurses and the Work They Have to Do*, London, Ward and Lock.

PEMBER-REEVES, M. (1914) *Round About a Pound a Week*, London. (Reprinted by Virago, 1981.)

POTTER, B. (1890) 'The Lords and the sweating system', *Nineteenth Century*, **XXVII**, June, p.885.

RATHBONE, E. (1924) *The Disinherited Family*, London, Edward Arnold.

ROWNTREE SEEBOHM, B. (1902) *Poverty: A Study in Town Life*, London, Nelson.

SEYMER, L.R. (1932) *A General History of Nursing*, London, Faber & Faber.

SHADWELL, A.M.D. (1906) *Industrial Efficiency*, London, Longman.

SHAFTS.

SHEAVYN, P. (1911) 'Professional Women', in her *The Position of Women: Actual and Ideal*, London, James Nisbet.

SMITH, C. (1908) 'The minimum wage', in TUCKWELL, G. (Ed.) *Women in Industry*, London, Duckworth.

SPRING-RICE, M. (1939) *Working Class Wives: Their Health and Condition*, London. (Reprinted by Virago, 1981.)

SQUIRE, R.E. (1927) *Thirty Years in the Public Service: An Industrial Retrospect*, London, Nisbet.

STEWART, I. (1890) 'Our hospitals: a practical view of nursing', *Murray's Magazine*, **8**, pp.162–9.

TENNANT, M. (1898) 'The women's factory department', *The Fortnightly*, **64**, pp.150–1.

TUCKWELL, G. (1898) 'Commercial manslaughter', *Nineteenth Centtury*, **44**, pp.253–8.

TUCKWELL, G. (1902) 'The more obvious defects of our factory code', in WEBB, MRS S. (Ed.) *The Case for the Factory Acts*, London, Grant Richards.

TUCKWELL, G. (Ed.) (1908) *Women in Industry*, London: Duckworth.

WEBB, B. (1902) 'Women and the Factory Acts', in *The Case for the Factory Acts*, London, Grant Richards.

WEBB, B. (Ed.) (1902) *The Case for the Factory Acts*, London, Grant Richards.

WEBB, S. and WEBB, B. (1894) *A History of Trade Unionism*, London, Longman and Co. (Revised editions in 1896, 1902, 1911 and 1920.)

WEBB, S. and WEBB, B. (1902) *Problems of Modern Industry*, London, Longman Green and Co.

WHITE, A. (1885) 'The nomad poor of London', *Contemporary Review*, **XLVII**, pp.714–26.

WOMEN'S HERALD.

WOMEN'S TRADE UNION JOURNAL.

THE WOMAN WORKER.

'Women workers': *Papers read at a conference convened by the Liverpool Ladies Union of Workers among Women and Girls, 1892.*

'Women workers': *Proceedings of a conference convened by the Bristol and Clifton Ladies Association for the Care of Girls in 1892*, Bristol, J.W. Arrowsmith (1893).

'Women workers': *Official Report of a conference held in Glasgow, October 1894*, Glasgow, James McLeod and Sons.

Collections

ARCHIVES OF GIRTON COLLEGE, Girton College Library, Cambridge

BRITISH LIBRARY OF POLITICAL AND ECONOMIC SCIENCE, Violet Markham Papers, Lucy Deane Streatfield Papers, British Association for Advancement of Science (BAAS Papers).

CLARA COLLET AND LUCY DEANE STREATFIELD PAPERS, Modern Records Centre, University of Warwick.

FAWCETT LIBRARY, Guildhall University, London, Biographical Collection.

GERTRUDE TUCKWELL COLLECTION, Trades Union Congress Library, Congress House, London.

PUBLIC RECORDS OFFICE (PRO), Kew, Home Office Files: HO45, and Labour Office: LAB 14, 15.

TRADES UNION CONGRESS, Annual Reports for Period, Congress House London.

Secondary Sources: Books and Articles

ALEXANDER, S. (1976) 'Women's work in nineteenth century London', in MITCHELL, J. and OAKLEY, A. (Eds) *The Rights and Wrongs of Women*, Harmondsworth, Penguin.

ALLSOP, J. (1984) *Health Policy and the NHS*, London, Hutchinson.

ANDERSON, G. (1988) 'The white blouse revolution' in ANDERSON, T. (Ed.) *The White Blouse Revolution*, Manchester, Manchester University Press.

ANDERSON, G. (Ed.) (1988) *The White Blouse Revolution: Female Office Workers since 1870*, Manchester, Manchester University Press.

ANTHIAS, F. and YUVAL-DAVIS, N. (1983) 'Contextualising feminism – gender, ethnic and class divisions', *Feminist Review*, **15**, pp.62–75.

ARBER, S. (1991) 'Class, paid employment and family roles: making sense of structural disadvantage', *Social Science and Medicine*, **32**, pp.425–36.

ARMSTRONG, D. (1986) 'The invention of infant mortality', *Sociology of Health and Illness*, **8** (2), pp.209–33.

BAILEY, P. (1990) 'Parasexuality and glamour: the Victorian barmaid as cultural prototype', *Gender and History*, **2** (2), pp.148–72.

BALY, M. (1986) *Florence Nightingale and the Nursing Legacy*, London, Croom Helm.

BANKS, O. (1981) *Faces of Feminism*, Oxford, Martin Robertson.

BANKS, O. (1986) *Becoming a Feminist: The Social Origins of First Wave Feminism*, Brighton, Wheatsheaf.

BARRETT, M. (1988) *Women's Oppression Today: Problems in Marxist Feminist Analysis*, 2nd end, London, Verso.

BARRETT, M. and MCINTOSH, M. (1980) 'The "family wage": some problems for socialists and feminists', *Capital and Class*, **11**, pp.51–72.

BARRON, R.D. and NORRIS, G. (1976) 'Sexual divisions and the dual labour market', in BARKER, D. and ALLEN, S. (Eds) *Dependence and Exploitation in Work and Marriage*, London, Longman.

BARTLEY, M., POPAY, J. and PLEWIS, I. (1992) 'Domestic conditions, paid employment and women's experience of ill-health', *Sociology of Health and Illness*, **14** (3), pp.313–43.

BARTRIP, P. (1985) 'The rise and decline of workman's compensation', in WEINDLING, P. (Ed.) *The Social History of Occupational Health*, London, Croom Helm.

BEALE, J. (1982) *Getting it Together: Women as Trade Unionists*, London, Pluto Press.

BEECHEY, V. (1983) 'What's so special about women's employment?', *Feminist Review*, **15**, pp.23–46.

BEER, R. (n.d.) *The Match-girls Strike, 1888*, Labour History Museum, Pamphlet No. 2.

BENENSON, H. (1991) 'The "family wage" and working women's consciousness in Britain, 1880–1914', *Politics and Society*, **10** (1), pp.71–108.

BLAND, L. (1995) *Banishing the Beast: English Feminism and Sexual Morality*, Harmondsworth, Penguin.

BOHLIN-HART, P. (1989) *Work, Family and the State: Child Labour and the Organisation of Production in the British Cotton Industry 1780–1920*, Lund, Lund University Press.

BORNAT, J. (1986) ' "What about that lass of yours being in the union?" Textile workers and their union in Yorkshire', in DAVIDOFF, L. and WESTOVER, B. (Eds) *Our Work, Our Lives, Our Words*, London, Macmillan.

BRADLEY, H. (1989) *Women's Work, Men's Work: A Social History of the Sexual Division of Labour*, Cambridge, Polity in association with Basil Blackwell.

BRANCA, P. (1975) *Silent Sisterhood: Middle-class Women in Victorian England*, London, Croom Helm.

BRENNER, J. and RAMAS, M. (1984) 'Rethinking women's oppression', *New Left Review*, **CXLIV**, pp.33–71.

BROOKES, B. (1986) 'Women and reproduction *c.* 1860–1919', in LEWIS, J. (Ed.) *Labour and Love: Women's Experience of Home and Family*, Oxford, Basil Blackwell.

BURSTYN, J. (1980) *Victorian Education and the Idea of Womanhood*, London, Croom Helm.

BYTHELL, D. (1978) *The Sweated Trades*, London, Batsford.

CAINE, B. (1985) 'Beatrice Webb and the "women question"', *History Workshop Journal*, **15**, pp.25–42.

CANNING, K. (1994) 'Feminist history after the Linguistic turn: historicising discourse and experience', *Signs*, **19** (2), pp.368–404.

CARPENTER, M. (1980) 'Asylum nursing before 1914', in DAVIES, C. (Ed.) *Rewriting Nursing History*, London, Croom Helm.

CHEW, D. (1982) *The Life and Writings of Ada Nield Chew*, London, Virago.

CHINN, C. (1988) *They Worked all their Lives: Women of the Urban Poor in England, 1880–1939*, Manchester, Manchester University Press.

COOTE, A. and KELLNER, P. (1980) *Hear this Brother: Women Workers and Union Power*, London, *New Statesman*, Report No. 1.

COPELMAN, D.M. (1986) '"A new comradeship between men and women": family marriage and London's women teachers, 1870–1914', in LEWIS, J. (Ed.) *Labour and Love: Women's Experiences of Home and Family 1850–1914*, Oxford, Blackwell.

CORR, H. and JAMIESON, L. (Eds) (1990) *The Politics of Everyday Life: Continuities and Change in Work, Labour and Family*, London, Macmillan.

CORRIGAN, P. and SAYER, D. (1985) *The Great Arch: English State Formation as Cultural Revolution*, Oxford, Basil Blackwell.

CRAWFORD, R. (1977) '"You are dangerous to your health": the ideology and politics of victim blaming', *International Journal of Health Services*, **7**, pp.663–80.

DALE, J. and FOSTER, P. (1986) *Feminists and State Welfare*, London, Routledge and Kegan Paul.

DANT, T. (1991) *Knowledge, Ideology and Discourse: A Sociological Perspective*, London, Routledge.

DAVIDOFF, L. and WESTOVER, B. (Eds) (1986) *Our Work, Our Lives, Our Words: Women's History and Women's Work*, London, Macmillan.

DAVIES, C. (Ed.) (1980a) *Rewriting Nursing History*, London, Croom Helm.

DAVIES, C. (1980b) 'Making sense of the census in Britain and the USA: the changing occupational classification and the position of nurses', *Sociological Review*, **28**, pp.581–601.

DAVIES, C. (1988) 'The health visitor as mother's friend: a woman's place in public health 1900–1914', *Social History of Medicine*, **1** (1), pp.39–59.

DAVIN, A. (1978) 'Imperialism and motherhood', *History Workshop Journal*, **5**, pp.9–65.

DAVY, T. (1986) '"A cissy job for men: a nice job for girls": women shorthand typists in London 1900–1039', in DAVIDOFF, L. and WESTOVER, B. (Eds) *Our Work, Our Lives, Our Words*, London, Macmillan.

DELAMONT, S. and DUFFIN, L. (Eds) (1979) *The Nineteenth Century Woman*, London, Croom Helm.

DINGWALL, R. (1977) 'Collectivism, regionalism and feminism: health visiting and British social policy, 1850–1975', *Journal of Social Policy*, **6**, pp.291–315.

DINGWALL, R., RAFFERTY, A.M. and WEBSTER, C. (1988) *An Introduction to a Social History of Nursing*, London, Routledge.

DOHRN, S. (1988) 'Pioneers in a dead-end profession: the first women clerks in banks and insurance companies', in ANDERSON, G. (Ed.) *The White Blouse Revolution*, Manchester, Manchester University Press.

DONZELOT, J. (1980) *The Policing of Families*, London, Hutchinson.

DOUGHAN, D. (1987) 'Periodicals by, about the for women in Britain', *Women's Studies International Forum*, **10** (3), pp.261–76.

DOYAL, L. (with PENNELL, I.) (1979) *The Political Economy Of Ill-health*, London, Pluto Press.

DUFFIN, L. (1979) 'The conspicuous consumptive', in DUFFIN, L. and DELAMONT, S. (Eds) *The Nineteenth Century Woman*, London, Croom Helm.

DUSSAULT, G. and SHEIHAM, A. (1982) 'Medical theories and professional development: the theory of focal sepsis and dentistry in early twentieth centuiry Britain', *Social Science and Medicine*, **16**, pp.1405–12.

DWORK, D. (1987) *War is Good for Babies and Other Young Children*, London, Tavistock.

DYHOUSE, C. (1978) 'Working-class mothers and infant mortality in England 1895–1914', *Journal of Social History*, **12**, pp.248–67.

DYHOUSE, C. (1989) *Feminism and the Family in England 1880–1939*, Oxford, Basil Blackwell.

EHRENREICH, B. and ENGLISH, D. (1973) *Complaints and Disorders: The Sexual Politics of Sickness*, London, Writers and Readers.

FELTES, N.N. (1992) 'Misery or the production of misery: defining sweated labour in 1890', *Social History*, **17** (3), pp.443–52.

FEURER, R. (1988) 'The meaning of "sisterhood": the British women's movement and protective labour legislation, 1870–1900', *Victorian Studies*, **31** (2), pp.233–60.

FIGLIO, K. (1978) 'Chlorosis and chronic disease in nineteenth century Britain', *International Journal of Health Studies*, **8** (4), pp.589–617.

FIGLIO, K. (1982) 'Does illness mediate social relations?' in WRIGHT, P. and TREACHER, A. (Eds) *The Problem of Medical Knowledge*, Edinburgh, Edinburgh University Press.

FIGLIO, K. (1985) 'What is an accident?' in WEINDLING, P. (Ed.) *The Social History of Occupational Health*, London, Croom Helm.

FINLAYSON, G. (1990) 'A moving frontier: voluntarism and the State', *Twentieth Century British History*, **1**, pp.183–206.

FLINN, M.W. (Ed.) (1965) Introduction and Reprint of E. CHADWICK, *The Report on the Sanitary Conditions of the Labouring Population of Great Britain*, Edinburgh, Edinburgh University Press.

FOUCAULT, M. (1970) *The Order of Things: An Archaeology of the Human Sciences*, London, Tavistock.

FOUCAULT, M. (1979) *Discipline and Punish: The Birth of the Prison*, London, Tavistock.

FOUCAULT, M. (1980) *Power/Knowledge: Selected Interviews and Other Writings*, edited by GORDON, C., Brighton, Harvester Press.

FREIDSON, E. (1970) *Profession of Medicine: A Study in the Sociology of Applied Knowledge*, New York, Dodd Meade.

GOFFMAN, E. (1961) *Asylums*, Harmondsworth, Penguin.

GOLDMAN, L. (1991) 'Statistics and the science of Society in early Victorian Britain: an intellectual context for the General Register Office', *Social History of Medicine*, **4** (3), pp.415–34.

GORDON, E. (1987) 'Women, work and collective action: Dundee jute workers 1870–1906', *Journal of Social History*, **21** (1), pp.27–48.

GORDON, L. (1988) *Heroes of Their Own Lives: The Politics and History of Family Violence*, New York, Viking Press.

GORDON, L. (1990) Review of *Gender and the Politics of History*, by Joan Scott, and reply to Scott's Review of her *Heroes of their Own Lives: The Politics and History of Family Violence*, in *Signs*, **15** (4), pp.853–8 and 852–3.

GRAY, R. (1987a) 'The language of factory reform', in JOYCE, P. (Ed.) *The Historical Meanings of Work*, Cambridge, Cambridge University Press.

GRAY, R. (1987b) 'Medical men, industrial labour and the State in nineteenth century Britain', unpublished paper (cited with author's permission).

GRAY, R. (1988) 'Medical men, industrial labour and the State in Britain *c*. 1830–50', paper presented to the Annual Conference of the British Sociological Association, Edinburgh.

GRAY, R. (1991) 'Medical men, industrial labour and the State in Britain, 1830–50', *Social History*, **16** (1), pp.19–43.

HAKIM, C. (1979) *Occupational Segregation: A Comparative Study of the Degree and Pattern of Differentiation between Men's and Women's Work in Britain, the United States and other Countries*, London, Research Paper No. 9, Department of Employment.

HAKIM, C. (1980) 'Census reports as documentary evidence: the census commentaries 1801–1951', *Sociological Review*, **28** (3), pp.551–80.

HAKIM, C. (1985) 'Social monitors: population censuses as social surveys', in BULMER, M. (Ed.) *Essays on the History of British Sociological Research*, Cambridge, Cambridge University Press.

HALL, S. and SCHWARTZ, B. (1986) 'State and society 1880–1930', in LANGAN, M. and SCHWARTZ, B. (Eds) *Crises in the British State 1880–1930*, London, Hutchison.

HARRIS, B. (1986) 'Physical deterioration and the doctors', unpublished paper presented to the British Sociological Association Medical Sociology Conference, York.

HARRISON, B. (1989) '"Some of them gets lead poisoned": occupational lead exposure in women, 1880–1914', *Social History of Medicine*, **2**, pp.171–93.

HARRISON, B. (1990) 'Suffer the working day: women in the "dangerous trades"', in *British Feminist Histories*, a special issue of *Women's Studies International Forum*, **13** (1), pp.79–90.

HARRISON, B. (1991) 'Women's health or social control? The role of the medical profession in relation to factory legislation in late nineteenth-century Britain', *Sociology of Health and Illness*, **13** (4), pp.469–91.

HARRISON, B. (1993a) 'Are accidents gender neutral? The case of the industrial accident in Britain, 1880–1914', *Women's History Review*, **2**, pp.253–76.

HARRISON, B. (1993b) 'Feminism and the health consequences of women's

work in late nineteenth-century Britain', in PLATT, S., THOMAS, H., SCOTT, S. and
WILLIAMS, G. (Eds) *Locating Health: Historical and Contemporary Perspectives*, Andover: Ashgate.

HARRISON, B. (1995a) 'The politics of occupational health in late nineteenth-
century Britain: The case of the match-making industry, *Sociology of Health
and Illness*, **17** (1), pp.20–41.

HARRISON, B. (1995b) 'Women's health', in PURVIS, J. (Ed.) *Women's History,
Britain: 1850–1945*, London, University College Press.

HARRISON, B. (In press) 'Gender, the State and occupational ill-health: women
factory inspectors and the health of women at work 1893–1914', *Proceedings of
the International Conference on Nursing, Women's History and the Politics of
Welfare*, University of Nottingham, Nursing Policy Series.

HARRISON, B. and MOCKETT, H. (1990) 'Women in the factory: The State and
factory legislation in nineteenth-century Britain', in JAMIESON, L. and CORR, H.
(Eds) *State, Private Life and Political Change*, London, Macmillan.

HARRISON, BRIAN (1981) 'Women's health and the women's movement, 1840–
1940', in WEBSTER, C. (Ed.) *Biology Medicine and Society*, Cambridge, Cambridge University Press, pp.15–69.

HARRISON, BRIAN (1992) 'A different world for women: nineteenth-century women
campaigners', *Twentieth Century British History*, **3** (1), pp.76–83.

HARTMANN, H. (1976) 'Capitalism, patriarchy and job segregation by sex', *Signs*,
1, pp.137–69.

HARTMANN, H. (1979) 'The unhappy marriage of Marxism and feminism: toward
a more progressive union', *Capital and Class*, **8**, pp.1–37.

Health Visitor (1987) A special issue devoted to the history of health visiting,
60 (5).

HENNOCK, E.P. (1976) 'Poverty and social theory in England: the experience of the
eighteen-eighties', *Social History*, **1**, pp.67–91.

HEWITT, M. (1958) *Wives and Mothers in Victorian Industry: A Study of the Effects
of Employment of Married Women in Victorian Industry*, London: Rockliffe.

HIGGS, E. (1986) 'Domestic service and household production', in JOHN, A.V.
(Ed.) *Unequal Opportunities: Women's Employment in England 1800–1918*,
Oxford, Basil Blackwell, pp.125–50.

HIGGS, E. (1987) 'Women, occupation and work in nineteenth-century censuses',
History Workshop Journal, **23**, pp.59–80.

HOLCOMBE, L. (1973) *Victorian Ladies at Work: Middle-class Women at Work in
England and Wales 1850–1914*, Newton Abbot, David and Charles.

HOLLIS, P. (1979) *Women in Public: The Women's Movement 1850–1900*, London,
Allen and Unwin.

HOLLIS, P. (1987) *Ladies Elect: Women in English Local Government 1865–1914*,
Oxford: Clarendon.

HUMPHRIES, J. (1977) 'Class struggle and the persistence of the working-class
family', *Cambridge Journal of Economics*, **1** (3), pp.241–58.

HUMPHRIES, J. (1981) 'Protective legislation, the capitalist state and working class
men: the case of the 1842 Mines Regulation Act', *Feminist Review*, **7**, pp.1–33.

ILLICH, I. (1976) *The Limits to Medicine*, London, Marion Boyars.

INESON, A. and THOM, D. (1985) 'TNT poisoning and the employment of women workers in the First World War', in WEINDLING, P. (Ed.) *The Social History of Occupational Health*, London: Croom Helm.

INKSTER, I. (1977) 'Marginal men: aspects of the role of the medical community in Sheffield, 1790–1850', in WOODWARD, J. and RICHARDS, D. (Eds) *Health Care and Popular Medicine in Nineteenth–Century England*, London, Croom Helm.

JALLAND, P. and HOOPER, P. (1986) *Women From Birth to Death: The Female Life Cycle in Britain from 1830–1914*, Brighton, Harvester Wheatsheaf.

JAMIESON, L., and CORR, H. (Eds) (1990) *State, Private Life and Political Change*, London, Macmillan.

JESSOP, B. (1990) *State Theory: Putting the Capitalist State in its Place*, Cambridge, Cambridge University Press.

JOHANSSON, S.R. (1978) 'Sex and death in Victorian England: an examination of age-specific death rates 1840–1910', in VINCINUS, M. (Ed.) *A Widening Sphere: Changing Roles of Victorian Women*, Bloomington, Indiana University Press.

JOHN, A.V. (1981) 'Letters', *Feminist Review*, **9**, pp.106–9.

JOHN, A.V. (1984a) *Coalmining Women*, Cambridge, Cambridge Educational Press.

JOHN, A.V. (1984b) *By the Sweat of their Brow: Women in Victorian Coalmining*, London, Routledge and Kegan Paul.

JOHN, A.V. (Ed.) (1986) *Unequal Opportunities: Women's Employment in England 1880–1918*, Oxford, Blackwell.

JONES, H. (1985) 'An inspector calls: health and safety at work in inter-war Britain', in WEINDLING, P. (Ed.) *The Social History of Occupational Health*, London, Croom Helm.

JONES, H. (1988) 'Women health workers: the case of the first women factory inspectors', *Social History of Medicine*, **1** (2), pp.165–82.

JOYCE, P. (Ed.) (1987) *The Historical Meanings of Work*, Cambridge, Cambridge University Press.

KLEINBERG, S.J. (Ed.) (1988) *Retrieving Women's History: Changing Perceptions of the Role of Women in Politics and Society*, Oxford, Berg.

LAMBERTZ, J. (1985) 'Sexual harassment in the nineteenth-century English cotton industry', *History Workshop Journal*, **19** (Spring), pp.29–61.

LAND, H. (1985) 'The introduction of family allowances: an act of historic justice?' in UNGERSON, C. (Ed.) *Women and Social Policy*, London, Macmillan.

LANGAN, M. and SCHWARTZ, B. (Eds) (1986) *Crisis in the British State 1880–1930*, London, Hutchinson.

LEE, W.R. (1964) 'Robert Baker: the first doctor in the factory department, Part I 1803–1858, Part II 1858 onwards', *British Journal of Industrial Medicine*, **21**, pp.85 and 167.

LEE, W.R. (1973) 'The emergence of occupational medicine in Victorian Britain', *British Journal of Industrial Medicine*, **30**, pp.118–24.

LEVINE, P. (1988) *Victorian Feminism 1850–1900*, London, Hutchinson Education.

LEVINE, P. (1990a) *Feminist Lives in Victorian England: Private Roles and Public Commitment*, Oxford, Basil Blackwell.

LEVINE, P. (1990b) ' "The humanising influences of five o'clock tea": Victorian feminist periodicals', *Victorian Studies*, **33**, pp.293–306.

LEVINE, P. (1993) 'Consistent contradictions: prostitution and protective labour legislation in nineteenth-century England', *Social History*, **19** (1), pp.17–35.

LEWENHAK, S. (1977) *Women and Trade Unions: An Outline History of Women in the British Trade Union Movement*, London, Ernest Benn.

LEWIS, J. (1980a) *The Politics of Motherhood: Child and Maternal Welfare in England 1900–1939*, London: Croom Helm.

LEWIS, J. (1980b) 'The social history of social policy: infant welfare in Edwardian England', *Journal of Social Policy*, **9**, pp.463–86.

LEWIS, J. (1984) *Women in England, 1870–1950*, Brighton, Harvester Wheatsheaf.

LEWIS, J. (1986a) *What Price Community Medicine? The Philosophy, Practice and Politics of Public Health since 1919*, Brighton, Harvester Wheatsheaf.

LEWIS, J. (Ed.) (1986b) *Labour and Love: Women's Experience of Home and Family 1850–1940*, Oxford, Blackwell.

LEWIS, J. (1986c) 'The working class mother and State intervention', in LEWIS, J. (Ed.) *Labour and Love: Women's Experiences of Home and Family 1850–1940*, Oxford, Blackwell.

LEWIS, J. (1988) 'Women clerical workers in the nineteenth and early twentieth century', in ANDERSON, G. (Ed.) *The White Blouse Revolution*, Manchester, Manchester University Press.

LEWIS, J. and DAVIES, C. (1991) 'Protective legislation in Britain, 1870–1990: equality, difference and their implications for women', *Policy and Politics*, **19** (1), pp.13–25.

LIDDINGTON, J. and NORRIS, J. (1978) *One Hand Tied Behind Us*, London, Virago.

LIDDINGTON, J. (1979) 'Women cotton workers and the suffrage campaign: the radical suffragettes in Lancashire 1893–1914', in BURMAN, S. (Ed.) *Fit Work for Women*, London, Croom Helm.

LOWN, J. (1983) 'Not so much a factory, more a form of patriarchy: gender and class during industrialisation', in GARMARNIKOW, E., MORGAN, D., PURVIS, J. and TAYLORSON, D. (Eds) *Gender Class and Work*, London, Heinemann Education Books.

LOWN, J. (1990) *Women and Industrialisation: Gender at Work in Nineteenth Century England*, Cambridge, Polity Press.

MACKINNON, C. (1989) *Toward a Feminist Theory of the State*, Cambridge, Mass., Harvard University Press.

MCFEELY, M.D. (1986) 'The lady inspectors: women at work 1893–1921', *History Today*, **336**, pp.47–53.

MCFEELEY, M.D. (1988) *Lady Inspectors: The Campaign for a Better Workplace 1893–1921*, Oxford, Basil Blackwell.

MCKEOWN, T. (1971) 'A historical appraisal of the medical task', in MCLACHLAN, D. and MCKEOWN, T. (Eds) *Medical History and Medical Care*, Oxford, Nuffield Provincial Hospital Trust.

MCKINLEY, J. (1974) 'A case for refocusing upstream: the political economy of illness', in *Applying the Behavioural Sciences to Cardiovascular Risk, Proceedings of the Conference of the American Heart Association*, Seattle.

MCLAREN, A. (1977) 'Women's work and the regulation of family size: the question of abortion in nineteenth century', *History Workshop Journal*, **4**, pp.48–70.

MAGGS, C. (1980) 'Nursing recruitment to four provincial hospitals', in DAVIES, C. (Ed.) *Rewriting Nursing History*, London, Croom Helm.

MAGGS, C.J. (1983) *The Origins of General Nursing*, London, Croom Helm.

MALCOLMSON, P. (1981) 'Laundresses and the laundry trade in victorian England', *Victorian Studies*, **24** (4), pp.429–62.

MAPPEN, E. (1985) *Helping Women at Work: The Women's Industrial Council, 1889–1914*, London, Hutchinson.

MAPPEN, E. (1986) 'Strategists for change: social feminist approaches to the problems of women's work', in JOHN, A.V. (Ed.) *Unequal Opportunities: Women's Employment in England 1800–1918*, Oxford, Basil Blackwell, pp.235–59.

MARK-LAWSON, J. and WITZ, A. (1988) 'From "family labour" to "family wage"? The case of women's labour in nineteenth-century coalmining', *Social History*, **13** (2), pp.151–73.

MARLAND, H. (1993) 'A pioneer in infant welfare: the Huddersfield Scheme, 1903–1920', *Social History of Medicine*, **6** (1), pp.25–50.

MARVEL, H. (1977) 'Factory regulation: a reinterpretation of the English experience'. *Journal of Law and Economy*, **20**, pp.379–402.

MEIKLEJOHN, A. (1963) 'The successful prevention of lead poisoning in the glazing of earthenware in the North Staffordshire potteries', *British Journal of Industrial Medicine*, **20**, pp.169–80.

MELLING, J. (1992) 'Welfare capitalism and the origins of welfare states: British industry, workplace welfare and social reform, c. 1870–1914', *Social History*, **17** (3), pp.453–78.

MIDDLETON, C. (1983) 'Patriarchal exploitation and the rise of English capitalism', in GARMARNIKOW, E., MORGAN, D., PURVIS, J. and TAYLORSON, D. (Eds) *Gender Class and Work*, London, Heinemann Educational Books.

MOCKETT, H. (1988) '"A danger to the state": women and factory legislation, 1830–1850', unpublished paper presented to the Annual Conference of the British Sociological Association, Edinburgh.

MORGAN, C. (1992) 'Women, work and consciousness in mid-nineteenth-century English cotton industry', *Social History*, **17**, pp.23–41.

MORRIS, J. (1986a) 'The characteristics of sweating: the late nineteenth-century London and Leeds tailoring trade', in JOHN, A.V. (Ed.) *Unequal Opportunities: Women's Employment in England 1800–1918*, Oxford, Basil Blackwell, pp.95–121.

MORRIS, J. (1986b) *Women Workers and the Sweated Trades*, London, Gower.

MORT, F. (1986) 'Purity, feminism and the State: sexuality and moral politics 1880–1914', in LANGAN, M. and SCHWARTZ, B. (Eds) *Crises in the British State 1880–1930*, London: Hutchinson.

MURRAY, J.H. (1984) *Strong Minded Women: and Other Lost Voices from 19th-Century England*, Harmonsworth, Penguin.

MURRAY, J.H. and CLARKE, A.H. (1985) *The English women's Review of Social and Industrial Questions: An Index (with Introduction)*, New York, Garland.

NICHOLSON, L. (1986) *Gender and History: The Limits of Social Theory in the Age of the Family*, New York, University of Columbia Press.

OAKLEY, A. (1984) *The Captured Womb: A History of the Medical Care of Pregnant Women*, Oxford, Clarendon.

OMORI, M. (1986) 'British factory inspectorate as a women's profession, 1893–1921', *Saga University Economic Review*, **19** (1), pp.41–64.

OREM, L. (1974) 'The welfare of women in labouring families, England 1860–1950', in HARTMAN, M. and BANNER, L.W. (Eds) *Clio's Consciousness Raised: New Perspectives on the History of Women*, New York, Harper & Row.

OSTERUD, N.G. (1986) 'Gender divisions and the organisation of work in the Leicester hosiery industry', in JOHN, A.V. (Ed.) *Unequal Opportunities: Women's Employment in England 1800–1918*, Oxford, Blackwell.

PENNINGTON, S. and WESTOVER, B. (1989) *A Hidden Workforce: Homeworkers in England 1850–1985*, London, Macmillan.

PETERSON, M. (1978) *The Medical Profession in Victorian London*, Princeton New Jersey, Princeton University Press.

PORTER, D. (1991) '"Enemies of the race": biologism, enviromentalism and public health in Edwardian England', *Victorian Studies*, **34** (2), pp.159–78.

POSNER, E. (1973) 'John Thomas Arlidge (1822–1899) and the potteries', *British Journal of Industrial Medicine*, **30**, pp.266–270.

PURVIS, J. (1989) *Hard Lessons: The Lives and Education of Working-class Women in Nineteenth-Century England*, Cambridge, Polity Press.

PURVIS, J. (1991) *A History of Women's Education in England*, Milton Keynes, Open University Press.

PURVIS, J. (1992) 'Using primary sources when researching women's history from a feminist perspective', *Women's History Review*, **1** (2), pp.273–306.

RAMAZANOGLU, C. (1989) *Feminism and the Contradictions of Oppression*, London, Routledge.

RICE, F. (1981) 'Madness and industrial society: a study of the early growth and organisation of insanity in mid-nineteenth-century Scotland, 1830–1870', unpublished PhD Thesis, Strathclyde University.

RILEY, D. (1988) *'Am I that Name?': Feminism and the Category of 'Women' in History*, London, Macmillan.

ROBERTS, E. (1984) *A Woman's Place: An Oral History of Working-Class Women 1890–1940*, Oxford, Blackwell.

ROSE, M.E. (1971) 'The doctor and the industrial revolution', *British Journal of Industrial Medicine*, **28**, pp.22–7.

ROSE, S.O. (1987) 'Gender at work: sex, class and industrial capitalism', *History Workshop Journal*, **21**, pp.113–31.

ROSE, S.O. (1988) 'Gender antagonism and class conflict: exclusionary strategies by male trade unionists in nineteenth-century Britain', *Social History*, **13** (2), pp.191–208.

ROSE, S.O. (1992) *Limited Livelihoods: Gender and Class in Nineteenth-Century England*, Berkely, University of California Press.

ROSEN, G. (1952–3) 'Charles Turner Thackrah in the agitation for early factory reform', *British Journal of Industrial Medicine*, **9/10**, pp.285–7.

ROSS, E. (1986) 'Labour and love: rediscovering London's working-class mothers 1870–1918', in LEWIS, J. (Ed.) *Labour and Love: Women's Experiences of Home and Family 1850–1940*, Oxford, Basil Blackwell.

RUBENSTEIN, D. (1986) *Before the Suffragettes: Women's Emancipation in the 1890s*, Brighton, Harvester Press.

RUBENSTEIN, D. (1991) 'Millicent Garrett Fawcett and the meaning of women's emancipation, 1886–1899', *Victorian Studies*, **25**, pp.365–80.

SATRE, L. (1982) 'After the match girls strike: Bryant and May in the 1890s', *Victorian Studies*, **25**, pp.7–31.

SCHMEICHEN, J.A. (1984) *Sweated Industries and Sweated Labour*, London: Croom Helm.

SCHWARTZ, B. (1986) 'The corporate economy 1890–1929', in LANGAN, M. and SCHWARZ, B. (Eds) *Crises in the British State 1880–1930*, London, Hutchinson.

SCOTT, A.E. (1986) 'Industrialisation, gender segregation and stratification theory', in CROMPTON, R. and MANN, M. (Eds) *Gender and Stratification*, Cambridge, Polity.

SCOTT, J. (1976) 'On language, gender and working-class history', *International Labour and Working-class History*, **31**, pp.1–13.

SCOTT, J. (1988) *Gender and the Politics of History*, New York, Columbia University Press.

SCOTT, J. (1990) Review of *Heroes of their Own Lives: The Politics and History of Family Violence* by Linda Gordon and a response to Gordon in *Signs*, **15** (4), pp.848–52 and 859–60.

SEECOMBE, W. (1986) 'Patriarchy stabilised: the construction of the male breadwinner norm in nineteenth-century Britain', *Social History*, **11**, pp.53–76.

SHORTER, E. (1983) *A History of Women's Bodies*, Harmonsworth, Penguin.

SHOWALTER, E. (1987) *The Female Malady: Women, Madness and English Culture 1830–1980*, London, Virago.

SMILEY, J. (1971) 'Some aspects of the early evolution of the appointed factory doctor service', *British Journal of Industrial Medicine*, **28**, pp.315–22.

SMITH, D.E. (1985) *The Everyday World as Problematic*, Milton Keynes, Open University Press.

SMITH, D.E. (1990) *Texts, Facts and Femininity: Exploring the Relations of Ruling*, London, Routledge.

SMITH, F.B. (1979) *The People's Health, 1830–1914*, London, Croom Helm.

SMITH, F.B. (1982) *Florence Nightingale Reputation and Power*, London, Croom Helm.

SMITH-ROSENBERG, C. (1972) 'The hysterical woman: sex roles and role conflict in nineteenth-century America', *Social Research*, **39**, pp.25–42.

SOLDEN, N. (1978) *Women in British Trade Unions 1874–1976*, London, Gill and Macmillan.

SONTAG, S. (1977) *Illness as Metaphor*, New York, Farrar, Straus and Giroux.

SONTAG, S. (1990) *AIDS and its Metaphors*, New York, Doubleday.

STANLEY, L. (1990) 'Recovering Women in history from feminist deconstructionism', *Women's Studies International Forum*, **13** (1/2), pp.151–9.

STEARNS, P. N. (1973) 'Working-class women in Britain 1890–1914', in VINCINUS, M. (Ed.) *Suffer and be Still: Women in the Victorian Age*, Bloomington, Indiana University Press.

STEDMAN-JONES, G. (1984) *Outcaste London: A Study of the Relationships Between the Classes in Victorian Society*, 2nd edn, London, Allen Lane, Penguin.

STRACHEY, R. (1923) *The Cause*, London. (Reprinted by Virago 1978.)

SWINDELLS, J. (1985) *Victorian Writing and Working Women*, Cambridge, Polity Press.

SZRETER, S. (1988) 'The importance of social intervention in Britain's mortality decline *c*. 1850–1914: a reinterpretation of the role of public health', *Social History of Medicine*, **1** (1), pp.1–38.

SZRETER, S. (1991) 'The GRO and the historians', and, 'The GRO and the public health movement', *Social History of Medicine*, **4** (3), pp.435–64.

THANE, P. (1982) *The Foundations of the Welfare State*, London, Longman.

THOM, D. (1986) 'The bundle of sticks: women, trade unionist and collective organisation before 1918', in JOHN, A.V. (Ed.) *Unequal Opportunities: Women's Employment in England 1800–1918*, Oxford, Basil Blackwell, pp.261–289.

TILLY, L.A. and SCOTT, J.W. (1978) *Women, Work and the Family*, New York, Holt Reinhardt and Winston.

TURNBULL, A. (1994) '"An isolated missionary": the domestic subjects teacher in England 1870–1914', *Women's History Review*, **3** (1), pp.81–100.

TURNER, B. (1987) *Medical Power and Social Knowledge*, London, Sage.

VALVERDE, M. (1988) '"Giving the female a domestic turn": the social, legal and moral regulation of women's work in British cotton mills 1820–1850', *Journal of Social History*, **21**, pp.619–36.

VERBRUGGE, M. (1985) 'Gender and health: an update on hypotheses and evidence', *Journal of Health and Social Behaviour*, **26**, pp.156–82.

VERBRUGGE, M. (1988) *Able-Bodied Womanhood: Personal Health and Social Change in Nineteenth-Century Boston*, Oxford, Oxford University Press.

VINCINUS, M. (1985) *Independent Women: Work and Community for Single Women*, London, Virago.

WADDINGTON, I. (1984) 'The development of medicine as a modern profession', in PIATELLI-PALMARINI, M. (Ed.) *A Social History of the Bio-medical Sciences*, Milan, Franco Maria Ricci.

WALBY, S. (1986) *Patriarchy at Work*, Cambridge, Polity.

WALBY, S. (Ed.) (1988) *Gender Segregation at Work*, Milton Keynes, Open University Press.

WALBY, S. (1990a) 'From private to public patriarchy: the periodisation of British history', *Women's Studies International Forum*, **13**, pp.91–104.

WALBY, S. (1990b) *Theorising Patriarchy*, Oxford, Basil Blackwell.

WEINDLING, P. (1985) 'Linking self help and medical science: the social history of occupational health', in WEINDLING, P. (Ed.) *The Social History of Occupational Health*, London, Croom Helm.

WEINDLING, P. (Ed.) (1985) *The Social History of Occupational Health*, London, Croom Helm.

WESTOVER, B. (1986) '"To fill the kids' tummies": the lives and work of Colchester tailoresses, 1880–1918', in DAVIDOFF, L. and WESTOVER, B. (Eds) *Our Work, Our Lives, Our Words*, London, Macmillan.

WHIPP, R. (1983) Pot bank and union: a study of work and trade unionism 1900–1925 unpublished PhD. thesis, University of Warwick.

WHITEHEAD, M. (1986) *The Health Divide*, London, Health Education Authority.

WITZ, A. (1992) *Professions and Patriarchy*, London, Routledge.

WOHL, A. (1983) *Endangered Lives: Public Health in Victorian Britain*, London, J.M. Dent.

WOODS, R. I., WATTERSON, P.A. and WOODWARD, J. (1988) (1989) 'The causes of rapid infant mortality decline in England and Wales, 1862–1921 Part I', *Population Studies*, **42**, pp.343–66; 'Part II' *Population Studies*, **43**, pp.113–32.

WOODWARD, J. (1984) 'Medicine and the City: the nineteenth-century experience, in WOODS, R. and WOODWARD, J. (Eds) *Urban Disease and Mortality in Nineteenth-Century England*, New York, St Martin's Press.

ZIMMECK, E. (1986) 'Jobs for the girls: the expansion of clerical work for women 1850–1914', in JOHN, A.V. (Ed.) *Unequal Opportunities: Women's Employment in England 1800–1918*, Oxford, Basil Blackwell, pp.153–77.

Index

abortion 90, 237
Abraham (later Tennant), May 36, 54, 129, 168
  protective legislation 155
  white lead industry 62
  women factory inspectors 185–6, 188–9, 192–4
accidents 11, 13, 35, 54, 59
  machinery 59–60, 226
  medical practitioners 166, 167, 168, 177
  schools 122–3
  women factory inspectors 186, 193
aerated water bottling 39, 43, 59
age 5–8, 10, 51, 63, 106
Anderson, Adelaide 7, 25, 56, 58, 129
  hours of work 34, 35
  lead 60, 90
  maternity 84–5, 86, 90
  office work 117–18
  sanitary conditions 38, 39
  women factory inspectors 186–9, 191–6
anthrax 54, 58–9
Anti-Sweating League 97–9, 158, 214
Arlidge, Thomas 40, 52, 151, 166, 167, 176
Armstrong, D 86
arsenic 14, 54
asbestos 14, 58, 192, 228
Ashley MP, Lord 27, 225
Asquith, Lord 82–3, 184, 185, 194

Bailey, P 114
Baker, Robert 165, 166, 169, 173

Banks, Olive 201, 208
barmaids 28, 106, 113–14
Barrett, M 232–3, 234
Barrett, M and McIntosh, M 230, 236
Besant, Annie 66
birth control 90, 142, 158, 218
bisulphide of carbon 57
Black, Clementina 182
  domestic service 110
  pay 21, 27
  protective legislation 141, 158, 202, 204, 212, 214, 217
  shop work 113, 114
  sweated trades 94–5, 97, 100
Blackburn, Helen 202, 206
Bodichon, Barbara Leigh Smith 202
Bondfield, Margaret 113, 114, 115
boot-and-shoe manufacturing 12
Booth, Charles 96, 107, 112, 125, 205
Bornat, J 108
bottle-sighting 151
Bottomley, Horatio 111
Boucherett, Jessie 202, 203, 206, 209, 210, 216
Bowley 23
brass-finishing 58
Brenner, J and Ramos, M 233, 235
brick-making 12
Broadhurst, Henry 181–2
bronchitis 33
Bronte, Charlotte 121
bronzing 58
Brownlow, Jane 206
Bryant and May 66–70, 149, 173–4, 211

DATE DUE

NOV 2 3 2008			
			Printed In USA

HIGHSMITH #45230